Ethnographies of Breastfeeding

Ethnographies of Breastfeeding

Cultural Contexts and Confrontations

Edited by
Tanya Cassidy and Abdullahi El Tom

Bloomsbury Academic
An imprint of Bloomsbury Publishing Plc

B L O O M S B U R Y
LONDON · OXFORD · NEW YORK · NEW DELHI · SYDNEY

Bloomsbury Academic

An imprint of Bloomsbury Publishing Plc

50 Bedford Square	1385 Broadway
London	New York
WC1B 3DP	NY 10018
UK	USA

www.bloomsbury.com

BLOOMSBURY and the Diana logo are trademarks of Bloomsbury Publishing Plc

First published 2015
Paperback edition first published 2016

© Tanya Cassidy and Abdullahi El Tom, 2015

Tanya Cassidy and Abdullahi El Tom have asserted their right under the Copyright, Designs and Patents Act, 1988, to be identified as Authors of this work.

British Library Cataloguing-in-Publication Data
A catalogue record for this book is available from the British Library.

ISBN: HB: 978-1-47256-925-7
PB: 978-1-4742-9444-7
ePDF: 978-1-47256-927-1
ePub: 978-1-47256-926-4

Library of Congress Cataloging-in-Publication Data
Ethnographies of breastfeeding : cultural contexts and confrontations / edited by Tanya Cassidy and Abdullahi El Tom.
pages cm
Summary: "Studies of breastfeeding have proliferated over the last decade. Breastfeeding is an intimate and deep-rooted bodily practice and yet also a highly controversial sociocultural process, invoking strong reactions from advocates and opponents. Whilst breastfeeding practices and experiences vary greatly in different parts of the world, reducing infant mortality is a pressing international goal for governments and societies. Representing cross-cultural concerns of researchers, policy-makers and mothers, this important book takes a rich ethnographic survey of breastfeeding all over the world. Breastfeeding is shown to highlight various links between gender, power and resources in culture. Each chapter covers a new topic and ethnic or national group, and major topical themes of research such as the rise of milk banks, mother-to-mother sharing networks facilitated by social media, breastmilk and HIV are explored"– Provided by publisher.
Includes bibliographical references and index.
ISBN 978-1-4725-6925-7 (hardback) – ISBN 978-1-4725-6926-4 (epub) – ISBN 978-1-4725-6927-1 (epdf) 1. Breastfeeding–Cross-cultural studies. 2. Ethnology. 3. Women–Social conditions–Cross-cultural studies. I. Cassidy, Tanya. II. Tom, Abdullahi Osman El- editor.
RJ216.E78 2014
649'.33–dc23
2014019352

Typeset by Fakenham Prepress Solutions, Fakenham, Norfolk, NR21 8NN

Contents

Notes on Contributors

Dr. Valérie Adt is a sociologist and member of the research group in the Interdisciplinary Institute of Contemporary Anthropology at the Edgar Morin Centre (IIAC, EHESS-CNRS) in Paris, France. She is a specialist in food socialization and French school lunches, and a member of the inter-ministerial committee Plaisir à la cantine program. She has researched (visual anthropology) thousands of French kids taking their lunch in school cafeterias throughout the Paris area (2011–12).

Chiara Alfieri (M.Sc.) is an ethnologist who has carried out extensive studies among the Bobo and Dioula in Bobo-Dioulasso (south-west Burkina Faso). During the last ten years, she has worked on health topics such as infant and child disease, breastfeeding and infant feeding, HIV, and women's and mothers' relationships with health facilities. She also worked in the areas of children and rituals and children's play. In 2013 she began a new research program on children and antiretrovirals.

Dr. Katherine Carroll is a medical sociologist and Australian Research Council fellow at the Centre for Health Communication, Faculty of Arts and Social Sciences, at the University of Technology, Sydney. In 2011 she was awarded a three-year Australian Research Council (ARC) postdoctoral fellowship to establish the place of donor human milk (DHM) in Australia's "tissue economy." She has also been awarded an Endeavour Research Fellowship to examine the sociocultural elements that support the best practice use of DHM in the U.S.A. Her recent work has investigated breastmilk donation for use in neonatal intensive care units using ethnographic and video-ethnographic methods.

Dr. Tanya Cassidy is a Cochrane Fellow in the Department of Anthropology at the National University of Ireland, Maynooth, and is also Adjunct Assistant Professor in the Department of Sociology, Anthropology, Criminology at the University of Windsor in Canada. She is a sociologist trained at the University of Chicago in social psychological cross-cultural theories with a specialty in medical issues. Born in Canada, she has lived and worked in Ireland, where she has also become a citizen, since completing her doctorate. Her transatlantic duality is linked to her long-standing theorization of consumption and identity, particularly in relationship to gender and alcohol in Ireland, now being extended to issues related to breastmilk and premature birth.

Dr. Rossella Cevese currently works as a medical anthropologist at Caritas Italiana, an Italian religious charitable organization. In 2011 she completed her Ph.D. in anthropology at Verona University, where she worked on the topic of health, gender, and migration. Her fieldwork was about practices of familiar health and representations about the body among a group of Moroccan women in Italy. She started studying reproductive health in 2003, and for her dissertation did fieldwork in Bolivia about practices of childbirth among Guaraní women (2003). She has a master's degree in cultural mediation, and in 2007 received a certificate from a CIEH (Centre International d'Écologie Humaine) from the Université d'Aix-Marseille. Her research interests focused on migrants' practices of health and urbanscapes.

Professor Gervaise Debucquet is an Associate Professor and an agronomist engineer at the National Institute of Agronomy (Paris-Grignon) with a doctorate in the socio-anthropology of food. She is currently professor and researcher at the Audencia School of Management (Nantes). She has carried out research for ten years into the socio-anthropology of food, analyzing the link between food representations and food habits and preferences. Her research topics focus on the mechanisms of the perception of food risks (GMO, microbiological, and parasitical risks) and, more widely, on the process of formation of gust and disgust. Recently, she has been working on consumers' perception and uses of nutritional and health claims. Following this research, since 2008 she has been involved in a national research project (NUPEM)—including biologists, nutritionists, neonatologists, and sociologists—to analyze the specific case of perinatal nutrition.

Professor Alice Desclaux (M.D., Ph.D.) is a medical anthropologist. She was Professor of Medical Anthropology at Université Paul Cézanne d'Aix-Marseille, where she founded the Centre de Recherche Cultures, Santé, Sociétés. She works now as a social scientist in UMI 233, an international research unit (Cameroon–Senegal–France) of the Institut de Recherche pour le Développement. At the Centre de Recherche et de Formation de Fann (Dakar, Senegal), her main areas of research include social experience of

HIV infection, vulnerability, children and HIV, pharmaceuticalization of public health, and the anthropology of medical research in Africa.

Dr. Abdullahi Osman El Tom has published extensively on the peoples of the Sudan. He was recently chair of the Department of Anthropology at the National University of Ireland, Maynooth (NUIM). Following the successful hosting of the 2010 EASA bi-annual conference at NUIM, he was elected to the EASA executive board. He has published extensively on both medical and political anthropological topics ranging from female circumcision to genocide in Darfur. He received his doctoral training as a social anthropologist from the Department of Anthropology at the University of St. Andrews in Scotland, prior to which he had conducted master's-level work in Northern Ireland. Both postgraduate projects originated with his professional research on the Berti peoples of northern Darfur.

Dr. Charlotte Faircloth is currently a Leverhulme Trust Early Career Fellow at the University of Kent, in the U.K. Prior to this she held a Mildred Blaxter post-doctoral fellowship from the Foundation for the Sociology of Health and Illness; her book *Militant Lactivism? Infant Care and Maternal Identity* is published by Berghahn Books. She completed her Ph.D. in the Department of Social Anthropology at the University of Cambridge. Her doctoral work looked at women's experiences of "full-term" breastfeeding and attachment parenting in London and Paris, with a focus on questions of kinship, identity, and the new "parenting culture." More broadly, her work explores notions of body, gender, and equality in care-giving, and has a theoretical focus on accountability and the constitution of knowledge claims.

Professor Vanessa Maher (Ph.D., University of Cambridge) is Professor in Cultural Anthropology at the University of Verona, where she also co-ordinates the anthropology curriculum of a Ph.D. program in history and anthropology. She taught in Turin for 18 years and helped to found the University Centre of Women's Studies there and in other Italian universities. In 1972 she was part of the London Women's Anthropology Collective. Born in Kenya, she spent her childhood and adolescence in Tanzania, and for a year was a voluntary teacher in Nigeria, near Onitsha. Her Ph.D. at Cambridge researched the Middle Atlas of Morocco.

Dr. Anne Matthews is a Lecturer in the School of Nursing, Dublin City University, Ireland. Prior to that she worked as a health professional (registered nurse and midwife) in healthcare policy and as a health researcher in

Ireland and Malawi. She has a B.Soc.Sc. (Social Policy, Information Studies) from University College Dublin (1995) and a M.Sc. (Econ.) in Social Policy and Planning from the London School of Economics and Political Science (1996). Her Ph.D. examined past and present perspectives on power and empowerment in midwifery in Ireland (2006). Her research interests are in health policy analysis, health workforce planning, and systematic reviewing of the effectiveness of maternity and other healthcare interventions. Her teaching interests are in health policy, and complementary and alternative therapies and research methods. She has co-edited two books on Irish social policy and has published policy and research articles in her areas of interest and experience. She was the co-ordinator for the Irish team within the RN4CAST European Framework 7 project 2009–10.

Dr. Birgitte Bruun Nielsen (M.D., Ph.D.) is an Associate Professor in the Department of Obstetrics and Gynaecology at Aarhus University Hospital in Denmark. She has been engaged in research in reproductive health in developing countries for 20 years. She is a specialist in obstetrics and gynaecology and, in the clinical department, takes care of pregnant women with chronic diseases. Her research interest focuses on maternal health, delivery care, sex selection, and cross-border reproductive care, and usually is also engaged in interdisciplinary research.

Dr. Aunchalee Palmquist is an Assistant Professor of Anthropology at Elon University in North Carolina, U.S.A. Before this, she was a GHI fellow from 2009–11 at Yale University. She has also completed a post-doctoral fellowship in the Social and Behavioral Research Branch at the National Human Genome Research Institute. She was awarded her Ph.D. in medical anthropology from the University of Hawaii-Manoa. Her dissertation on migration, social change, and health transitions was based on ethnographic research conducted in the Republic of Palau. She specializes in medical anthropology and the anthropology of food. She has conducted ethnographic fieldwork in Thailand, the Republic of Palau, Hawaii, and the continental U.S. Her current research addresses health disparities, infant and child feeding beliefs and practices, food insecurity, immigrant health, and indigenous health.

Professor Tulsi Patel is a Professor of Sociology in the Delhi School of Economics at Delhi University, New Delhi. She was Rotating Chair, India Studies at Heidelberg University, Germany for a full semester (2005–6). An Honorary Research Associate at the Department of Sociology, University of

Manchester (2001–4), she has also undertaken teaching assignments at the London School of Economics and the Royal Holloway College of the University of London (1996–7). She has previously taught at Jamia Millia Islamia, New Delhi and Miranda House (University of Delhi). Her areas of interest include gender, anthropology of fertility and reproduction, medical sociology, sociology of the family, and old age. She has authored *Fertility Behaviour: Population and Society in a Rajasthan Village* (1994, 2nd edn 2006) and edited *The Family in India: Structure and Practice* (2005). In addition, she has published several articles in national and international journals.

Dr. Sunita Reddy is an Assistant Professor at the Center of Social Medicine and Community Health, School of Social Sciences, Jawaharlal Nehru University, New Delhi, India. She taught briefly at the Indian Institute of Technology, New Delhi and Department of Sociology, Delhi School of Economics, Delhi University before joining JNU in 2004. She is an anthropologist, specializing in medical anthropology. She has researched on various issues of women's and children's health: breastfeeding practices, tribal women's health, child-birth, and child-rearing practices among the tribes. She has researched on disaster issues from social science perspectives and published *Clash of Waves: Post Tsunami Relief and Rehabilitation in Andaman and Nicobar Islands* (2013) with Indos, New Delhi. This book is based on a longitudinal study using anthropological research techniques. Her current area of research is medical tourism and reproductive tourism and surrogacy issues.

Dr. Alanna Rudzik is an International Junior Research Fellow, working in the Parent/Infant Sleep Lab at Durham University in the U.K. Before coming to Durham she held a SSHRC post-doctoral fellowship at the University of Toronto, working with Professor Daniel Sellen, in which she investigated cultural norms of infant feeding and mothering among Torontonian women. She obtained her Ph.D. in anthropology from the University of Massachusetts, Amherst in 2010. Her doctoral research with women from São Paulo, Brazil, focused on the effects of stressful life circumstances on breastfeeding duration in the early post-partum period, employing both biological and ethno-graphic research methods. She was awarded a doctoral fellowship from the Canadian Social Sciences and Humanities Research Council (SSHRC) to fund her Ph.D. research.

Malene Tanderup is a medical student in the Institute of Clinical Medicine, Aarhus University, Denmark. She has a Bachelor of Medicine and Bachelor of Surgery degree and is now completing her master's degree in medicine and surgery. She is part of the research project Reproductive Tourism in India: A Description of Surrogate Mothers and their Offspring, which is an interdisciplinary project within medicine, sociology and medical anthropology and cross-cultural studies, with researchers from Denmark and India. She is also a board member of the development workers union Dialogos and Dialogos Youth Group, which works primarily in Uganda, Nepal, and Bolivia.

Professor Penny Van Esterik is Professor of Anthropology at York University in Toronto, Canada where she teaches nutritional anthropology, in addition to undertaking research on food and globalization in south-east Asia. She is a founding member of WABA (World Alliance for Breastfeeding Action) and writes on infant and young child feeding. Her work includes the book *Beyond the Breast–Bottle Controversy*. She continues to publish extensively and to organize important cross-cultural discussions on breastmilk issues, especially in light of HIV/AIDS. She was recently awarded Food Anthropologist of the Year by the AAA Society for the Anthropology of Food and Nutrition.

Preface

Ethnographies of Breastfeeding: Cultural Contexts and Confrontations

Tanya M. Cassidy and Abdullahi El Tom

This volume originated from a workshop at the 2010 European Association of Social Anthropologists (EASA) held at the National University of Ireland, Maynooth (NUIM), the institutional affiliation of both of the editors of this volume. In keeping with the conference theme of "Crisis and Imagination," we organized a panel that dealt with explorations of alternative imaginations regarding global concerns, and the crisis circumstances of when a mother's own breastmilk is not available. Entitled "The 'Breastmilk Problem'," we put out a call for papers to contribute to a workshop that treated the problematization of breastmilk globally, illustrating traditions of milk banking and sharing. We further argued that such initiatives are at a critical phase, experiencing unprecedented opportunities and challenges, inviting a reimagining of global health within a flexible maternal economy.

The editors participated in this workshop, as did Professor Gervaise Debucquet, Dr. Rossella Cevese, Professor Alice Desclaux, Dr. Anne Matthews, and Professor Vanessa Maher, our discussant. Although the original meeting had a European orientation, both of the editors enjoy long-standing links with other parts of the world, including North America, Australia, and Africa, so as a result additional contributions were commissioned from international researchers at all levels of their careers. We are also including a foreword by Professor Penny Van Esterik, who was unable to join the original EASA workshop, but who has been a mentor for many years.

We wish to sincerely thank Professor Fiona Dykes at Lancaster University and Dr. Mark Maguire, as well as the entire Department of Anthropology at the NUIM, and the Department of Sociology, Anthropology, Criminology at the University of Windsor in Canada. We also wish to thank Louise Butler and Molly Beck at Bloomsbury, as well as all of the contributors to this volume, whose contributions have been invaluable. In addition, we would also like to thank Joseph and Drenda Vijuk, whose financial support helped this project to move forward in this age of austerity. We would also like to thank Dr. Conrad Brunström for all of his support and help throughout this project.

Finally, we would like to dedicate this volume to Gabriel and Liam, whose separate but interrelated journeys with breastmilk were the catalysts for this project.

Foreword

What Flows Through Us: Rethinking Breastfeeding as Product and Process

Penny Van Esterik

It is a pleasure to offer a few comments to introduce this collection of papers on breastmilk, or human milk, as I prefer to call it. (After all, we don't call cows' milk udder milk—why stress the container over the species?) I have been interested in human milk since the 1970s, as an anthropologist, feminist, and advocate for breastfeeding. In the years since I first published on the subject of breastfeeding, my ideas have constantly changed as a result of increased contact with mothers in different parts of the world, new research, and my continuing attempts to bring the interpretation of breastfeeding into play with broader concepts in the social sciences.

In 1989, I argued that the interpretation of breastfeeding often involved a shift from a process to a product interpretation. "Process models emphasize the continuity between pregnancy, birth, and the process of lactation. The adoption of the biomedical model with its accumulated scientific evidence about the nutrient content of breastmilk and breastmilk substitutes is a product-oriented model" (Van Esterik 1989: 5). The product model is compatible not only with biomedical control of infant feeding, but also with the commoditization of food, and encourages the comparison of different kinds of milks and other infant foods. A key point that I saw only later with increased attention to milk banks, HIV infections, and feminist performance art (cf. Van Esterik 2010, 2008a) is that human milk is incommensurable, a singular product with unique properties that are still being uncovered. How do you compare products that are in essence not comparable? Human milk, like all kinds of mammalian milk, "reflects 200 million years of symbiotic co-evolution between producer and consumer" (Hinde and German 2012: 2219).

If, in my earlier work, I had referred to the process of breastfeeding instead of the process of lactation as part of the continuity of care, perhaps I would have seen how deeply product and process are intertwined—how they are two inseparable sides of the same coin, intertwined like the two sides of a Mobius strip. We simply cannot separate the product component from the process component. The product and the process gradually turn an infant into a flourishing Thai, Lao, Mexican, Italian, American, or Somali person. We might call the first six months of "person making" that occur in particular locations the social womb.[1] This social womb is where the nurturing that turns the infant into a social and cultural being occurs. The embodied co-dependence of the breastfeeding mother and infant intensifies this "personing" process, assisted by physiological products such as hormones. Of course, millions of infants have become functioning persons without the help of human milk.

Process language is better at capturing the embodied nature of nurturing experiences like breastfeeding; the complex symbiotic relation between mother and infant has communication and co-regulation functions that extend far beyond nutrition. In the ethnographic literature, human milk is rarely thought about outside the maternal nursing relationship, with some exceptions, such as using human milk as a cure for eye diseases, or stories in the early 1980s of young men diagnosed with HIV who tried to use human milk to treat their symptoms. In 2012, researchers found that the milk of women with higher than median-level concentrations of the milk sugars, oligosaccharides containing immunologically bioactive components, reduced the risk of HIV transmission to their infants (Bode et al. 2012). The following year, 2013, researchers at Duke University isolated a protein in human milk, tenascin-C, that appears to disable the HIV-infected cells (Fouda et al. 2013 or www.dukehealth.org). One cannot help wondering if perhaps those gay men in New York knew something that scientists would not discover for another 30 years. At least they were open to the possibility that human milk could treat rather than cause HIV. And for that reason they attended to human milk outside the maternal breastfeeding relationship.

The papers in this book present new ways of dealing with human milk out of the breast and address the challenges this brings to national and international policy-making. They demonstrate what follows from acknowledging the entanglement of product and process. Why does this matter? Does the distinction between product and process, exclusive breastfeeding and mixed feeding, humanized or human milk matter to people other than epidemiologists and researchers? Does it matter to mothers or only to academic researchers?

Recent attacks on breastfeeding advocacy, scientific research, and on aspects of breastfeeding *per se* by Wolf (2010),[2] Barston (2012), and

Williams (2012a) are widely cited in the media. Breastfeeding advocates have been known to circle the wagons and shoot inward, leaving those with different opinions wounded, and the public less able to appreciate the advantages of breastfeeding. As Tara Moss argued on her blog (2013):

> On breastfeeding, for example, the evidence is in ... yet every opinion piece that begins with "I support breastfeeding, but", and then goes on to list reasons why women shouldn't breastfeed, or why breastfeeding doesn't have any "real" benefits, or why breastfeeding will be an awful experience for you (because it was for the writer), undermines decades of research, important health messages and hard facts.

Wolf in particular argues that medical research does not prove that "breast is best," and that confounding variables make it difficult to isolate the protective powers of breastmilk, stating that many publications in the best medical journals conclude that breastfeeding has no medical benefits (Wolf 2010: 84–5). This is patently untrue, but is a position that circulates widely in North American popular culture. This backlash comes at a time when important new properties of human milk are just being discovered. Wolf does make a useful methodological point here. But it is not that confounding demonstrates that human milk has no advantages over artificial milk products, but rather that it is near impossible to separate the effects of the product, human milk, from the process of breastfeeding. When we read in the literature that human milk has known health benefits for the infant's gut or brain, how can we know whether the benefit was due to the process of breastfeeding rather than the product, human milk, or indeed the context in which infants were fed? In studies that compare infants fed human milk with those fed infant formula, we cannot always know if the difference is product or process related unless one experimental group is bottle-fed with expressed human milk. It is possible to imagine experimental conditions where such a comparison could be made, but they would not be ethical because of the known advantages of human milk over all commercial replacements. Now that we know that even premature, sick, and HIV-positive infants thrive on human milk, it may be possible to observe the effects of the product, human milk apart from the process of breastfeeding, as some of the papers in this volume demonstrate. It is worth asking how often product replaces process in research studies. Since breastfeeding makes mothers and infants more interdependent, perhaps this intensifies the "personing" process, which might accelerate brain development quite apart from what human milk does nutritionally. More importantly, "Formula-feeding is by definition the experiment" (Weisinger

2012: 7); infants who are not breastfed are always the experimental group, while breastfed infants are controls, whether the researcher acknowledges this in the research design or not.

More interesting than the false claims that human milk is over-rated are the gaps in the literatures where human milk and breastfeeding should be found. Why has human milk and breastfeeding been erased from all the important discussions taking place around childhood obesity, diabetes, autism, allergies, and breast cancer? In an interview entitled "Just what's inside those breasts?" on NPR (National Public Radio) online, discussing her book on the history of breasts, Florence Williams (2012b) points out:

> We know far more about red wine than we know about human breast milk. But the things they're discovering are sort of amazing. We used to think that breast milk was just a food and that it was filled with fats and proteins and vitamins and that formula companies were successfully able to mimic this. But we now know that there are substances in breast milk that exist almost at the same levels that are not digestible by infants. So what are they doing there? It turns out they're digestible by beneficial bacteria. So over millions of years, the mother has been creating a substance that will recruit useful bacteria into her infant's gut, and this sets her infant up for life. So as much as breast milk is a food, we also now understand that it's also a medicine. (Williams 2012b)

Recently I was listening to a scientific presentation on the wonders of stem cell research and the potential miracles offered by these live cells. I mentioned to my colleague that there are living cells in human milk, but that no one seemed very impressed by the fact that living cells pass from mother to infant and survive in the intestinal tract of infants for several months until the infant gut is fully populated, or as long as new cells keep coming in from the mother (Mannel et al. 2008: 304). The Human Microbiome project, for example, did not consider human milk. Until recently, stem cell research ignored the research potential of pluripotent stem cells in human milk, but that situation is changing rapidly.

Foeini Hassiotou and her Australian colleagues (Hassiotou et al. 2013) published research that has argued that "breastmilk is a novel source of stem cells with multi-lineage differentiation potential." Interviewed for a discussion on "Stopping Multiple Sclerosis" by the University of Cambridge's *The Naked Scientist*, she said:

> So we've been examining stem cells in human milk. We find them in all the milk samples that we've analysed so far, which is hundreds and hundreds of them.

What we think is happening is that some of these stem cells come from the mother's breast tissue and some come from the mother's blood. So the question is, how they get into the milk, and what they do as soon as they are ingested by the baby ... From an immunological perspective, you do see a lot of things happening in the breast-fed babies, beneficial things that would not see them in formula-fed babies—for example, breast-fed babies don't really get allergies,[3] whereas formula-fed babies do. Breast-fed babies are protected from infections, so there are benefits, and these that can be facilitated through biochemical factors, molecules in the milk, but also by the cells—immune cells, but also, maybe, the stem cells, so that's what we're trying to find out. (Hassiotou 2013)

In addition, at Lund University, Sweden, Professor Catharina Svanborg and her research team have been working on a substance discovered in human milk known as HAMLET (Human Alpha-lactalbumin Made LEthal to Tumour cells), which has been shown to kill cancer cells (Gustafsson et al. 2009; Ho 2013). Although human milk has been used by a number of cancer patients for a number of years, the clinical trials associated with HAMLET are now showing great promise.

Although pasteurization kills many of the bioactive components of human milk, it leaves behind a product infinitely better than commercial formulas. Some living cells in human milk could be destroyed by freezing, boiling, and heat treatments, but human milk is still better than any alternative. It took thousands of generations to develop the perfect food for newborn humans (and the perfect food for newborn calves, for that matter), and we cannot reduce the importance of what a newborn human infant is fed to a lifestyle choice mothers make at birth and soon forget. The implications of these feeding decisions reach into adulthood and even to future generations.

Only recently has there been attention paid to the constituent properties of human milk outside of the maternal breastfeeding relationship. Often this interest is driven by the need to improve the composition of commercial human milk substitutes. Every component of human milk plays some medicinal role in addition to a nutritional role in the development of a human infant. While human milk as medicine cannot solve all health problems, we are reminded of the errors of thinking that separates food from medicine as two distinct categories, a mistake driven by Cartesian dualistic thinking that complementary medicine is working hard to correct. This tension between food and medicine, between the product that heals and poisons (cf. Derrida 1981), is fueled by the fact that so much can flow through human milk, including chemotherapy drugs, PCBs, HIV, TB, leprosy, the spirits of the ancestors, viral fragments of mother's diseases—but not necessarily the diseases themselves (just the fragments that leave traces that can act like vaccinations, protecting newborns from the diseases their mothers carry).

Recent research, including some of the discussions in this volume, suggests that we should be looking for new ways to think about human milk and breastfeeding. Historically, there have always been substitutes for maternal nursing, but these alternative strategies were not always passed from generation to generation because the outcomes were not good. In the past, most attempts to provide alternatives to human milk failed. In the last few decades, more at-risk infants who never received any human milk survive because they were given modern infant formula in a hygienic setting. While there is no artificial substitute for blood, infant formula was developed as an acceptable substitute for human milk. From that innovative product development in the late 1800s came the slow creep to the modern assumption that the two products are comparable and equivalent.

Can we say that infant formula is analogous to human milk or that bottle feeding is analogous to breastfeeding? There is no suitable analogy that reveals the full complexity and power of the product or the process. But that has not stopped us from making more or less suitable analogies for the product—wine, blood, semen, urine, yogurt, liquid gold. What would happen if human milk were really treated like liquid gold? What accommodations would be made for it and for its producers? We can begin to see the power of analogies and metaphors by comparing the use of a term like liquid gold to phrases that treat human milk as analogous to urine, and breastfeeding as a process analogous to urination, to be accomplished in the world's bathrooms. These indignities are further reinforced by signs that direct nursing mothers to bathrooms with baby facilities. Ironically, many of the public bathrooms are identified by pictures of feeding bottles, not nursing mothers.

While there are many analogies used to describe the product, human milk, it is harder to find analogies for the process of breastfeeding that do not simply rename the process. El Guindi (2012) distinguishes sucking from suckling, stressing that the latter is a deliberate act between a woman and an infant to accomplish something. This process has nothing to do with the product itself, but everything to do with re-categorizing kin (El Guindi 2012: 10). In the case of milk siblingship, the relation between the one act of suckling to establish an incest taboo and continuous acts of maternal nurture are culturally structured and complex.

One naturopathic doctor finds breastfeeding scary, a "sobering issue." After lauding the benefits of breastfeeding, she stresses the down-loading of "our inventory of environmental chemicals" into our babies, noting that if women could cleanse themselves of toxins before conceiving, "Subsequent generations would not accumulate the toxins from the previous generation" (Kaur 2003: 21). She advises women to express as much milk as possible between nursings in the first few months and discard it, pump and dump after each feed. Pump and dump is an increasingly common way to talk about the process of ridding the maternal body of excess milk as well as environmental toxins. But although the phrase is common in American public culture, perhaps because of its pleasing rhyme, it contradicts the idea that human milk is a precious gift, a resource that should never be wasted.

Pump and dump is also an insult to the women who produce this incredible product and pass it to infants through the process of breastfeeding or through other means. Assisted by helpful devices such as supplementary feeders or breast pumps, human milk reaches infants in need. This fact of contemporary practice creates another slippery slope, as new mothers are targeted by advertising messages from stores such as Babies R Us, urging them to purchase "breastfeeding essentials" (cf. Sobonya 2013). Mothers may then accumulate consumer goods in anticipation of future breastfeeding problems. How does pumping change women's perceptions of the product, human milk, and the process of breastfeeding? Practices implicated in milk banking and milk sharing will no doubt stimulate research to answer these questions. What we learn from these papers is that mothers are bricoleurs who seek all possible ways to maximize infant survival.

These papers also draw attention to the power of human milk to connect people across time and space, revealing some of the range of social solutions to the predicable and unpredictable problems of life with an infant, including the provision of human milk from someone other than the mother; these strategies include the use of donor milk banks, community milk banks, relatives, and neighbors who provide a casual, comfort feed to bridge the occasional gap between feeds; the more formal wet-nursing relations of past and present; the regular shared feeding among friends; surrogate feeding in emergency situations such as medical crises, war, and natural disasters that leave infants without their mother's milk; and milk siblingship that sets up a complex kinship relationship between families.

Less well explored are the linkages created through time, as human milk flows from one generation to the next. How is this important information exchanged? Through inheritance systems that link grandmothers to granddaughters? Or through taste regimes that socialize infants to their future food traditions?

Human milk is unlike the new range of "silver bullets" designed to "solve" the problem of infant and child malnutrition by providing highly processed baby foods and ready-to-use therapeutic foods (RUTF) such as Plumpy'Nut. These products emerge from the new public–private partnerships between industry, UN agencies and large NGOs that implement child feeding programs. Rather than seek silver bullets, the papers here demonstrate the complexity of the problem of how to feed and nurture a newborn. There are no simple solutions offered here, no technical solutions to replace nurture. In fact conditions that fully support mothers and infants often challenge gender hierarchies and basic capitalist principles. There are few problems in the modern world more difficult to address than gender hierarchies and economic inequities.

Even these "silver bullets" cannot save every child. Nor can human milk. But the papers emphasize the importance of finding ways to increase access to human milk, not access to a commercial alternative to human milk. The more we know about the product, human milk, the more we can contribute to making infant formula safer, if not safe. It is important not to confuse commercial efforts to make infant formula safer with marketing claims about humanizing cows' milk or suggestions that human milk and infant formulas are in any way equivalent.

Few women choose to use infant formula because they think the product is better than human milk; they choose it because they think—or people close to them think—that it is better than *their* milk. Why do they think there are problems with their milk? Because they know or suspect that their diet is inadequate; because they are tired or emotionally stressed and these conditions will damage the milk; because they want to have sex, or because they have been coerced into having sex; because they cannot follow customs or rituals that will protect their milk. These are not conditions that can be changed by lectures that tell women "breast is best." And they cannot be addressed through global health policies that ignore the conditions in which women nurture their children.

Do we expect too much of the modern maternal body? How plastic is it? A woman who sits all day in an office in front of a computer is then supposed to be able to give her body over to breastfeeding? How can women shift from CEO or factory worker to earth mother in an hour? Perhaps we need to rethink how maternal bodies need to be reshaped in order to be successful at breastfeeding? Is the transition from worker to breastfeeding mother easier for a rice farmer than a dentist? These questions suggest that we need a better understanding of how women integrate their reproductive and productive lives, paying particular attention to the quality of life of the breastfeeding mother.

To paraphrase Lévi-Strauss, human milk is good to think. Ignored, attacked, undervalued, traded, sold, over- or under-regulated, or made into ice cream,[4] human milk is the foundation of mammalian life and at the heart of human nurture. Solving the problem of universal access to human milk requires supporting and valuing the providers of that milk. Policies and practices that accomplish these objectives might go a long way to addressing other problems of the modern world.

Introduction

Ethnographies of Breastfeeding: Cultural Contexts and Confrontations

Tanya M. Cassidy and Abdullahi El Tom

Babies are always nursed, and in the few cases where the mother's milk fails her, a wet nurse is sought among the kinsfolk. (Mead 1928: 21)

Argued to be one of the first ethnographic accounts that highlighted domesticity along with the normalcy of breastfeeding,[1] Margaret Mead's seminal, albeit controversial (see Geertz 1989), 1928 discussion of the young women of Samoa is an apt way to begin this twenty-first-century presentation of ethnographies of breastfeeding. Much later in life, Mead (1972) was to also tell us about the personal links these experiences had for her when she herself was expecting her own infant in 1939. Specifically, she told us that she had fully intended to hire a wet nurse if she experienced difficulties producing breastmilk[2] (Mead 1972: 265–82), something that the historian Janet Golden (1996: 1) observes would have been extremely difficult to achieve at that place and time in history. Furthermore, Mead's linking of breastfeeding to her foundational cross-cultural study of food (1943), along with her other writings, was to influence generations of social scientists, including many of those who have contributed to this volume. This volume begins and ends with contributions from two influential professors of the anthropologies of breastfeeding, Penny Van Esterik and Vanessa Maher, both of whom offer their lifelong ethnographic knowledge and some of their theoretical arguments to frame some of the debates discussed herein this volume (see for instance Van Esterik 1989; Maher 1992).

Ethnographic studies by social scientists have shown that breastfeeding throughout history and across different cultures is not only a nutritional exchange, but a complicated psychosocial cultural behavior. By considering the product, as well as the producer and the consumer (Van Esterik, Foreword, this volume), we are offering an anthropological discussion of breastmilk issues across space and time. As the chapters in this volume indicate, these issues are intimately tied to the production and consumption of alternative human milk distribution systems (wet-nursing) and/or alternative animal-based milk substitutes, both of which are linked to concerns regarding the spread of disease to infants and/or to the lactating women, as well as being linked ultimately to the reduction of infant morbidity and mortality rates, albeit with some economic incentive. Ethnographies are about spaces in time, and this volume moves around the world, looking forward and back while discussing the present. We move from Brazil to North America, over to Ireland and the U.K., and then into France and Italy, followed by a triangulation from Africa, before we go to India and end in Australia.

Ethnographies of Breastfeeding: Cultural Contexts and Confrontations is part of this long history in the social sciences of studying not only what the first foods infants around the world receive, but the sociocultural contexts and some of the conflicts associated with these foods and their practices. Penny Van Esterik (1989; 2008a) has argued that controversies associated with infant feeding can be traced back to the 1930s, although historians and those who use ethnographic historical discussions would argue these controversies have much longer roots (Cassidy 2012b; and Chapter 3). The global community at the dawn of the twenty-first century, as it was at the beginning of the twentieth century, is looking to the life-saving properties associated with human lactation. The World Health Organization (WHO) and United Nations Children's Fund (UNICEF) have jointly recognized the global infant nutritional importance of human milk for the first six months of life (Butte et al. 2002; WHO 2003a). Specifically, the WHO has recognized that in circumstances where an infant is unable to be breastfed, the next best option is to feed it expressed breastmilk from either the infant's own mother, or from a healthy wet nurse, or from a human milk bank (WHO 2003a: 10).

MAKING MEANINGS OF MOTHERS' OWN MILK

Throughout history mother's own milk has been considered the ideal nutrition for infants, but there are also many cross-cultural contradictions and conflicts associated with maternal breastfeeding around the world. For instance, there is a long history associated with conflicts surrounding colostrum itself, which medical evidence now suggests is a form of perfect food and medicine, but yet many cultures have advocated discarding due to cultural constructions that this often-yellow substance is "bad quality," with some arguing (incorrectly) that it is even harmful to infants (see Gunnlaugsson and Einarsdottir 1993). In addition, the issue of public breastfeeding also illustrates cross-cultural variants, especially in cultures where women's breasts have a primarily sexual framing (see for instance Dettwyler 1995b; Anderson 2012). The emotion of embarrassment is often discussed by mothers in cultures such as Ireland (Cassidy, Chapter 3). There is also no cross-cultural consensus associated with how long to breastfeed an infant, although the anthropologist and breastfeeding advocate Kathy Dettwyler (1995a; 2005) has argued that there is strong bio-cross-cultural evidence that infants continue to receive breastmilk until over the age of two and up to the age of seven. In addition, controversies associated with how often infants should receive breastmilk was also discussed by Mead, which have been recognized as part of the origins of on-demand feeding and associated attachment parenting ideals, and have been central to breastfeeding advocacy groups such as La Leche League (see Faircloth 2013; and Chapter 4). The timing and duration of breastfeeding has implications both for parenting issues and for female employment. Van Esterik (Van Esterik and Greiner 1981) and Mead (1970) have argued that if a global culture of breastfeeding is considered ideal, the work environments of the world need to accommodate mothers having access to their infants at all times for at least the first six months of life.

The ethnographic journey with breastmilk in our volume begins in Brazil, an area frequently discussed in terms of the anthropology of parenting, especially maternal, and child (Scheper-Hughes 1992). Brazil has undergone profound changes since the 1980s, and recently Nancy Scheper-Hughes (2013) has argued that these changes have directly affected the mother–child relationship and the extremely large reduction in infant mortality rates. Scheper-Hughes does not discuss the radical changes associated with breastmilk that have correspondingly occurred during this time as well (Ortiz 2012). Alanna Rudzik's chapter (which is based on her comparatively recent doctoral ethnographic work from São Paulo, Brazil) offers a contemporary discussion of mothers, process, and product, making use of some theoretical insights originally presented by Van Esterik (1996a). Rudzik applies these issues to her discussion of the embodied experiences of the women she talked to in Brazil, for whom these issues integrate both process and product of breastfeeding. Brazil is the world leader in donor human milk banks, having over 200. Along with this country's initiatives in milk banking, Brazil has also spearheaded the worldwide "milk donation day," which began on May 19, 2005. João Aprígio Guerra de Almeida, the advisor to the Brazilian government on human milk banking, assured that "on that day in 2005, the first agreement to create an international network of milk banks was signed by 13 countries and international organisations" (Ortiz 2012; Guerra de Almeida 2013, personal communication).

Discussion of the maternal meanings of mother's own milk continues with Charlotte Faircloth's comparative discussion between mothers in the U.K. and France, concerning their experiences of breastfeeding and expressing, and how this relates to a juxtaposition of a maternal body with a sexualized body. Faircloth's work, based on her doctoral studies published elsewhere, is linked to issues of parenting, and especially the influence of "attachment theories" (2013). The topic of breastmilk expression is also discussed with these mothers, something that has become an increasing feature of ethnographic and historical discussions (see for example Lepore 2009; Ryan et al. 2013).

France is an important ethnographic space historically as it employed a widespread wet-nursing system well into the twentieth century (Sussman 1982). Our discussion continues in France with Gervaise Debucquet and Valérie Adt, whose discussion of issues of maternal "choice" regarding breast-feeding versus bottle feeding makes use of Bourdieuian notions of class-based considerations of food. They argue that their breastfeeding mothers often discuss maternal milk in term of food education, such as increasing the child's issues of "taste," thus offering a more symbiotic vision. By contrast, bottle-feeding mothers often frame their discussions around knowledge and science, a more performative vision. These different presentations co-exist within French food cultures. Such variations in taste are perhaps related to a greater cultural acceptance, at least historically, of the use of other people's breastmilk, possibly one of the most contested breastfeeding issues cross-culturally, and one which often does not accommodate a maternal voice in the debates.

EMOTIONS, RISK AND IDENTITY ISSUES WITH OTHER MOTHERS' MILK

Using other mothers' breastmilk also has a long history and has occurred in most cultures around the world, albeit often secretively (Shaw 2004). These exchanges have different names and features throughout history and across various cultures, and to capture these differences Cassidy (Chapter 3) has offered the suggested use of the term "lactation surrogacy," which includes not only traditional wet-nursing, systems of milk kinship and fostering relationships of infants historically, but also the modern medicalized versions of human milk banking, cross-nursing between family and friends, as well as the more recent internet-based informal milk sharing, many of which are covered by authors in this volume.

Unfortunately, urbanization and other modern forms of living arrangements lead to loss of traditional community institutions supportive of wet-nursing

(El Tom, Chapter 7). Hence, modern milk banking becomes a necessity that cannot be ignored without risking the lives of premature babies. It is encouraging that several countries have now either established their milk banks or are on their way to doing so, and it is equally gratifying that supportive research is gathering apace in this field. By its very nature, milk banking requires the collaboration of diverse disciplines, including biomedicine, anthropology, sociology, law, ethics, biochemistry, history, etc.

Two separate chapters in this volume by Cevese and El Tom introduce another aspect of wet-nursing that is crucial for success of milk banking. They show how the cultural perception of milk is endowed with the power of connecting people and that it is enduring and capable of surviving current global conditions of mobility, emigration, and transnational coexistence. Among Muslim societies the connecting power of breastmilk stands side by side with that of marriage, with its agnatic and uterine associations. Breastmilk in particular is a powerful medium of relationship and is amenable to multiple uses of connecting people. It can be used to create friendship between two families, render undesirable potential suitors unmarriageable, and, through controversial adult breastfeeding, circumvent Islamic codes concerning veiling and privacy among strangers of the opposite sex (El Tom, Chapter 7). Furthermore, in Islamic culture (according to one vision) milk donors have to be carefully selected as they transmit their own characters through breastmilk. Human characters, so to speak, are then not learnt but conveyed through other channels such as heredity, genes, and breastmilk (El Tom, Chapter 7).

The connecting power of breastmilk poses a formidable challenge to milk banking in Muslim societies and, if not handled properly, may severely limit the commitment of Muslim women to milk donation. This is precisely the finding of Cevese among immigrant Moroccan women in Italy who refuse sharing of milk with unknown mothers. More often than not, milk banking depersonalizes milk, reasoning its individual agency, and transforms it into an ontological entity in the public space. It further introduces a new powerful set of actors in the guise of doctors, nurses, and milk bank staff who intervene between the givers and receivers. This process challenges kinship rules among Muslim societies and hence complicates use of services of milk banks. While this context points to some challenges that lie ahead, it should not imply that milk banking and Islamic cultures are incompatible.

Islam is quite categorical on the right of lactating mothers to be rewarded by the father of the babies for this service. However, Islam also leaves the room open for lactating mothers to offer their milk without expectation of direct reward (Ali 1983). This leaves ample room for milk banking to opt for some form of gift exchange (Maus 1923–4; Titmuss 1970) or commodity exchange or both without breaching Islamic codes. These suggestions afford milk banking plenty of space to manoeuver in the negotiation of milk banking within Islamic cultures. Moreover, more traditional cultural constructions of "milk kinship" (Clarke 2007) can easily accommodate alternative modern breastmilk exchange relations. However, it has been recognized in cases where suitable wet nurse breastmilk exchange relations are unable to be found that the use of artificial milk is borne (Shaikh and Ahmed 2006).

HEALTH CONSIDERATIONS AND "HUMANIZED" MILK

Recent archaeological evidence has indicated the use of non-human milk to feed infants in ancient times, which was clearly a major contributor to higher infant mortality rates (Powell et al. 2014). However, the history of specific combinations of products or "formulae" (claiming they are "imitating" or are the "next best thing" to mother's own milk) became increasing prevalent in the latter part of the nineteenth century and even more widespread in the twentieth century (Cassidy, Chapter 3). Like milk banking, the history of these infant-feeding formulae can be traced back to persuasive stories involving saving of premature infants' lives, as marketing evidence often proclaimed. For instance, it is argued that Henri Nestlé created a product which was a combination "of cow's milk, wheat flour and sugar in an attempt to develop an alternative source of infant nutrition for mothers who were unable to breastfeed." For some healthcare providers the answer to these transmission issues was (and still is) to advocate the use of artificial infant foods, although there is increasing evidence that human milk is particularly important for premature infants (Cassidy, Chapter 3). Alternative health considerations are those associated with pandemics such as syphilis historically and HIV/AIDS today (Cassidy 2013).

Today the overwhelming global problem associated with breastfeeding is the maternal transmission of HIV/AIDS through lactation. The use of infant formula continues to be the recommended choice by American and some European healthcare professional bodies for feeding infants whose mothers have HIV/AIDS, which is completely opposite to the recommendation in most African nations where clean water supplies are limited. The contributions by Matthews on Malawi in East Africa and the Desclaux and Alfieri discussion from West Africa take the debates set forth in this publication in a different direction. They deal with numerous issues surrounding feeding of infants whose mothers are HIV-positive and particularly in the context of developing countries. Research to date shows that HIV can be transmitted through breastfeeding. However, this transmission can be prevented or drastically reduced if antiretroviral therapy is used. Optimistic experts have talked about virtual elimination of mother-to-child transmission of HIV by the year 2015 (UNICEF/UNAIDS/WHO/UNFPA/UNESCO 2010; Desclaux and Alfieri, Chapter 8). Needless to say, anybody who is familiar with international promises to the developing world knows such a target is likely to prove a fairy tale that cannot be realized. The date 2015 itself is probably inspired by the Millennium Development Goals (MDGs) that are already off target.

Policies on HIV lactating mothers are also influenced by a major finding that mixed feeding increases chances of HIV transmission. Hence, exclusive breastfeeding is recommended in certain circumstances. Needless to say, this condition is also difficult to guarantee, as will be subsequently demonstrated. Key researchers (Desclaux and Alfieri, Chapter 8; Matthews, Chapter 9) pose formidable challenges to the WHO recommendations in this respect. They demonstrate that the research on which such recommendations are based is riddled with unanswered questions and can at best be described as inconclusive (Van Esterik 2010). These notions portray breastmilk as dangerous, poisonous, and lethal (Cassidy, Chapter 3; Matthews, Chapter 9).

Recommendations of the WHO in this field come across as confused as the research on which they are based. In what is described as a double standard (Desclaux and Alfieri, Chapter 8; Matthews, Chapter 9), the WHO recommends that HIV mothers in the developed world do not breastfeed, while HIV mothers in the developing world are instructed to exclusively breastfeed but to wean early (approximately at three months). This recommendation is taken to the extreme in Sweden whereby it is declared criminal for HIV mothers to breastfeed their infants (Matthews, Chapter 9). The discrepancy or double standard in the WHO recommendation is justified by certain realistic concerns. Thus, an earlier recommendation reads, "The WHO recommends HIV-infected women to breastfeed their infants exclusively for the first six months of life, unless replacement feeding is acceptable, feasible, affordable, sustainable and safe (AFASS) for their infants before that time" (Matthews, Chapter 9).

As a matter of empirical fact, these conditions cannot be met in most developing countries. That means breastfeeding still remains a better option for many mothers who are now demonized by the recommendation. There is now additional evidence from South Africa indicating that exclusive breastfeeding for the first three months is statistically the best health choice for infants with mothers who are HIV/AIDS positive (Cassidy 2013). This then tracks back to the wealthier nations now having to accommodate mothers who are HIV/AIDS positive who may wish to provide their infants with mother's own milk or render safe human milk from alternative mothers.

Ethnographic methods were the main presentation of the papers presented in 1992 by Professor Vanessa Maher in her edited volume entitled *The Anthropology of Breastfeeding* that also grew out of an EASA workshop on the same subject. As Professor Maher mentions in this volume (Chapter 12), the latter part of the 1990s saw the publication of Edith White's book on issues related to HIV/AIDS and breastfeeding. In 2006, Professor Penny Van Esterik, a longstanding anthropological researcher (Van Esterik 1989) within the field of infant feeding, organized a conference in Canada and produced a report on issues related to HIV/AIDS, infant feeding, and gender. All of these discussions have contributed to this work, which is designed to add to the cross-cultural evidence, and to potentially help to frame policies in the future.

BUILDING BRIDGES WITH BREASTMILK

Building bridges with liquids is part of an important 1893 experiment conducted by Sir William Armstrong, who originally filled two wine glasses full of purified water and placed a cotton thread between them. Armstrong applied a high-voltage charge to the glasses, removed the thread, and a water bridge was retained between the glasses. "Floating water bridge between two beakers" was web-published as part of a teaching exercise by academics in Austria in 2007; this was then picked up and republished on YouTube, where the surprising image of building a bridge with liquid went viral. We use this analogy here to illustrate the fluidity of bridge building, as well as the surprising forms that this can take, which we believe is apt to a global consideration of human milk in all its surprising forms of exchange.

Many continue to argue that one of the most contentious issues globally continues to be related to infant feeding practices. These issues are further complicated when we are discussing international reproductive surrogacy. Reddy and her colleagues (Reddy et al., Chapter 10) discuss the contentious issues associated with breastmilk and reproductive surrogacy—a question linked to fears and concerns regarding bonding—but also maternal mental health, which is intimately linked to global bodily exploitation. Although social scientists and cultures around the world argue for the pre-eminence of mother's own milk, strategies for when this is not available have been the concern of mothers and medical practitioners for centuries. Integral to these discussions are the dominant roles of female relatives and friends regarding breastfeeding practices. In other cultures, it was this community that helped to feed infants, and cross-nursing was a normal and expected exchange between maternal bodies and infants of the community. The isolating features of a modern maternal–infant dyad has often resulted in the loss of intergenerational knowledge and the associated practices of this female embodied behavior, which has formed part of gender-based socialization in many cultures. Furthermore, it has also lost potential sources of trusted alternatives. However, the economics of breastfeeding work has historical examples of exploitation, and such exchanges between non-family or close friends, if not regulated, could result in similar abuses.

It has been argued that the world goal to increase breastfeeding rates would be helped by the establishment of donor human milk banks cross-culturally, a call to which internet-based human milk sharing groups have also offered a response (see Carroll, Chapter 11; Palmquist, Chapter 2). Furthermore, it has also been recognized that the widespread availability of human milk banks may contribute to increased rates of breastfeeding in the communities generally, while helping mothers of preterm infants until their own lactation is fully established (Torres et al. 2010). A neonatal nursing editorial tells us it is time we stopped treating infant nutrition as a "life-style choice rather than a health choice" (Worden 2007: 4).

This volume also builds bridges between cultural and social anthro-pologists, by offering sociocultural interpretations of breastfeeding, but also between those trained in departments of anthropology versus those with similar sociocultural approaches trained in departments of sociology. Recent American flagship journals in both anthropology and sociology have highlighted breastfeeding, the former using ethnographic methods to discuss bio-cultural factors associated with breastfeeding interactions in Africa (Fouts, Hewlett, Lamb 2012), and the latter considering the costs associated with exclusive and intensive mothering involved in long-term commitments to breastmilk feeding infants (Rippeyoung and Noonan 2012). Although these two disciplines might approach some of the debates associated with human milk from different perspectives, there is a relationship between those who prioritize ethnographic methods to study these issues.

Human milk comes with its own baggage. It is not only a nutritional substance and its function is not restricted to the physical survival of the baby. Breastmilk, as indeed breastfeeding, is steeped in the expressive and symbolic configuration of every society, old and new, traditional and modern. It defines motherhood, femininity, class, and status and creates kinship, affinal, and enmity relationships. This volume offers an opportunity to consider anthropological issues when we look at how we imagine infants have been, are being, and will be fed when they are not given milk from their mother's own breast. Such questions are addressed by considering the problematization of breastmilk globally, illustrating traditions of milk banking and sharing. Such initiatives are at a critical phase and are experiencing unprecedented opportunities and challenges, inviting a reimagining of global health within a flexible maternal economy.

Finally, it is key to remember that ethnography is the study of lived experiences, and those experiences are conveyed through narratives (Marcus and Cushman 1982; Clifford and Marcus 1986). The link between personal experiences and research has resulted in more explicitly reflexive connections between the researchers and their research, a methodological approach that has been labeled "autoethnography" (Reed-Danahay 1997; Ellis and Bochner 2000). Within the medical social sciences, narrative analysis, and in turn autoethnographic methodological practice is being increasingly presented (see for instance Ellis and Bochner 1999; Ellis 1999; Foster et al. 2006). *Ethnographies of Breastfeeding* has very personal auto-ethnographic origins for the editors (Cassidy and El Tom 2010), as well as offering innovative internet-based ethnographic and historical ethnographic work, along with more traditional ethnographies that all offer maternal voices from around the world. These papers continue this tradition of using ethnographic methods to discuss cross-culturally not only maternal experiences such as embodiment, sexuality, and reproduction, but how these experiences are mediated within varying systems of human milk exchanges, and how all of these issues continue to be mediated globally by public health concerns such as HIV/AIDS.

-1-

The Embodied Experience of Breastfeeding and the Product/Process Dichotomy in São Paulo, Brazil

Alanna E.F. Rudzik

While global health experts and medical professionals widely promote the benefits of breastfeeding—and breastmilk—women's breastfeeding practices are shaped by biology, cultural context, and individual experience (McDade and Worthman 1998; Sellen 2001; Rudzik 2012). Human milk, lactation, and breastfeeding are now widely researched topics. However, attention to experience is still overshadowed by research into outcomes and determinants (Van Esterik 2012), especially in contexts outside of North America and Europe, such as Brazil. Meanwhile, fueled by this research emphasis, breastfeeding promotional strategies focus on the *product* rather than the *process* of the embodied breastfeeding encounter.

The recommendation of the World Health Organization is that all women exclusively breastfeed their infants for at least six months, with continued breastfeeding thereafter to two years and beyond (World Health Organization, UNICEF 2003). Yet exclusive breastfeeding rates in Brazil remain far below the universal recommendation (Scavenius et al. 2007; Venancio et al. 2010) after decades of intensive promotion of infant formula by domestic and international industries (Bosi and Machado 2005), and despite the Brazilian Ministry of Health launching the world's most extensive breastfeeding promotional campaign in 1981 (Rea 1990). Research in Brazil has shown that women's choices about breastfeeding have long-term impacts on the health and wellbeing of their children (Victora et al. 2005) and there is a widespread and genuine commitment among healthcare professionals to improve breastfeeding rates (Bosi and Machado 2005; Scavenius et al. 2007). Most breastfeeding promotional materials in Brazil rely heavily on a "technologized discourse" (Demetrio et al. 2013) or biomedicalized understandings of breastfeeding. Medical arguments that champion breastmilk as the "best" choice for infant feeding emphasize the immunological and nutritive content of breastmilk, and women internalize these, rather than other benefits related to breastfeeding (Scavenius et al. 2007; Demetrio et al. 2013). As Scavenius and colleagues maintain, "if breastfeeding is to succeed, mothers must understand the *process* of breastfeeding, either intuitively, or rationally, or as part of a mother's culture of maternity" (2007: 678).

THE PRODUCT/PROCESS DICHOTOMY

Among breastfeeding researchers, a distinction between *product* and *process* with regard to breastfeeding is well established. The act of breastfeeding is an inter-subjective embodied process, "a holistic activity that is embedded in local practices in complex and patterned ways" (Van Esterik 2012: 58). In order to establish breastfeeding and to maintain sufficient supplies of breastmilk, particularly in the early weeks, a breastfeeding woman must feed her infant on demand and around the clock. Biologically, frequent emptying of the breast is required to properly stimulate milk production. Emotionally, breastfeeding requires "an embodied commitment accomplished on a constant basis" (Stearns 2013). In contrast, breastmilk as a substance is decontextualized and has become medicalized, commodified, and disembodied (Dykes 2002; 2005; Ryan, Todres, and Alexander 2011).

In early work on the emerging "insufficient milk syndrome" diagnosis in four developing countries, Van Esterik found that in contexts where women viewed breastfeeding as a process with intrinsic difficulties they observed variation in their milk quantity or quality and managed these variations through appropriate cultural means, rather than concluding that they were suffering from a "syndrome." In contexts where women's breastfeeding style emphasized breastmilk as a product rather than breastfeeding as a process, they were more inclined to interpret breastfeeding problems as evidence that they were suffering from insufficient milk (Van Esterik 1988). More subtle links between early supplementation with infant formula, reduced stimulation of the breast, and diminished milk production tended to be overwhelmed by a biomedicalized reading of the situation (Greiner, Van Esterik, and Latham 1981).

The medicalization of breastmilk and its conceptual separation from the maternal body allows for it to be viewed as simply a product to be provided by any caregiver (Blum 1993). This view of breastmilk has been accelerated by the growth in recent years of a robust personal breast pump industry, which has technologized the breastfeeding experience for many women. Pumps allow women to provide their infants with breastmilk when breastfeeding is not possible. Expressing breastmilk by pumping is attractive to some women precisely because it reduces the role of the body in transmitting breastmilk to the infant (Clemons and Amir 2010; Johnson et al. 2012). While pumps offer the potential for a breastfeeding woman to maintain a greater degree of separation from her infant, for work, social, or family reasons (Dykes 2002; Ryan, Team, and Alexander 2013), they remove breastmilk from the context of a maternal–infant dyad and introduce a mechanical "third party" into the breastfeeding process.

In affluent countries, research regarding the use of breast pumps has found that this introduction can lead to the breastfeeding relationship being framed as dysfunctional and in need of technological support (Ryan, Team, and Alexander 2013). Their use can also heighten the degree to which women imagine their bodies as machines, and potentially malfunctioning ones at that (Dykes 2002; Ryan, Team, and Alexander 2013). Examining the quantity and quality of breastmilk extracted through breast pumping allows for regular "inspection" of the machinery, that tends to reinforce rather than allay women's fears about supply (Dykes 2002).[1] In addition to these interventions in the breastfeeding *process*, pumping has also had an impact on societal views of the *product*. When we focus on the breastmilk removed by the pumps, rather than on the interaction between women and their babies, provision through the breast, bottle, or cup are all seen as equivalent (Auerbach 1991). From there:

> it is an easy step to thinking in terms of the production, manufacture and use of substitutes whose list of properties might lead one to believe that substance B (infant formula) is very much like substance A (breast milk). Such "likeness" then supports "equivalence" and from there is developed the notion that there is "really no difference" between the properties initially identified. (Auerbach 1991)

In Brazil, pumping breastmilk to feed your own baby is less common, as adequate electrical pumps are too expensive for general use. Pumped breastmilk largely exists in the context of donation to the large network of milk banks that provide human milk to premature and sick infants (Estevez de Alencar and Fleury Seidl 2009). Brazilian women who donate their milk focus on the special qualities and nutritional benefits of human milk in direct comparison with infant formulas (Estevez de Alencar and Fleury Seidl 2009). Research in the U.K. likewise found that women commodified and commercialized their breastmilk, viewing it as a consumer commodity similar, though superior, to formula (Ryan, Team, and Alexander 2013).

The international and local formula industry influenced Brazilian cultural norms with respect to infant feeding and is largely responsible for the decontextualization and product view of breastmilk (Bosi and Machado 2005). Through the twentieth century the industry marketed its products to doctors and other medical professionals, who prescribed infant formula indiscriminately to mothers, emphasizing the reliability of their product in implicit comparison to breastfeeding (Bosi and Machado 2005). Where breastmilk and infant formula are compared as competing products, breastmilk "can become a scarce resource or one which mothers cannot produce in sufficient quantity to assure adequate feeding" (Auerbach 1991: 115). In her landmark ethnography *Death Without Weeping*, Nancy Scheper-Hughes describes the way women's mistrust of their bodily capacity to produce milk played out in their breastfeeding experiences, ultimately leading to formula feeding and formula-related deaths of many children (Scheper-Hughes 1992). Conceptual distancing and alienation of women from their bodies, breasts, and breastmilk is particularly powerful when breastfeeding problems arise (Dykes 2005).

In Western culture in general and biomedicine in particular the mechanical metaphor for the human body is pervasive. The body is seen as a machine that can break down, be repaired, and have components swapped in and out without affecting the essence of the individual (Martin 1989; Davis-Floyd 1994). In the case of breastfeeding, this mechanistic reduction means that women's bodies producing breastmilk come to be seen as equivalent to factories processing cows' milk into infant formula, but far less reliable (Dykes 2005; Van Esterik 2012). Via its legacy in biomedicine, mind–body dualism underlies the reductionist diagnosis of "insufficient milk syndrome" (Greiner, Van Esterik, and Latham 1981; Scheper-Hughes and Lock 1987). The origins of this philosophy lie with Descartes, who postulated that the subject is an essence of mind, detached and separable from the biological body, that "our being ... is a conscious mind which is independent of the world of matter, even of the body" (Matthews 2002). The subject stands *outside* the world of experience and imposes meaning on that world (Matthews 2006).

THE PHENOMENOLOGICAL APPROACH TO BREASTFEEDING RESEARCH

A corrective can be found in the phenomenological approach to breastfeeding research, focused on the lived experience or embodiment of women where breastfeeding has been widely used (Stearns 2013). In particular, Merleau-Ponty's *Phenomenology of Perception* (1981) develops a phenomenology in which existence is analyzed as both embodied and gendered (Spencer 2008). Merleau-Ponty rejected the supposed separation of the mind from the body/world, and the subject from the object (Dreyfus 2000). Merleau-Ponty's move away from a Cartesian view of the body allows for the development of a powerfully anthropological take on breastfeeding, in which women's experiences are of both the body and the individual—more precisely, of the embodied individual. This is particularly needed as research exploring women's experiences with breastfeeding is still lacking (Regan and Ball 2013). The data presented below will explore the embodied breastfeeding experiences of a group of women from São Paulo, Brazil.

Location and Background

The qualitative data presented here are drawn from a larger research project which investigated the impact of daily life stressors on breastfeeding practice and duration among low-income women in six neighborhoods of São Paulo (Rudzik 2012; Rudzik, Breakey, and Bribiescas 2014). The participants were between 15 and 38 years old and were all becoming mothers and breast-feeding for the first time. Semi-structured interviews were carried out with each woman. One interview took place prior to the birth of the baby, in the last trimester of pregnancy. This interview gathered information about the women's plans for and expectations regarding breastfeeding. After birth, up to six interviews were conducted with each participant, lasting between half an hour and one-and-a-quarter hours. All interviews were conducted in Portuguese by the researcher and were digitally recorded with permission.

Antenatal Expectations

As mentioned earlier, Brazil has one of the world's most extensive breast-feeding promotion campaigns, wherein health professionals and the ministry of health dedicate a great deal of time to increasing breastfeeding rates and educating women. Campaigns and health workers are a "push" factor in getting mothers to breastfeed (Scavenius et al. 2007). However, the means of promoting breastmilk as the perfect food tends to objectify the milk, focusing on the product, rather than the process of breastfeeding. In the health clinics where I carried out my research, the displays and the discourse focused on milk, the food, rather than on breastfeeding, the action.

When women were first interviewed for the study, towards the end of their pregnancies, and were asked "Why do you want to breastfeed your baby?" embodied, inter-subjective reasons for wanting to breastfeed were very uncommon. Only three women gave such reasons as their initial response when asked why they planned to breastfeed. These women held the idea that breastfeeding was a tangible way to demonstrate love for their child. Anita (19) said she wanted to breastfeed "for the contact of the mother with the baby. For the love you give when giving the breast." Eva (16) felt that "Breastfeeding, the baby will have your attention, your love." A few other participants who mentioned a biomedical reason as their first response, afterwards added that breastfeeding also offered an enhanced link or feeling of connection with the baby. One participant explained: "You're more connected to the baby as well ... The love, the touch. Feeling the baby. It's very important" (Sonia, 28). Another felt "it's a privilege to be breastfeeding your child ... it's the best contact of anything. He's there feeling your warmth, the warmth of his mother" (Ana, 26).

The vast majority of women, more than three-quarters, responded that they wanted to breastfeed because of health or development benefits for the baby. Their responses reflected the product-oriented nature of breast-feeding education in the health sector. Some answers given were: "The baby is healthier" (Bete, 38); "They say that it helps the baby avoid sickness" (Carolina, 19); and "I think it's important because the baby grows up strong and less sick" (Josilene, 24). Fully a quarter of the participants empha-sized some component of breastmilk that they felt was important, such as "vitamins," "antibodies," "minerals," and "protein"; they did not give any additional or more complex reason for wanting to breastfeed when prompted. Clearly, the biomedical understanding of breastmilk, the product, had been absorbed by these future mothers, though some expressed it in more specific and others in more general terms. These echoed findings of other researchers in Brazil, where women stated that "breast milk is good because it makes the child healthy, it works like a vaccine" (Demetrio et al. 2013), and in the U.K., where women discussed their decision to breastfeed with regard to breastmilk constituents being beneficial to the baby's health (Dykes 2005). Taking biomedicalization of reasons for breastfeeding to the extreme, two participants reported that they planned to breastfeed purely because they had been told to by their doctor. While instructions from health professionals may influence women's pre-partum breastfeeding intentions (Demetrio et al. 2013), given the lack of success of most breastfeeding education, the extent to which this type of motivation influences actual breastfeeding practice is questionable (Kukla 2006).

Breastmilk had important vitamins and minerals. Breastmilk had antibodies. But in their responses, breastmilk did not seem to have much to do with the women themselves. Few if any of the participants gave answers that implicated bodily process in producing and providing the magical liquid. When asked what factors might interfere with breastfeeding many women said they could think of nothing that would interfere: "I think nothing … there's nothing that can interfere, no" (Pietra, 16). Rosinha (18) answered: "Ah, I don't know. I don't think anything can. What's important is your child." While these answers show a strong faith in breastfeeding, they do not reflect the lived reality of the breastfeeding process (Dykes and Williams 1999). The women seem to have been well aware of the biomedical rationale for breastfeeding, but were not prepared for its physical reality.

Women's view of breastfeeding as merely a way to transfer breastmilk, the product, to infants had implications for their pre-partum anxieties about breastfeeding. Participants alluded to the idea of breastmilk running out, drying up or simply proving inadequate, as though in a presence/absence scenario: "Things that can interfere? If you don't have milk. Only that" (Jacira, 18); "Only if it dries up. If not, I'll give it until 6 months" (Amaracleia, 18).

This concern was salient enough in the minds of five other participants who, when asked about how long they planned to breastfeed, responded that it would depend on the milk, they would breastfeed "while I have milk." In common with breastfeeding women from elsewhere in Brazil, the possibility that breastmilk would prove insufficient was seen as a concern, but the steps leading to that insufficiency—what Scavenius and colleagues refer to as a "debreastfeeding process"—were not recognized as the underlying cause (Scavenius et al. 2007). Women who ultimately weaned their infant before three months of age were particularly likely to have held a pre-partum idea that a woman's breastmilk might be inadequate to sustain the infant, either in quantity or quality.

Postnatal Experiences

There was a difference in focus between the pre-partum interviews and those that took place after the baby was born. In strong contrast to the pre-partum interviews, women spoke not about antibodies and vitamins, but about the experience of using their body to breastfeed their child. Women's first attempts at breastfeeding were the first conflict with their conception of milk as a product essentially stored in the body, to be found either present or absent. Marina's notion of her breastmilk is reminiscent of turning on a tap. She said:

> I only had milk at exactly the moment that [the baby] latched on to my breast. [The nurse] said "Go ahead, you can give it to her" and I said "But I don't have milk!" and she said "Put her on your breast" and I let her and she sucked and all I saw was milk going into her mouth, and I said "Ah, there is milk." (Marina, 24)

Rosalia's maternity nurse introduced her to the idea of breastfeeding as a process when she began to breastfeed for the first time, following the birth:

> I thought that I didn't have milk. [I thought] how am I supposed to have milk for this boy when I don't even have milk, and he's going to be dying of hunger here with me ... I said "There's no milk" and [the nurse] said "How do you mean there's no milk? It's only with him sucking that there will be milk." I was worried that there wasn't milk for him to nurse ... but then when he started to suck, my breast began to fill with milk and got full and so it was fine. (Rosalia, 18)

Participants reported surprise, both positive and negative, at the embodied nature of breastfeeding. Débora (24) found that breastfeeding was a positive pleasure: "Ah, the satisfaction of breastfeeding [was a surprise] because for me it's good, I feel good breastfeeding." But many of the new mothers felt negatively about the intrinsic sensation involved in the breastfeeding encounter. Kelly, who struggled to breastfeed and switched to formula at about four weeks, felt that "It was more difficult. I thought it would be like automatically she would suck and the milk would come. But no, first came out that watery stuff." Claudinha also felt breastfeeding was more difficult than she'd expected: "I thought that it would be normal and that when I put her there I wouldn't feel anything. It was more difficult than I expected." Kelly's use of the word "automatically" is suggestive here, along with Claudinha's expectation that breastfeeding would "normally" involve no feeling. Distancing and alienation from the body also may lead to breastfeeding being problematic, when women are unprepared for the bodiliness of breastfeeding (Dykes 2005).

It was particularly noticeable that women who had not planned to become pregnant were very vocal about the negative sensations they experienced with breastfeeding (Rudzik 2012). Claudinha had trouble defining her dislike of breastfeeding: "I don't know why but I didn't like it at all. It's a thing that makes you feel strange. Her there [at the breast] ... It's strange. I don't know how to explain myself, you know? I don't feel very good." Neuma (19) also disliked breastfeeding her baby, though she had difficulty describing why: "Oh I don't know, I think it's strange. I don't like it at all. She stays there sucking the breast [pause] Sometimes it hurts." When asked whether breastfeeding was pleasant, she responded "Well I don't think ... it isn't ... the sensation doesn't ... there isn't ... I don't think so.'

These quotes speak to psychological discomfort tied to the presence of the baby at the breast and the physicality of the breastfeeding encounter. Kelleher has argued that among breastfeeding women emotional and psychological states were linked to their physiological condition (Kelleher 2006). Women in industrialized countries report this discomfort with the act of breastfeeding as an invasion of bodily limits (Schmied and Lupton 2001; Marshall, Godfrey, and Renfrew 2007) or an unwanted sense of physicality (Britton 1998). Among women in São Paulo, women's discomfort with motherhood due to the unplanned nature of their pregnancies shaped the way that physical discomforts were perceived. Previous findings from the project have reported on the connection between unplanned pregnancy and maternal ambivalence regarding breastfeeding (Rudzik 2012).

A woman's embodied experience of breastfeeding can unsettle her perceptions of herself (Chodorow 2003; Sandre-Pereira 2003). In the case of the participants discussed here, many were very young women who were undergoing a rapid transition from adolescent to mother. The transition was underscored by a change in accepted use of the body, particularly the breasts. When asked about how her life had changed since her daughter's birth, Maria José's very first comment was "Now my breasts aren't just for me, you know?" Her breastfeeding meant that she had to share her body with her baby. When asked how breastfeeding had affected her idea of her breasts Claudinha (16) said:

> Now ... well, I don't want to say that it's public! [laughs] It's not. But ... it's not an intimate thing for anyone. If there's someone in the house, you have to just take it [the breast] out, and that's it! Any place. I was embarrassed until [the baby] was about a month old. My mum was mad because I was hiding from her. She said everything that I have she has, so why hide?

Though Claudinha's mother was trying to be supportive, to help her become comfortable breastfeeding, what she had asserted was that as a woman breastfeeding a baby Claudinha did not have the prerogative to decide who would see her breasts and when. Claudinha's account suggests that she felt her body boundaries and her privacy were infringed upon as a function of her role as a breastfeeding mother. The potential for family members to impinge on women's breastfeeding and bodily practice is a common theme among experiential studies of breastfeeding (Mahon-Daly and Andrews 2002; Marshall, Godfrey, and Renfrew 2007).

The intensity of breastfeeding contact in the early weeks was obvious in many women's narratives: "At night she keeps the nipple in her mouth the whole time. She doesn't take the pacifier, she just keeps the nipple there" (Claudinha, 16). Women described feeling compelled to breastfeed even if they didn't want to. Gilderlene (16) in trying to convince another young mother to breastfeed, said: "And I tell her 'Even if I don't want to, I give [the baby] the breast. There's no problem.'" Rosinha (18) described having to get used to that demand:

> [At first] I said that if I was in the street I wasn't going to give [the breast], no way … I would just let him cry until I arrived home. [AR: What changed?] What changed? I had to get used to it. I had to give it. When he wanted it I had to give it.

The "calling" of the infants and response of the mothers characterizes the inter-subjective nature of the breastfeeding relationship (Ryan, Todres, and Alexander 2011). Some women were also able to achieve "fulfillment" or a sense of unity through breastfeeding (Ryan, Todres, and Alexander 2011). Sonia (27) felt that in breastfeeding "[my daughter] and I are the same person. I don't want to be far from her." Débora thought that breastfeeding was a special time and a special connection:

> It's a moment just for you two, mother and child. It's really a moment of connection … It's a way to be closer because since [my son's] no longer in the belly, I think breastfeeding is the way to have him closer to me. Because when I gave birth to him, I missed my belly … when he came out it felt like he didn't belong to me … So when I'm breastfeeding, it's a sensation that I'm protecting him … as though he were still [pause] that there's a part of him that's still inside me.

For Débora, the on-going physicality of the breastfeeding process felt positive, continuing the embodied connection with her child that she had valued in pregnancy. As one of the few mothers to recognize the inter-subjective nature of breastfeeding prenatally, this connection did not come as a surprise to her.

Discussion

Prenatally, most first-time mothers in the periphery of São Paulo lacked an appreciation of the embodied nature of breastfeeding. Although all participants stated an intention to breastfeed for at least three months, few were cognizant of the intensity of embodied interaction required to maintain the breastfeeding process. Since breastfeeding is the single task that requires the most time and effort from mothers in the first months of a baby's life, and as the only task that cannot be directly shared with another, it actively requires the maternal body to be available (Stearns 2013). As Stearns argues, "being a breastfeeding mother is not only or simply a decision that merits one a potentially positive judgment about her mothering abilities; it is also an embodied commitment accomplished on a constant basis" (2013). Many women find that breastfeeding requires a different level of dedication than they are prepared for when they state that they want to breastfeed "for the health of the child." While some women in the study were aware of pain as a possibility, most were altogether unprepared for the ongoing intense physicality of the process of breastfeeding. This was particularly troublesome for women who had unplanned pregnancies, who were more ambivalent to breastfeeding overall (Rudzik 2012).

In order for pregnant women to be properly prepared for the experience, breastfeeding needs to be a social and cultural embodied practice of a woman within a family and in complex networks of social relationships (Demetrio et al. 2013). However, following the precipitous decline of breast-feeding in Brazil, as elsewhere, and the consequent loss of intergenerational embodied knowledge of breastfeeding, passed on from grandmothers, mothers, aunts, and *comadres*, the women I interviewed in São Paulo lacked a strong community to draw on. What remained—what has been put in place through great effort—is breastfeeding promotion and educational programs provided by the health sector. These generally highlight the vital importance of breastmilk, down to its component parts, for infant health. Unfortunately, the milk is often presented out of context of the biological and emotional aspects of the mother–infant relationship. Without a breast-feeding community to counterbalance the *product* emphasis, women who are becoming mothers and breastfeeding for the first time construct a mecha-nized, factory-model understanding of breastmilk's presence in the body. The *process*, the embodied connection between a women and her infant and the dance of request and provision that maintains breastmilk supply, is hidden. Women are then confronted with the sometimes overwhelming physicality of breastfeeding in the early hours, days, and weeks of breastfeeding. Among the participants discussed here, some women were able and willing to embrace this largely unsuspected aspect of breastfeeding, and maintain the practice. Others found it to be too great a burden, and the common expla-nation that they "lacked milk" or the "milk had dried up" was borne out as their process shaped their supply of "product."

Demedicalizing Breastmilk: The Discourses, Practices, and Identities of Informal Milk Sharing

Aunchalee Palmquist

Milk sharing is an emergent infant-feeding practice in which a breastfeeding mother[1] nourishes a child who is not her own biological offspring through privately negotiated altruistic breastmilk gifts. Altruistic milk sharing is often called "informal"[2] milk sharing, to distinguish it from breastmilk donations that are processed and distributed by a human milk bank. It is distinct from "milk selling," which involves marketing breastmilk for profit. While wet-nursing, cross-nursing, co-nursing, and other forms of co-operative breastfeeding have a long history in the United States (Golden 2001), it was the use of internet social networking sites on Facebook that catapulted milk sharing into the public gaze, transforming it into a *bona fide* modern social phenomenon (Akre, Gribble, and Minchin 2011; Geraghty, Heier, and Rasmussen 2011; Cassidy 2012a; Gribble and Hausman 2012).

There is no question that milk sharing is first and foremost about babies and breastmilk. Yet, the giving and receiving of breast is much more than simply a means to feed a baby (Shaw and Bartlett 2010). Milk sharing is at once personal and political. It simultaneously involves individuals and communities and is intrinsically biocultural, involving a symbiotic relationship between mothers, babies, and others. The act of milk sharing carries both symbolic meaning and tangible significance. Milk sharing is part of our ancient history, and with the aid of the internet it has been reimagined and reinvigorated in the twenty-first century. The focus of this chapter is on the ways in which milk sharing reflects processes of demedicalization, specifically the demedicalization of expressed breastmilk.

The chapter is based on analyses of content posted on two public Facebook social networking pages that host non-profit milk sharing connections, Eats on Feets (EOF) and Human Milk 4 Human Babies (HM4HB), from April 2011 to March 2013. A total of 1249 posts were archived and categorized during this timeframe. Analysis of the posts followed a two-step process, the first a categorical analysis and the second a thematic analysis. Categories included requests for milk, notifications of milk to donate, general breastfeeding support and information, and links to news articles, blogs, and other media. Themes reflected the variety of reasons for donation, reasons for requesting breastmilk, milk sharing philosophies and ideologies, discourses of milk sharing in the popular media, testimonials about the positive experiences of milk sharing, resources for breastfeeding, and information on the various strategies for collecting, storing, and delivering breastmilk. Interpretations of these data are enriched by my own experience as a breastmilk donor, my training as an International Board Certified Lactation Consultant (IBCLC), and conversations with donors, recipients, breastfeeding professionals, and other breastfeeding advocates. Illustrative quotes drawn from the data that reflect processes of demedicalization are presented throughout verbatim.

MEDICALIZATION, DEMEDICALIZATION, AND RESISTANCE

Medicalization refers to the manner by which normal physiological, behavioral, or emotional aspects of the human condition become pathologized by medical institutions and their practices (Conrad 2007). Conversely, demedicalization refers to the process by which previously defined medical conditions come to be accepted as normal states of being (Conrad 1992). Although commonly treated as separate and distinctive processes, medicalization and demedicalization often operate simultaneously (Halfmann 2012). Conrad (2013) identifies several key characteristics of medicalization. He describes medicalization as the way in which problems come to be defined as medical categories. Medicalization may occur in varying degrees along a continuum, and medical categories may expand or contract. Because medicalization is an artifact of broader sociocultural processes, it is not driven solely by medical institutions. Patients may also push for greater medicalization of particular issues. Finally, he notes that medicalization is bi-directional. Likewise, Halfmann (2012) argues that medicalization and demedicalization converge and diverge in unpredictable ways. He proposes examining the discourses, practices, and identities involved in medicalization and demedicalization as a way to better understand their simultaneity.

According to Halfmann (2012), discourses include biomedical vocabularies, models, and definitions that are involved in medicalizing the body and are often part of the first steps toward increased medicalization at a conceptual level. Practices refer to actions and behaviors that are nested within a biomedical paradigm and further reify discourses. Examples include forms of biomedical testing, surveillance, risk assessment, diagnostics, and treatment. It also involves the establishment of new biomedical professions that are born out of a niche that is filled with creating new pathologies. Halfmann (2012) uses the concepts of identities or actors to mean both individuals and groups who become increasingly invested in both biomedical discourses and practices in constructing identities and fulfilling social and cultural expectations associated with those identities. Processes of demedicalization often involve discourses, practices, and identities that diverge from the biomedical paradigm. Halfmann (2012) uses the case of abortion in the U.S. to illustrate the intersecting spheres of medicalization and demedicalization.

Medicalization of women's reproductive health has been the subject of numerous anthropological studies. These studies demonstrate the ways biomedicine has pathologized normal processes, such as menstruation, pregnancy, childbirth, and menopause, in the U.S. and globally (Ehrenreich and English 1978; Bell 1987; Martin 1987; Scheper-Hughes and Lock 1987; Ginsburg and Rapp 1991; Davis-Floyd 1992; Lock 1995; Davis-Floyd and Sargent 1997; Ferguson and Parry 1998; Browner 2000; Rapp 2000; Finkler 2001; Lock 2001; Rapp 2001; Inhorn 2003a, 2006; Cheyney 2011). The pathologizing influences of science and technology on women's bodies have received attention by scholars interested in the medicalization of breastfeeding (Apple 1987; Van Esterik 1996a; Hausman 2006; Tapias 2006; Moran and Gilad 2007; Jansson 2009; Thulier 2009; Avishai 2011; Hausman 2011; Lee 2011; Andrews and Knaak 2013; Ryan, Team, and Alexander 2013). Yet, even in this literature, there are very few studies that describe processes of demedicalization.

A recent exception is Torres (Torres 2013, 2014), who contributes to this literature by focusing on the emergence of new health professionals devoted to supporting breastfeeding in clinical settings in a paradoxical effort to "demedicalize" breastfeeding. While not specifically focusing on demedicalization, Cheyney (2010, 2011), Miller (2012), as well as Miller and Shriver (2012), describe home birth practices in the United States as active protests against the medicalization of birth. Because demedicalization begins with medicalization, examinations of demedicalization intrinsically call attention to the liminality of these co-existing processes as they intersect. Efforts to demedicalize already medicalized conditions such as pregnancy and childbirth often begin with practices of actors in their everyday lives (Halfmann 2012). These collective acts of resistance are small, but significant, gestures that can often incite broader social movements of demedicalization that "trickle up," leading to changes in biomedical practices and policies (Halfmann 2012). Understanding demedicalization as acts of resistance is also important in refocusing attention on the ways individuals exercise agency and seek empowerment despite hegemonic influences; a focus on demedicalization leads to an understanding of the everyday practices of resistance to medicalization (Lock 2001). This analysis is one of the ways in which milk sharing is enacted to demedicalize women's bodies, the fluids they produce, and the babies they nourish.

MEDICALIZATION OF BREASTMILK

The medicalization of breastmilk refers to the manner by which breastmilk has been defined as a medical substance that requires scientific testing, surveillance, and regulation (Conrad 1992). In the United States the inception of medicalized breastmilk coincided with the rise of pediatrics, around the turn of the twentieth century. Doctors during this time became increasingly aware that infants fed with breastmilk substitutes were less likely to survive (Wolf 2001). Pediatricians were divided on whether to address this problem by improving breastfeeding rates or increasing the quality of bovine milk used in breastmilk substitutes (Apple 1987; Wolf 2001). Wet-nursing was one potential solution to breastmilk shortages, although at the time it was unpopular because of how difficult it was to maintain some semblance of quality control over eligible wet nurses (Swanson 2009). As a compromise, doctors began collecting expressed breastmilk, both for medical use and research purposes (Golden 2001).

Human milk banks were the earliest repositories of expressed breastmilk in the United States. The first milk bank was established at the Boston Floating Children's Hospital in 1910. Swanson (2009: 25) describes the floating hospital as "a boat that cruised Boston harbor daily in the summer months, taking infants and children and their mothers out into the fresh air and providing medical services to those on board." Prospective wet nurses on shore were put through various screening practices to ensure that the breastmilk collected for the floating hospital came from physically healthy and morally suitable donors (Golden 2001). Women were paid by the ounce for their milk, which was then bottle-fed to the babies on board (Swanson 2009).

Using the Boston Floating Children's Hospital as a model, "mother's milk stations" sprung up across the country (Golden 2001; Wolf 2001). Depending on the locale of the mother's milk station, paid wet nurses were subjected to various clinical milk expression protocols, such as having their breasts scrubbed with boiled water and soap, being dressed with medical gowns, caps, and surgical masks, and having their hands scrubbed for ten minutes prior to expressing milk into sterilized bottles (Swanson 2009). Disembodied breastmilk from individual donors was then pooled together to create a nutritionally uniform product and pasteurized utilizing the same procedures to treat bovine milk. On the surface at least, all traces of the women who were part of creating this life-saving elixir had been eradicated (Hassan 2010). The final product, sterile human milk, was only available by a doctor's prescription.

Pediatricians were the first to capitalize on emergent science and technology in efforts to deliver expressed breastmilk to medically fragile infants (Wolf 2001). Increasingly, they began to think of breastmilk as raw material for neonatal therapies and human milk-based formulas, a new type of "therapeutic merchandise" (Golden 2001: 179). Breastmilk was subjected to boiling, freezing, drying, and reconstitution in efforts to extend its shelf life and expand its medical applications (Swanson 2009). The primary limiting factor in successfully developing and sustaining the production of promising new human milk technologies was, of course, a reliable supply of breastmilk. As breastfeeding rates declined in the wake of wildly popular bovine milk-based infant formulas, the pool of lactating women who were willing and available to contribute to milk banks waned (Wolf 2001). Between 1946 and 1956 breastfeeding rates fell 50 percent and by 1971 only 21 percent of women initiated breastfeeding (Fentiman 2009).

Milk banks rebounded along with a rise in breastfeeding promotion and advocacy in the 1970s (Blum and Vandewater 1993; Jones 2003). In the 1980s concerns about disease transmission via breastmilk were heightened with the emergence of HIV/AIDS, further galvanizing the rationale for medical surveillance and control over milk collection and distribution (Hausman 2011). Milk banks across the country shut down in the absence of methods for reliably screening for HIV. In 1985 the Human Milk Banking Association of North America (HMBANA) was established as a non-profit organization devoted to collecting human milk from healthy donors, pasteurizing and testing it for safety, and dispensing it by prescription to those babies with a documented medical need (Updegrove 2013a: 503). Clinician demand for banked human milk in hospital neonatal intensive care units (NICU) steadily intensified, following substantial evidence for significantly higher rates of fatal necrotizing enterocolitis (NEC) among pre-term infants fed with breastmilk substitutes. Currently, HMBANA has 11 milk banks in operation across the nation, and in 2011 they dispensed an estimated 2.15 million ounces of human milk (Updegrove 2013b).

Breastfeeding rates in the U.S.A. have steadily risen in recent years, though are far below other nations in both breastfeeding initiation and exclusive breastfeeding at three and six months (CDC 2012). One advantage of more breastfeeding mothers is the new pool of potential human milk bank donors (Updegrove 2013a). More donor milk means that more lives are saved. It also means greater opportunities for innovation in human milk technologies. For example, the company Prolacta has successfully developed and marketed human milk-based fortifiers to enhance the nutritional value of breastmilk fed to premature infants in the NICU (Fentiman 2009; Hassan 2010).

The medicalization of breastmilk is most pronounced in hospital NICUs. For example, mothers who deliver infants that are immediately sent into the NICU are encouraged to start expressing their colostrum and breastmilk within six hours post-partum (Renfrew et al. 2009; Mannel, Martens, and Walker 2013). Pumping is required every two hours throughout the day and night to stimulate a mother's breasts in the absence of a suckling infant. Hand expression is also used in the early days post-partum to provide additional stimulation and more effectively collect colostrum. Many mothers of NICU babies experience difficulty establishing and maintaining a breastmilk supply post-partum due to a variety of factors. A traumatic birth experience, excessive blood loss, medications, post-partum separation, post-partum depression and anxiety, and lack of breastfeeding support are just a few of the common factors that may contribute to difficulties in successfully establishing lactation.

The use of banked donor milk in NICU settings is highly regulated and dispensed with the same care as pharmaceuticals. Donor milk feedings are described as a medical therapy in NICUs. Neonatal pediatricians, NICU nurses, dieticians, and IBCLCs are all trained in various protocols used to prepare and deliver donor milk to NICU babies safely. Among the most premature and medically fragile NICU babies, donor milk is delivered through a nasogastric tube and is closely monitored with highly specialized computerized technologies. Various monitors and sensors are used to ensure the proper amount and rate of delivery and to track infants' physiological responses to the feedings. Older and more robust infants on donor milk may be fed using a variety of breastfeeding technologies, including bottles, syringes, tubes, nipple shields, and supplemental nursing systems.

The medicalization of breastmilk is also evidenced by the continued intensification of breastmilk research. Human milk labs have popped up across the country. The University of Massachusetts Breastmilk Lab,[3] for example, collects donor milk to better understand the links between lactation and breast cancer. Many HMBANA milk banks also undertake research to better understand the effects of storage and handling practices on the quality of banked milk (Updegrove 2013b). Human milk research over the past decade has provided a rich evidence base describing the molecular characteristics, nutritional composition, and clinical uses of breastmilk, and health benefits of breastfeeding in mothers and infants (Mannel et al. 2013).

Once medical professionals embraced breastmilk as a therapeutic tool, a variety of emergent discourses, practices, and identities served to reify breastmilk as a powerful medicine. Today, the medicalization of breastmilk is most pronounced in biomedical settings, but breastmilk science has been thoroughly integrated into the design of national public health policies and localized breastfeeding campaigns alike (Fentiman 2009). Most women who choose to breastfeed describe doing so for the health benefits (Fischer and Olson 2013; Labbok 2013; Street and Lewallen 2013; Tully and Ball 2013; Bernie 2014). Recent studies have found that breastfeeding mothers also regularly express their breastmilk (Van Esterik 1996b; Avishai 2004; Labiner-Wolfe, Fein, Shealy, and Wang 2008; Ryan et al. 2013). Even breastmilk expression in the home has been subjected to medicalization with the recent Academy of Breastfeeding Medicine (ABM) protocol for the handling, storing, and feeding expressed breastmilk for full-term infants (ABM 2010).

At the same time, biomedical discourses and practices define breastmilk as a potential biohazard, sending a clear message that breastmilk is not intrinsically safe (Hausman 2006, 2011). Despite the fact that the American government Centers for Disease Control and Prevention (CDC) states healthcare professionals are not required to use universal precautions while handling breastmilk, milk banks still treat it as a biohazard. HMBANA has adopted the same screening and testing protocols used for human blood banks, despite the fact that some diseases which are transmitted through blood are not also transmitted through human milk. Milk banking safety protocols are used expressly to protect already vulnerable infants from the "inadvertent exposures" (Updegrove 2013b: 504) and "inherent dangers" (Updegrove 2013b: 507) of feeding breastmilk. The discourses of risk tied up in breastmilk safety protocols, while directed at human milk donors, inadvertently antagonize breastfeeding women generally. For instance, upon passing the screening protocol for HMBANA, eligible donors receive a letter stating that:

> As a member of the Human Milk Banking Association of North America, we believe it is important for you to know that acceptance as a donor does not indicate that your milk is safe to share with individuals outside the Mothers' Milk Bank. HMBANA banks take several steps to assure the safety of donor milk

BEYOND the health screening of the donor; there is no guarantee of safety of a donor's milk for a recipient if it has not been processed by a HMBANA donor human milk bank.

Clearly, this letter discourages milk sharing. Yet, perhaps without intending to, this type of language implies that a mother's raw breastmilk is not quite fit to share even with her own child unless it has been processed by a HMBANA milk bank.

It is important to note that the idea of breastmilk as a pollutant predates the HIV/AIDS era. Historically, it was not only a woman's health behavior that was viewed as a potential risk factor in giving her breastmilk to others; her moral character was also called into question. A substantial feminist literature describes the ways various cultural beliefs regarding the capacity of women's bodies and bodily fluids to harbor filth have led to social institutions and practices designed to harness, control, and purify them (Fildes 1988; Bramwell 2001; Golden 2001; Giles 2002, 2004; Shaw 2004; Hassan 2010; Muers 2010; Obladen 2012). Anxieties about the potential for harming one's own child through breastfeeding have historically been a major barrier in breastfeeding promotion and continue today (Apple 1987; Wolf 2001; Hausman 2006).

Milk sharing generates the greatest controversy at the intersection of "breastmilk-as-medicine" and "breastmilk-as-pollutant" (Gribble and Hausman 2012). The discourses, practices, and identities of milk sharing collide with this paradoxical vision of breastmilk in ways that disrupt medical authority and empower women. A metaphor of resistance is often invoked to illustrate how people protest, cast off, and otherwise express their discontent with oppressive social structures and institutions in their everyday lives. The ways in which these forms of resistance are situated in bodies is an important aspect of medical anthropological inquiry (Scheper-Hughes and Lock 1987; Van Wolputte 2004; Desjarlais and Throop 2011). Resistance to medicalization is an integral process of demedicalization (Lock 2001).

Discourses of resistance in online milk sharing networks refer to the mission statements, philosophies, and online exchanges that contest the framing of milk sharing as fundamentally dangerous. Practices of resistance are enacted through the everyday activities of milk sharing. Identities of resistance are the ways in which those engaged in milk sharing define themselves through their involvement in milk sharing.

DEMEDICALIZING BREASTMILK THROUGH MILK SHARING DISCOURSES

Compassion and empathy for babies and their families is what brings us all together. Women are reclaiming their breastmilk, fully recognising its value, and are willing to share it freely with the babies and children of their communities. We desire a paradigm shift back to our biological roots, so that babies and children are being nourished by breastmilk. (http://HM4HB.net/about.html)

Milk sharing has always been part of the breastfeeding landscape in the U.S. Prior to e-mail Listservs and popular social networking sites like Facebook, milk sharing occurred behind closed doors, beyond the public gaze. While the historical record suggests that milk sharing was not a mainstay of modern-day mothering in the mid- to late twentieth century, it has likely always been a part of breastfeeding culture throughout the world (cf. Shaw 2007; Thorley 2008; Shaw and Bartlett 2010).

The internet has transformed the face of milk sharing globally. Eats on Feets (EOF) and Human Milk 4 Human Babies (HM4HB) are two online sites created to facilitate altruistic milk sharing connections. Each site hosts a global page as well as local community pages representing every state in the U.S. and 52 countries. Through EOF and HM4HB, families in need of breastmilk can easily locate breastfeeding mothers with milk to share. Exchanges that take place on these sites are explicitly non-commercial, unlike other internet sites hosting breastmilk classifieds. Women, many of whom had never heard of milk sharing or had never considered that they could give their surplus of breastmilk to feed other babies, started logging on to Facebook to find their "milky match" in the fall of 2010 (Cassidy 2012a). This is when breastmilk began flowing as never before across county lines, state borders, and even national boundaries. Not only did these internet sites catapult milk sharing into mainstream consciousness, they ignited a social movement to normalize breastfeeding and sharing breastmilk (Cassidy 2012a). Milk sharing relies on a few key ideas that are important to its demedicalizing effect: altruism, informed choice, and safe breastmilk.

Milk sharing is sustained by generosity. By definition it does not involve the exchange of money. Selling breastmilk is actively discouraged, both by site administrators and members of EOF and HM4HB online communities. The act of giving breastmilk freely is tied up with idealized conceptualizations of breastmilk as something that one cannot easily put a price tag on, something that transcends individualism and individual profit, and should be made available to every baby in need:

> To me, milksharing is a political act, and a spiritual one. It says: no child is more precious than another, and all children deserve the food that is designed for them. It says, we may have different stories, different customs, different breasts, but we are all mothers to our children. It says that together, we have the power to feed our children what they need, and we will not be deceived, scared, placated or undermined into thinking or acting otherwise.

Non-profit models of donation are theoretically safer than for-profit models, which have been associated with questionable storage, handling, and delivery practices, and potentially harmful bacterial contamination (Geraghty et al. 2013; Keim et al. 2013). According to the EOF home page:

> Community breastmilk sharing works because mothers, fathers, professionals, communities, caring citizens and people just like YOU are joining together to help ensure that babies have access to commerce-free breastmilk. Babies need breastmilk to maintain optimum health. Parents and professionals know this! Every day, women from around the world selflessly donate thousands of ounces of breastmilk directly to babies. With Eats On Feets, these donations are commerce-free, just as nature intended, and they are making a huge difference in the lives of babies and their families.

Milk sharing participants also note the intrinsic safety mechanisms in altruistic models of donation:

> I would be much more concerned with the safety of milk that's been PURCHASED and not donated! When people are making money off milk, there's more incentive to do things like dilute milk (to make it look like more) or withhold information that could turn a family off from buying (like taking potentially harmful drugs).

Removing moneymaking incentives ideally eliminates economic barriers to accessing donor breastmilk. Medicalized breastmilk is expensive and, because of its scarcity, must be carefully distributed to those infants who have the greatest medical need. In contrast, shared milk flows freely from donors to recipients.

The idea that decisions about what to do with one's breastmilk and what to feed one's own child should rest firmly in the hands of the adults involved is at the heart of milk sharing discourses. Since their inception, informal milk sharing sites HM4HB and EOF have promoted safe milk sharing based on principals of informed choice. HM4HB defines informed choice as:

... a choice made by competent individuals, free from coercion, that takes into account sufficient information to make a decision. This information should include benefits and risks of a course of action, as well as taking into account what alternatives are available, and an individual's intuitive feelings on the subject.

EOF describes informed choice as a decision "made by examining all credible, verifiable and relevant information available and using it to objectively weigh options as well as potential consequences." Milk sharing is based on the principle that healthy breastfeeding mothers can safely share their breastmilk with other babies, and that all individuals entering into milk sharing relationships should exercise informed choice. Discourses of informed choice are used to respond to criticism that milk sharing is haphazard, unsafe, and unnecessarily places babies at risk of illness and death:

HM4HB is built on the principle of informed choice: we trust, honour, and value the autonomy of families and we assert they are capable of weighing the benefits and risks of milksharing in order to make choices that are best for them. We hold the space for them and protect their right to do what is normal, healthy, and ecological.

Medicalized systems of breastmilk donation strip away the relationships between donors and recipients. Conversely, informed milk sharing restores these relationships and gives greater agency to those who are involved.

Much of the concern about milk sharing practices stems from perceptions that milk sharing is conducted without consideration of the potential health risks. Critics claim that even individuals using their best judgment to screen and follow recommended safety protocols are not able to safeguard against the 'unknowns' of milk sharing—inadvertent exposures to toxins and pathogens, things milk banking screening can control—and this makes it unjustifiably risky. On November 27, 2013, Kim Updegrove, Executive Director of Mother's Milk Bank of Austin and President of HMBANA, described her concerns with milk sharing on NPR (National Public Radio): "Sharing a body fluid, with all of its potential bacteria and viruses, is dangerous. And it is playing Russian roulette with your child's life." In her blog devoted to breastfeeding advocacy, Amber McCann, IBCLC writes that during a FDA meeting she attended in which an expert panel was appointed to review federal guidelines to regulate donor milk, one of the participants had this to say about informal milk sharing: "These women ... these women who are doing this are going to hurt even kill their babies" (McCann 2013).

While critics tend to generalize milk sharing risks based on what is known about breastmilk contamination and infant illness, those intimately familiar with milk sharing view risk quite differently (Gribble 2014a). With internet-facilitated milk sharing, the contexts of risk are renegotiated with each milk sharing event. Blanket statements about the risk of "taking milk from strangers" is often described as irrelevant by those involved in milk sharing, because they develop relationships of trust—through screening practices and exercising informed choice—with their milk sharing counterparts (Cassidy 2012b). People engaged in milk sharing discuss risk reduction strategies and encourage each other to gather all the information they need from a prospective donor or recipient prior to making a final milk sharing decision. They use online spaces to share research articles and helpful information on safety and risk reduction strategies.

Informed choice is not monolithic and not completely centered on disease risks. It implies that there is full disclosure by both donors and recipients of any information that each of the involved parties wishes to know before giving or receiving breastmilk. The information may be related to medical history, but there are other issues people are interested in such as diet, motivations for milk sharing, information about the donor's or recipient's child, and general lifestyle factors. Because the agreements between donors and recipients are highly contextual—meaning they are made on a case-by-case basis—there is not a one-size-fits-all approach to practicing informed choice, and it certainly appears from the popularity of milk sharing that disease transmission is part of, but not at the center of, decisions made in milk sharing encounters (Gribble 2014a).

Although milk sharing discourses promote the demedicalization of breastmilk, milk sharing is not a rejection of biomedicine, *per se*. In fact, a scientific evidence base often informs milk sharing decisions. Donors and recipients share information regarding what types of diseases to consider for donor screening, the safe handling, storing, and feeding breastmilk, and the many health benefits of breastmilk over formula. Milk sharing advocates have even called upon health authorities to assist them in making milk sharing even safer:

> There are risks associated with milk sharing just as there are with feeding babies formula. It is thus a question of weighing and managing relative risk, minimizing potential harm, and maximizing benefit. Rather than resisting and dismissing milk sharing, the constructive approach would be for health authorities and health care professionals to engage with mothers in ways that help make the practice as safe as possible, such as providing reliable information on donor screening, milk collection, storage, pasteurization, and feeding practices, and expediting voluntary sharing of medical records.

Embedded deep within the controversies around the risks of milk sharing is a fundamental difference in how milk sharing critics and advocates perceive infant formula (Gribble and Hausman 2012). Infant formula is probably the most highly medicalized form of infant feeding and for that reason it has long been considered the safest alternative to mother's own milk. However, milk sharing discourses reflect the WHO (2003) recommendation that breastmilk from a healthy donor is the preferred first alternative for infant and young child feeding in the absence of mother's own milk:

> We want milksharing and wet-nursing to be commonplace and babies to be fed at women's breasts whenever and wherever they need it. We dream of a world where mothers from previous generations pass on the tradition of breastfeeding and are a wealth of knowledge and support. We can foresee a time when women protect each other and help one another feed their babies so that every mother feels whole and no mother feels broken or that her body is failing her. We imagine a world where family members, friends, lactation consultants, doctors, and midwives do not hesitate to recommend donor milk when it is needed. We envision a future where families come together to raise this generation, and the next, by nourishing human babies everywhere with human milk and unconditional love.

A rejection of infant formula, or formula intolerance, are two major factors that bring donors and recipients together on milk sharing pages. Those engaged in milk sharing describe human milk as being considered the best possible form of nourishment for a baby. Moreover, raw breastmilk from a healthy donor is considered far more beneficial to the developing gut and immune system of recipient babies. Pasteurization, while necessary for medically fragile infants, is seen as unnecessary when milk comes from a healthy donor and is being fed to a healthy term infant.

The increased demand for donor milk in NICUs leaves HMBANA milk banks struggling with frequent shortages. Because human milk banks provide milk to the most medically fragile babies—babies who may not survive, in fact, without the pasteurized donor milk they receive from a milk bank—questions have arisen as to why more milk sharing donors are not giving to milk banks. Gribble (2013) explored this question with an international sample of donors and recipients engaged in milk sharing on EOF and HM4HB sites. She concluded that, in reality, many donors and recipients had attempted to either donate or procure milk from a milk bank, but that insurmountable barriers on both sides prevented them from taking this route. Women who were not eligible to donate to a milk bank chose milk sharing in the hope that another baby in need might benefit from their milk. Recipients who had no other alternatives and were not able to afford the high cost of banked donor milk found milk sharing as an answer to their infant feeding dilemmas. Thus, milk sharing fills a unique niche in the non-medicalized demand for breastmilk.

Biomedicine is often criticized for being overly individualistic and reductionist. If milk banks are viewed as institutions that dehumanize breastmilk through medicalization, then milk sharing, one could argue, seeks to humanize milk sharing through processes of demedicalization. The language of milk sharing is also distinctive from descriptions of breastmilk found in the medical literature, which are reductionistic, scientific, and technical. When donors and recipients describe breastmilk and milk sharing, they use language that not only reflects its healthful properties but also its symbolic social significance:

> Breastmilk, the biologically normal sustenance for humankind, is a free-flowing resource and mothers of the world are willing to share it. Milksharing is a vital tradition that has been taken from us, and it is crucial that we regain trust in ourselves, our neighbors, and in our fellow women.

Breastmilk is called "liquid gold," "a gift," and "a miracle." The following is a recipient's description of her son's bottle of breastmilk, which was obtained through milk sharing: "… every time I see his 'bottle' it is a bottle of Love and Selflessness …"

NAVIGATING MEDICALIZED AND DEMEDICALIZED INFANT FEEDING THROUGH MILK SHARING PRACTICES

> Governments cannot be relied upon to institute the measures that are needed to nurture and protect breastfeeding and breastmilk at the speed and to the degree that is necessary to address national and global health crisis. Therefore, it is imperative that NGO's, networks, groups, families and individuals take matters into their own hands. (Shell Walker[4] 2010)

The ways in which the values, ideologies, and principals of informal milk sharing are translated into practice push the demedicalization of breastmilk. Milk sharing is a liminal practice, situated betwixt and between the extremes of medicalization and demedicalization.

Most donors and recipients are engaged with biomedicine throughout their lives. Risk discourses are familiar and embodied, particularly among women during the perinatal and post-partum periods (Cheyney 2011; Davis-Floyd 1992; Martin 1987). Recipients may be drawn to milk sharing precisely because of medical diagnoses, clinical experiences, and other health-related concerns, which have intense meaning in their highly medicalized post-partum lives. A child's failure to thrive, a mother's insufficient glandular tissue, infant allergies and sensitivities, and formula intolerance are pervasive in posts requesting donor milk online. Parents may even consult with their healthcare providers for information about informal milk sharing:

> Our pediatrician didn't seem fazed at all that I was using donated breastmilk— and she even encouraged it. She brought up the fact that women with new babies have been tested for infectious disease during their prenatal care—so the risks are very low. She was very comfortable with us feeding my daughter donated breastmilk, which made me even more comfortable myself!

All of these activities reflect the highly medicalized context in which demedicalized milk sharing practices are situated.

This liminality is salient, particularly, in descriptions of donor screening practices. Medicalized risk discourses are found throughout discussions of how to conduct milk sharing "safely":

> There are definitely risks, just like everything else in life. Not only are you trusting a mama to be disease and medication free (or fully disclosed), but also that she properly cleans her pumping parts, washes her hands, didn't leave the milk in the fridge too long before it got into the freezer, didn't have a power outage while in the freezer, etc. There's plenty of risk, and it's important to know that before you make the decision. I am totally for milk sharing, but "informed consent" is key.

The concept of breastmilk as potentially pathogenic can be found in the ways milk sharing actors approach milk sharing. Donors report that they provide pregnancy records, blood test records, evidence of having been screened by a human milk bank, and other medical records documenting their health status in the process of informed milk sharing:

> I'm a donor and provide my blood test results to any potential recipients. I have them scanned in and on a web site, so I can just send them the link. I don't have a baby (I was a surrogate), but I wouldn't spend four hours a day on pumping and bagging milk if I had ANY doubt about my health! I take donating very seriously.
> I offered the mommas a medical release signed by my doctor/midwife staying I had no communicable diseases or any condition that could potentially harm their child/children and it also contained the medicine I was on.

Likewise, recipients describe the various donor screening measures they take. Donor screening is highly contextual and the specific information that recipients require are largely dependent on their unique circumstances and the specific type of relationship they have with prospective donors. For example:

> Our donor is a close friend, and she had all the tests—she had just had her own baby—and still offered copies, a letter from her midwife, etc. It can't hurt.
>
> I'm a recipient and my son has SMA, which they recently found comes with a fatty oxidation disorder. I always ask mothers if they are on medication, drink caffeine, have been screened for contagious illness, or take in dairy. Also meeting the mother and getting to know her helps make me more comfortable.

Recipients note that when a donor is breastfeeding her own child many concerns they might have about the safety of milk sharing are assuaged: "Most of the time, if it's safe for their own baby, it's probably safe to share." Thus, unlike banked donor milk, they are defining the safety and quality of shared breastmilk not simply achieved through science, but through the personal relationships of trust cultivated by milk sharing practices. Milk sharing donors know where their milk is going and recipients know the people who give them milk:

> Today I got to meet a little one that I donate milk to. It was really neat to see another baby thriving off of your milk. I am not the most sentimental person in the world, but it was pretty amazing to meet this sweet baby girl! What a sweet mommy and Angel baby :-) this is beautiful.

The importance of trusting relationships in fostering attitudes about milk sharing safety further demedicalizes breastmilk:

> There is a risk to just about everything in life! But that never stopped me from seeking donor milk for my babies! I just used wisdom and followed my instincts. The benefits clearly outweighed the risks or turning to using formula.
>
> I personally donated to a mom who felt that as long as I was still breastfeeding my baby, she felt comfortable accepting my milk for hers, because she knew I wouldn't do anything to myself that could even potentially harm my own baby. We met, and became friends, and she felt even more comfortable with my milk after that.

It is precisely these immeasurable, non-empirical, unscientific parameters of milk sharing that fuel critics' antagonism. Critics argue that science is the only thing that will save mothers from themselves, because decisions based on trust and informed choice do not provide empirical measures of safety. Thus, the devaluation of informed choice, agency, trust, and benevolence—principals that serve as the foundation of safe milk sharing—by science further deepens the gulf between milk sharing and its medicalized counterpart. Milk sharing actors are willing to embrace milk sharing as a medically risky practice, but many health authorities do not agree that informed choice and trusting relationships will protect infants. Medicalized breastmilk is crucial to saving the lives of the most vulnerable patients, and milk sharing actors agree that milk banks are essential.

Yet, milk sharing is powerful because it is nested within communities and unites families:

> I'm friends with my recipient mom. She actually posted her need on the HM4HB page the day my son was born, and, we delivered at the same hospital and had the same surgeon perform our unplanned csections. Her daughter is 5 weeks older than my son. It's like it was meant to be!!

Milk sharing connects people in ways that are impossible to replicate under current medicalized milk donation rubrics. When donors and recipients are turned away from milk banks, milk sharing offers them a way to fulfill their parenting goals while connecting with others:

> There's a necessary openness and vulnerability, but that's part of the beauty. You connect with another mother that way, you connect with humanity.

MILK SHARING IDENTITIES AT THE INTERSECTIONS OF MEDICALIZATION AND DEMEDICALIZATION

The growth of milk sharing has inspired emergent identities that serve as important forces driving the demedicalization of breastmilk. There are numerous identities that are tied in with milk sharing activities: the founders of milk sharing organizations, internet site administrators, doulas, midwives, and other professional brokers of breastmilk, milk sharing advocates, milk sharing researchers, spouses/partners, and other family members of donors and recipients. However, the two most salient and arguably most important are donors and recipients. Milk sharing is primarily compelled by the needs of recipients and the ability and willingness of donors to meet those needs (Gribble 2014b, 2014c). Donor and recipient identities are constructed by the expectations they fill and roles that they play.

Breastmilk donors enjoy a special status in the milk sharing world. They are the producers and purveyors of a highly valued resource, the "liquid gold" that is breastmilk.

While donor is a label that has been widely appropriated by those engaged in milk sharing discourses, it is clear that the identity of someone who gives breastmilk to another carries far richer symbolic meaning than simply the act of giving breastmilk. Words that are used to describe those who give breastmilk through informal milk sharing include "milky mama," "milk mother," and "sisters," all of which denote a profound interpersonal connection between the acts and identities of donors:

> I currently donate to a baby girl with special needs she as her mom calls her is my milk daughter and their family is now a part of ours. It is a blessing to be able to donate milk and I work hard at it. I pump and or Hand express every day every two to three hours. And I work tue-fri baby sit and have three of my own. I love helping and wouldn't change it for the world. Tomorrow we got to see my milk daughter and deliver 160 ounces of milk.

These terms that give kin-like affinities indicate the powerful social bonds that are created through the act of sharing breastmilk:

> I have donated to 3 ladies, one of them I donated to regularly and we became friends. I met her baby girl the first time I donated to her and it really put it in perspective for me what I was doing and she gave me a card signed with her daughter's name and it said "thank you for helping me grow!" Made me cry! I donated roughly 1000 ounces all together and it was a great experience. I was extremely happy and blessed to have an oversupply and able to donate.

Donors often enter milk sharing after trying to donate to a milk bank. In Gribble's (2013) study of milk sharing donor and recipients, approximately half of all donors surveyed indicated that barriers such as location and the inability to meet eligibility criteria precluded them from giving milk to a milk bank. The strict eligibility requirements are in place to ensure that donors are healthy and not taking pharmaceuticals or galactagogues that might negatively affect already compromised premature infants (Updegrove 2013b). Ironically, the herbal galactagogues that many donors take to increase their breastmilk supply enough to donate to milk banks are the very same grounds for exclusion:

> The local milk bank won't accept 300 ounces because I was drinking an herbal nursing support tea.

Medicines that are safe for mothers to take while breastfeeding their own babies also make many would-be donors ineligible:

> I would like to tell SOMEBODY that the ONLY reason I don't give to milk banks is they won't take my milk due to taking thyroid meds ... That is why most women milk share: the rules are too stringent!

Milk sharing donors recognize that their surplus of breastmilk may be used for other primarily healthy, term babies, and have found this a rewarding way to contribute to society, even if their primary motivating desire was to help the most vulnerable of children.

Donor identities are also negotiated through in the ways they prioritize among a number of possible recipients. Because donors know recipients and the circumstances that bring them to milk sharing, they are in a unique position to decide where their milk goes. Milk sharing provides opportunities for donors to exercise agency in ways that also tie into their milk sharing identities:

> I try to prioritize my milk donations to babies that NEED Breastmilk, especially newborns that are adopted or have Mothers who can't breastfeed for medical reasons. It's hard because there are so many families desperate for milk and I would like to help more than I am able to.
>
> I've always done it first come, first serve. But in the future I think I'll want to know some about the family.
>
> I like donating to moms who adopt.

While milk sharing would not be possible without donors, recipient families play an equally important role in processes of demedicalization of breastmilk. Recipient parents/caregivers play a powerful role in milk sharing. They are the actors whose identities most directly subvert the medicalized discourses of breastmilk exchange. Each feeding reinforces the trust they have in their donors, their belief that the shared breastmilk is safe, and their identity as parents/caregivers who are doing the best they can for their child.

Recipients have various reasons for engaging in milk sharing. They are breastfeeding mothers who simply may not produce enough milk to feed their baby:

> I have mammary hypoplasia / IGT and am physically incapable of producing the amount of milk an infant requires. My daughters are 4 and 18 months now, and the younger daughter has had breastmilk for every day of her life (aside from

about two days when we ran out). She has received milk from nearly 50 donors, and the generosity of these women has been nothing short of profound. i have made a couple of very dear friends who I otherwise would not know. Milksharing has opened my heart to trust. It has been a difficult road for me, with all the grieving I did about my IGT and having to swallow my sadness and put all of that aside to seek out donor milk for my daughter, to give her what was best for her. I will never forget what these women have given to our family.

They are also adoptive parents, surrogate parents, foster parents, parents in blended families, grandparents, and other non-biological kin who seek to provide what they view is the best possible source of nourishment for their children:

Sweet milk donors, please message me if you have milk to donate. We adopted a baby girl who was born 10 weeks premature, she is not 6 months old. We are eager to locate breastmilk, she does tremendously better on breastmilk than on formula and given her background, we really want to give her the best of everything this first year, we believe it really makes a difference.

Some are simply seeking any source of breastmilk because their child is formula-intolerant and they simply have no other options:

My daughter was born without a pancreas and several other medical issues, including drug addiction. She has been drinking donated breastmilk since she was a few months old. It literally saved her life. She couldn't digest any kind of formula and was not thriving. My son was also born drug addicted with major digestive issues and we were able to put him on donated breastmilk as well at around 4 months old. Both babies began to thrive within days of being on the donated milk.

Some have moral and political objections to infant formula (Gribble 2013, 2014c). Others still view milk sharing as an extension of their general commitment to breastfeeding advocacy and one of the many ways they seek to normalize the idea that breastmilk is the absolute best form of nutrition for all babies, biological kin and non-biological kin alike:

My philosophy has and always will be that women who are selfless enough to give of their body and time to ensure another baby has the BEST milk/nutrition possible are heaven sent. They are giving milk to another baby that they are feeding to their own child; therefore it has to be pure and perfect. Besides, I'm not sure there is anything at all in their milk that could even come close to the garbage in formula. I will also honestly tell you from my heart that the only issue I had with using another mother's milk was the guilt I was feeling for not being able to provide for my baby myself.

Medicalized breastfeeding discourses are almost always constructed around the definition that breastfeeding is a biological act of motherhood, which is confined to her biological offspring. Milk sharing challenges the idea that breastfeeding and feeding breastmilk is the sole domain of women and mothers. Fathers and other caregivers whose roles, sex, and gender identities do not conform to hetero-normative standards now have greater access to breastmilk. Milk sharing enables them to enact emergent identities and create novel expressions of caregiving that unsettle the notion that breastfeeding and feeding breastmilk is a strictly a womanly art (Zizzo 2009; MacDonald 2012).

Although they may not seem likely agents of medicalization or demedicalization, recipient babies are key actors in milk sharing as well. One could argue that the reason for medicalizing breastmilk in the first place was, and remains to this day, to nurture and protect the health of babies. Healthy human babies thrive on human milk, often in dramatic contrast to when they are fed infant formula (Gribble and Hausman 2012). Parents read their babies' behaviors and other signs of growth and development to make determinations about how, when, and what to feed them (Ryan, Todres, and Alexander 2011; Lupton 2012). Babies who thrive on shared donor milk motivate their parents to continue milk sharing.

Recipient–donor milk sharing identities are symbiotic. Compared with donors, however, recipients are often in a more vulnerable position; they have the most to lose if they are not able to find a source of breastmilk or if their child suffers any negative consequences of milk sharing. By the very nature of this vulnerable position, the act of feeding a child breastmilk procured through informal milk sharing serves as a powerful display of resistance to medicalized rhetoric against milk sharing, and one that becomes an integral part of the recipient milk sharing identity. When parents of infants who have been nourished by breastmilk describe the undeniably positive affect it has had on their lives, it becomes quite clear that milk sharing will not be extinguished simply because the medical establishment discourages it.

I just remember that I know the source of the donor milk, I met the face of the mother it came from and saw the sweet face of her baby that is eating the same milk. I never saw the face of the cow or the faces of the factory workers who made that formula in the can. I was nervous with the first bottle, but once I saw the improvement in my son and how happy he was, all my nervousness seemed to vanish. Now we're 13 months in to our milk sharing journey with no end in sight! You have to trust yourself to make the wise choice in picking your donor, and you have to have some faith in the goodwill of that mother willing to share her liquid gold! :)

CONCLUSION

Milk sharing is associated with discourses, practices, and identities that reveal processes of demedicalization. A close examination of these three dimensions illustrates the complexities of demedicalization, particularly the interplay between highly medicalized and non-medicalized ideas and practices. Milk sharing discourses, practices, and identities challenge, in varying degrees, medicalized definitions of breastmilk as a dangerous biosubstance that must be tested, regulated, and controlled within the confines of medical institutions. Discourses that define breastmilk as whole, natural, and normal serve to distance milk sharing from medicalized breastmilk, which is dispensed in clinical settings by healthcare professionals who are treating sick infants. Milk sharing actors make decisions about giving and receiving breastmilk based on particular contexts, which change with each new connection and new situation. They are aware of the potential risks and alter their behavior depending on specific contexts of risk. Risk of disease is but one of many considerations in milk sharing practices. Milk sharing has created a space where emergent identities sustain the ebb and flow of demedicalized breastmilk. Donor identities are formed through acts of generosity, while recipient identities are formed through acts of gratitude.

Women across the U.S. are being encouraged to breastfeed, and never before has so much money and energy been poured into supporting them to succeed. Health authorities and other milk sharing critics who define breastmilk as a dangerous bodily fluid and potential biohazard that "should not be shared" walk a fine line between promoting public health safety and creating anxiety around breastfeeding generally. Prospective milk bank donors and milk sharing donors alike are almost always healthy breast-feeding mothers who are happily "sharing breastmilk" with their own infants. The dissonance between medicalized discourses saying "breast is best" and then "breast is dangerous" is a fundamental issue that ultimately threatens to impede breastfeeding promotion and the growth of milk banking.

–3–

Historical Ethnography and the Meanings of Human Milk in Ireland

Tanya Cassidy

The Australian researcher Karleen Gribble (Gribble 2007; Berry and Gribble 2008) argues that in a world in which breastfeeding is not "best" but "normal" we would have a natural recognition of all forms of women feeding other women's children. Historical and cross-cultural researchers have long recognized the existence of a similar system of communal milk sharing (Wickes 1953a, 1953b; Fildes 1988). More recent medicalized constructions of these exchanges have helped to fuel the debates regarding the need for human milk for human babies, not just as nutrition, but also potentially as a life-saving medicinal substance (Cassidy 2010; Panczuk et al. 2014). Ireland has long been praised for its maternal and infant healthcare (Earner-Byrne 2007) and continues to be one of the safest places in Europe to give birth (Zeitlin et al. 2013), although there continues to be controversy stemming from the influence of the Catholic Church, especially outside of urban centers (Lazenbatt 2013).

In this chapter I employ what Sharon MacDonald calls a "multidirectional temporal practice" (2003: 97) ethnographic analysis, engaging as Fenske (2007) argues the micro (small-scale, often face-to-face interactions), macro (structural, large-scale features), and agency (behavioral interactions) associated with maternal milk sharing in Ireland. At the same time, this is an autoethnographic story (Ellis and Bochner 2000), deliberately bringing emotion into a narrative that has a personal aspect to the overarching medical frame (Ellis and Bochner 1999). Specifically, this chapter tells a story about women in Ireland helping other women to feed their infants through the use of their breastmilk, which encapsulates not only wet-nursing and forms of milk kinship associated with foster-nursing, but also more casual forms of cross-nursing and modern milk sharing, as well as the more medicalized donor milk banking; one might suggest that all of these exchanges can be termed "lactation surrogacy" of one kind or another.

MULTIDIRECTIONAL TEMPORAL MEANINGS OF MILK

Making lactation surrogacy a normal part of a global breastfeeding culture would not only mean that all infants would have a greater probability of receiving breastmilk, but it would also mean that mothers would truly have "choice" as to what their infants are fed. If women feel they have a choice regarding their infants' feeding, whether in Ireland or in most cultures around the world today, their choice is generally seen to be between their own breastmilk or artificial milk, either from animal or vegetable sources, but not from other humans.

In some cultures, including Ireland (at least until recently), other women's breastmilk was a real and often-preferred "choice" for some mothers. Irish women are no different from mothers transnationally or transhistorically: they all want their infants to have the very best. Ireland is different, however, in terms of the statistical fact that it currently has one of the lowest rates of breastfeeding in Europe, although this rate has been slowly improving over the last two decades (WHO 2003a). Ireland is also different in that its dairy industry is the world's largest producer of "infant nutrition products, producing 15% of the world's powdered infant formula" (Irish Business and Employers' Confederation 2007; More 2009). At the same time, Ireland is also distinctive because it has the only community-based donor human milk bank in the U.K., and one of the very few in Europe, although community-based banks are more common in Africa and the United States. The community nature of the bank is extremely important in terms of the way in which the facility operates, in turn related to the long history of Irish women altruistically helping other women to feed their infants.

The extreme crisis birth, which is associated with prematurely born infants, can make such choices literally a matter of life and death, as this author has experienced and discussed elsewhere (Cassidy and El Tom 2010). At the same time, mothers of premature infants often have delayed or sometimes severely limited lactational capabilities. In such circumstances, choice may be reduced to the use of specially produced formula for premature infants. However, this statistically increases an infant's chances of contracting the leading cause of death among the prematurely born, necrotizing enterocolitis (NEC).

Lactationally challenged mothers of premature and low birth weight infants are left with a high sense of guilt at not being able to give their child the nutrition/medicine that they desperately need. In some parts of the world, mothers of premature infants in such lactational difficulties may be offered milk from a donor milk bank. In 2006 in the *BMJ* a medical practitioner argued, without evidence, that such circumstances create scenarios in which a mother may simply choose not to improve her own lactational capabilities, and instead simply use other people's breastmilk (Modi 2006). The availability of donor milk risks undermines breastfeeding rates, in other words. Gillian Weaver (2006), the chair of the UK Association of Milk Banking (UKAMB) and vice president of the European Milk Banking Association (EMBA), argues in response that the vast majority of women feel the need for a stopgap until their own milk comes in, which may take up to a week. If, in the meantime, their infant is given breastmilk, not formula, then extreme maternal anxieties may be alleviated, making subsequent maternal lactation easier (Gillian Weaver personal communication). The limited stores available in most of the not-for-profit milk banks around the world mean that these mothers know that this milk is limited, and that if they wish their infants to receive breastmilk for any extended period, then they must make every effort to produce the milk themselves. There is now one donor human milk bank in Ireland, located in County Fermanagh, in Northern Ireland, but situated close to the border between the north and the south, allowing easy access and exchange around the island of Ireland as a whole. This bank receives donations from women across Ireland as a whole and provides milk to infants in need regardless of which side of the border they reside. It is, without doubt, one of the most impressive examples of cross-border health co-operation that exists on the island.

Surrogate, as a noun, is an ancient word referring to the substitute of a person or thing (*OED* 2011). The noun "surrogacy" is much more modern, dating back only to the 1980s, and has been used primarily in the United States to refer to "the practice of surrogate motherhood" (*OED* 2011). Accepting this definition, my term "lactation surrogacy" would specifically move the surrogate notion of motherhood beyond the womb to include the biological production of infant nutrition, specifically breastmilk, whether by milk sharing, wet-nursing, and/or human milk banking, thus capturing all forms of breastmilk production by one female for another female's infant. The term "lactation surrogate" removes the gendered and individualized biological agency associated with surrogacy, and therefore should include not only the above alternatives to mother's own milk, but also infant nutrition derived from other sources, whether animal or vegetable.

HISTORY AND LANGUAGE OF MILK IN IRELAND

Despite contemporary concerns surrounding shared breastmilk, a number of sources argue that at various points in history, Ireland normalized such communal relationships. For instance, in both William Shaw's 1780 and Edward O'Reilly's 1817 *Irish English Dictionary* we are told that the term "bean-chioch" is translated as "wet nurse." Literally, "bean" is Gaelic for woman, whereas "chioch" refers to breastfeeding, but Irish speakers have told me that this way of referring to wet nurse is now common.

More recent historical cultural studies, such as Koch's five-volume historical *Encyclopedia of Celtic Culture*, point to old Irish traditions of fostering, and explain that the term "muime" is used synonymously for foster mother and wet nurse, as nursing was an "optional first step in the fostering process" (Koch 2006: 771). Koch also points out that this equating of wet nurse and foster mother is common in a number of languages. The long historical tradition of fostering can be found in old Irish law narrative detailing the entire process and, not unlike the Islamic milk kinship relationship, muime is also understood to be a term of affection. Irish dictionaries today, including the *Electronic Dictionary of the Irish Language* (eDIL), list "muim(m)e or buim(m)e" as a nurse or foster mother. In a seventeenth-century translation of an old Irish poem entitled "On the Humility of His Wisdom and the Brilliancy of His Faith" we are told that

> Humility is wisdom's nurse; so authentic lore attests;
> Hers the claim to foster it: anxious though its rearing be
> Foster-nurse humility: let not wisdom leave her arms,
> Suckles it at breast replete: with the doctrine of the truth. (MacErlean 1912)

Celtic mythology contains at least one story that argues that the fairies steal women to feed their infants because the milk of an Irish mother is considered the best. A Christian version of this tradition is linked to Saint Brigid, the patron saint of County Kildare in Ireland, who is said to have been a wet nurse to the Christ Child.

The link with foster mothering brings to mind the ingrained cultural system associated with Islamic law, unsurprisingly when considered in such a fashion. Other more contemporary references inform us that the complicated fostering system that existed in Ireland probably into the early part of the twentieth century was linked to the age of the infant, and for those under one year of age included a form of wet-nursing (Kelly 1988; Koch 2006). The southern African–American figure of the "mammy," which has been argued to enjoy more positive implications along with some other pejorative characterizations (see Pilgrim and Middleton 2002), is also often linked to foster nursing, and would offer an interesting topic of comparison with the Irish situation, especially considering the influence of Irish immigrant culture.

MEDIA AND THE MEANINGS OF MILK

The specific data I wish to discuss in detail in this chapter is linked to systematic searches of the *Irish Times* archives from 1859 to the present, and the Irish Newspapers Archives (INA), which includes publications as far back as 1763. The INA currently has 17 publications that span the island, and includes not only the *Irish Independent* (1905–) as well as the *Freeman's Journal* (1763– mid- to late nineteenth century, reissued), but also the *Nation* (nineteenth century to early twentieth century), as well as other more local newspapers such as the *Connaught Tribune* (1909–) and the *Donegal News* (1980–2001).

When I searched for "foster nurse" I found four hits, two of which were about a Mrs. Kilkelly, who had died in 1927 at the age of 94 and had formerly been the "foster nurse" of Miss Rosamond Ffrench of Monivea Castle. The other hits referred to someone whose name was "Foster" with the term or profession "nurse" following. When I searched for the phrase "wet nurse" I received 274 hits for the *Irish Times* and 175 hits for the Irish Newspaper Archives. The interesting differences, however, seem to be within the numerous references in the *Irish Times*, including the earliest reference, in which "wet nurse" is being used as a literary/political trope. For instance, discussions in newspapers from 1859 related to England and France, whereas the Irish Newspapers Archives are dominated by advertisements, the earlier ones being for placements, the earliest of which dates back to 1808, which may well be a selection feature of the dates available for the various newspapers. As I moved into the early twentieth century I found it interesting that the advertisements from mothers looking for wet nurses increased.

I performed systematic searches using exact phrase features and wildcard truncations within these archives. The relevant hits show important cultural changes from the latter part of the nineteenth century and throughout the twentieth century. When I saw the importance of the Rotunda Hospital, I also reviewed their annual reports for the twentieth century. However, this latter data need to be supplemented, and will form the basis of subsequent publications on this topic.

SUPPLY AND DEMAND OF IRISH WET NURSES IN THE NINETEENTH CENTURY

The Irish Newspapers Archives are dominated by advertisements, the earlier ones being for a placement dating back to 1808 in the *Freeman's Journal*, as the following classified advertisement indicates.

WANTS – A SITUATION as WET NURSE, a Young Woman, who can be well recommended by persons of the first respectability, — Letters addressed to M.R. at the Printer's of No. 2, South King-street, will be attended to. (*Freeman's Journal* 1808)

Wet-nursing was a common form of employment for both the urban and rural poor, as well as reinforcing familial ties, particularly in rural settings.

By the mid- to late nineteenth and early twentieth centuries I discovered that advertisements from mothers looking for wet nurses increased. In other words, fewer women were looking to be employed, but more women were still looking for breastmilk. I have also shown an early representation of this other form of advertising, again from the *Freeman's Journal*, but from 1872.

WET NURSE – Wanted Immediately a well tempered, healthy young Woman as Wet Nurse: applicants will please give reference as to character, &c. Address Y 40 Odice of this Paper. (*Freeman's Journal* 1872)

I began to ask the question: what mid-to-late nineteenth-century events caused this change in the market distribution of breastmilk? A much later advertisement from the 1950s provided me with what I believe to be the answer. The advertisement appeared on page 2 of the *Irish Times* in 1954, and is clearly drawing the reader/consumer back to thinking about historical issues related to infant feeding. The caption reads "How to choose a wetnurse":

Where the milk does not come in or for other reasons the mother cannot nurse her child, one should choose a wet-nurse who has the following appearance and habits. She must be neither too young nor too old. She should be well-built; her face healthy in appearance, tanned; and she should have a strong thick neck, strong, broad breasts, not too fat and not too thin. The wet-nurse should have good, praise-worthy habits. She should not be easily frightened or worried and not small-minded or prone to anger. (Bartholomaeus Mettinger [about 1450] in "The regime of your children")

The advertisement goes on to say:

Time have certainly changed. Nowadays the equivalent of the wet-nurse is probably the breast-milk bank. Or, as another perfectly good substitute for breast-feeding, the modern mother can turn to Trufood. Here is a range of balanced infant food which includes Humanised Trufood, the milk preparation nearest to breast milk. Trufood helps modern babies to grow into healthy, robust children who wouldn't know a wet-nurse if they saw one.

But as Harris (2002) has pointed out, part of the problem with these state-ments is that the term "wet-nurse" was not used until the seventeenth century, and that part of the duties of nurses that were hired by aristocratic women included breastfeeding. This, however, seems to have been such an accepted part of the arrangement that it is often not discussed. It is true that once the term wet-nurse is introduced, many birthing volumes, including Jane Sharpe's 1671 *Midwives Book, Or the Whole Art of Midwifery Discovered*, which was edited and republished by Elaine Hobby in 1999, discussed how to choose a wet-nurse, since there were many hazards "if great care is not taken in the choice of a nurse." However, the majority of these commentators also advocated maternal feeding in the first instance. This is not the place to discuss the fertility issues associated with class and wet-nursing historically in Britain and Ireland; suffice to say the above 1954 advertisement tells us more about Ireland in the 1950s than about wet-nursing in early-modern Europe.

"HUMANIZED," NOT HUMAN, MILK

The sociocultural historical changes associated with wet-nursing vary across countries and even regions. Wickes (1953a) argued that the heyday of wet-nursing in England occurred at the end of the eighteenth century, and that this profession increasingly disappeared during the nineteenth century, saying that by "1863 Routh was able to state that the safety of artificial feeding was sufficient to outweigh the moral disadvantages in the employment of a wet nurse," although Wickes goes on to point out the casual reference to one of Anthony Trollope's novels (*Dr Thorne* 1858), which discusses the use of a wet nurse, albeit by Lady Arabella, whose family was given "bosoms for show not for use" (Wickes 1953b: 418).

The use of animal milk has long been recognized by both mothers and their healthcare providers, and has included a number of different animals (Snyder 1908; Wickes 1953a; Cone 1976). Wickes points out that since the eighteenth century in Paris there was a hierarchy associated with milk from other animals, one recommending that if human milk is not available, the next best is "ass, goat, cow or ewe's milk in that order of preference based upon the size of the curd" (Wickes 1953a: 336). Wickes shows an image from Sadler (1895), which is now available from the Wellcome Trust Library, and is shown in Figure 1, of a child directly consuming milk from an ass's teat, the preferred method of delivery.

The middle of the nineteenth century marks the beginning of commercial exploitation of modified milk from cows, animals which fuel a longstanding

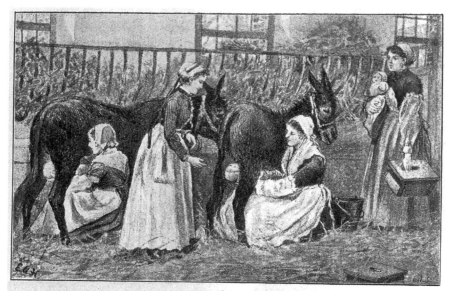

L'Allaitement des Nourrissons par les Ânesses à l'Hospice des Enfants Malades.

Figure 1. Child directly consuming milk from an ass's teat. Source: Wellcome Library, London. Copyrighted work available under Creative Commons Attribution only license CC BY 4.0. http://creativecommons.org/licenses/by/4.0/

commercial enterprise. One name synonymous with infant formula and the global market is Nestlé. On the international Nestlé website, the company details the history of this multinational leviathan, stating that "[t]he key factor which drove the early history of the enterprise that would become the Nestlé Company was Henri Nestlé's search for a healthy, economical alternative to breastfeeding for mothers who could not feed their infants at the breast" (Nestlé Corporation 2011). We are not told why the trained pharmacist used cows' milk in his "experiments," but the Canadian Nestlé website says that in 1867 Henri Nestlé was successful in developing the "world's first infant formula," which he used "to save the life of his neighbour's premature baby who can't tolerate breast milk" (Nestlé Canada 2011). Less than ten years later, in 1876, Nestlé was advertising on the front page of the *Irish Times*, with the following words:

NESTLE'S
MILK FOOD
FOR INFANTS
Prepared at Vevey, Switzerland, from the
Best Milk of Swiss Cows.

The reader/potential consumer is told that this milk food for infants is made from the "best" of Swiss cows. The *Irish Times* readership in the mid-nineteenth century was disproportionately located in the Dublin urban area, and we know that by the turn of the twentieth century the infant mortality rate in Dublin was the highest in Ireland, and one of the factors blamed for this was the "abandonment of breastfeeding" (O'Brien 1982: 108).

Commentators are aware of the fall in breastfeeding in Dublin, but we can also find advertisements for other artificial infant foods in newspapers from the countryside as well. Also in 1876 we see in the *Nenagh Guardian*, the weekly Tipperary paper, an advertisement for Giffey's Milk Food for Infants and Invalids, manufactured in Germany, with the statements that "Eminent Physicians Acknowledge that [Giffey's Milk Food] is the best substitute for Mother's Milk"; "is the most nutritious"; "is the most wholesome"; "is the most economical preparation ever introduced to the public"; "does not require milk or sugar"; "is worth a trial in any house, where a child needs extra nourishment beyond that supplied by the Mother"; and finally, "Giffey's Milk Food is sold throughout the Kingdom in tins containing ½ pound and 1s each" and by a London importer for wholesale distribution. Clearly there were indications of the potential profits available even at this early time.

It is of course impossible to ignore the level of poverty and malnutrition throughout Ireland in the mid- to late part of the nineteenth century, especially during the famine years (1845–8) and their aftermath. Research has shown that maternal malnutrition is directly related to a myriad of infant health-related issues, and can contribute to lactation supply problems. At the same time, more women, especially in cities, were working outside of the home, thus increasing the difficulty of breastfeeding for any length of time.

The medical profession at the turn of the twentieth century was divided in its opinions regarding the use of human versus other animal milk. Thus, in a 1904 paper read by Walter Smith to the Royal Academy of Medicine in Ireland, the author said that despite the fact that the "milk of various mammals has been employed for human nutriment, but practically we need consider only two—viz., woman's and cow's milk" (Smith 1904: 403). Part of this paper discusses the work done by Theodore Esterich (1857–1911) in Austria regarding sterilization and milk, whether human or bovine. This discussion is interesting because it comes five to six years before the first donor human milk bank was established in Vienna by Esterich and his team (1909). According to its modern definition, donor milk banking involves the "collecting, screening, processing, storing and distributing of donated human milk" (Weaver 2008). Hospitals and foundling homes had long employed wet nurses whenever possible. However, with this profession disappearing, an alternative answer to feeding premature infants was needed, especially when a significant proportion of these mothers had difficulty with lactation, at least initially.

MEDICAL MOTHER'S MILK

According to historian Janet Golden (1996), the first American human milk bank (in Boston) employed a majority of donors who were either Canadian or Irish. This author has argued that it was the Mother's Milk Bureau established in Detroit that in fact properly satisfies the modern definition of a modern medicalized milk system (Cassidy 2010). The use of the term "bank" was not common until the 1940s, and is linked to the contemporary establishment of blood banks, which first opened in Chicago (Watson 1941; Cassidy 2010).

Returning to my Irish newspaper searches, the earliest reference I found to mothers' milk bureaus comes from a 1937 *Sunday Independent* in which a narrative, complete with pictures, details the New York Mother's Milk Bureau and its workings. This story talks about the huge strides made by the medical profession. Although these pictures depict women, they are veiled in medical garb, and the milk itself looks more like medicine. There is a sense that this phenomenon is something unusual, and that it is not surprising that it is occurring in exotic faraway New York. This is not the place to go into the details of the New York milk system, but I should mention briefly that B. Raymond Hoobler, the physician who began the Detroit system, was in New York earlier and had earlier conducted what he called an "experiment," which in essence was the first milk bank exchange among women who did not identify themselves as wet nurses (Cassidy 2010).

In Ireland, we know that at least four or five years earlier, a similar system was in operation at the Rotunda Hospital in Dublin. The Rotunda Annual Report from 1932–3 states that "[b]reast milk has been our sheet-anchor for feeding the premature infants; where it has been impossible to obtain the mother's milk, a breastmilk pool has been made from other mothers willing to contribute" (Solomons 1934: 380). Although this milk banking/sharing/pooling was available at the Rotunda for premature infants, in 1944 the following "clinical observation" was offered, together with an extensive quote from the annual report:

> One clinical observation is of paramount importance. Not one of the babies who contracted enteritis (enteral or parental) and died was wholly or partially breast-fed. The bottlefed babies have their milk carefully sterilised and every precaution

is taken to avoid infection. The above phenomenon has been so constantly observed that we have formed the opinion that breastmilk contains some active principle that prevents neo-natal infection. Hence the importance of breast-feeding cannot be over emphasized. It is not enough to lecture the mothers, however, on their maternal duty and then to feel that all responsibility has been removed from us and to be conscience free if non-breast fed babies die in our hospital. Some mothers there are, no doubt, who could and yet refuse to try and breastfeed their babies, but many are unable to do so for different reasons, malnutrition being perhaps the most important. Hence antenatal care should lay great stress on preparing the mother for lactation, not only by giving her the usual medical care, but also seeing that her diet is adequate.

Further, we must now realize that the babies of mothers who cannot feed their babies are very open to neo-natal infection and need special protection. These mothers and babies should have no visitors and should receive special care and be isolated if possible. The greatest step forward in regard to the management of the immature and special groups in the nursery would be the introduction of a special breastmilk pool from which they could be fed. We are convinced that many lives could be saved by these methods.

The whole position is far too serious, however, for complacency or inaction. This year in the Rotunda Hospital we have lost the lives of 56 babies, born in the hospital, through infection. If instead of babies the deaths were those of mothers with puerperal sepsis there would be a world-wide outcry. (Falkner 1944: 355)

By 1958 the Rotunda annual report now refers to the Donor Milk Bank, which it says had a "reasonably satisfactory year," but goes on to lament the lack of donors:

In spite of all the propaganda and encouragement few mothers breast-feed for longer than six weeks, and a considerable number have never started or have given up before this time. Mothers who become donors will usually continue to lactate for 4–6 months, during which time they feed their own infants only, donating the excess to the Bank. Donors are hard to come by, few mothers being interested. The donor panel at any one time seldom exceeds 16, and not infrequently falls to as low as four donors. (Clinical Report of the Rotunda Hospital, 1958: 19)

It seems that the bank was to close shortly after this, as is evidenced by a sad story reporting from a 1966 *Irish Independent* that begins with an appeal for mothers' milk to save a baby at Galway Regional Hospital. The article reports a hospital spokesperson as saying that "[n]ot enough mothers were feeding their babies to enable a milk bank to be established on lines similar to that operated by the Dublin Rotunda Hospital some years ago," and the possibility of looking to Africa was being considered.

The story of the Irish breastfeeding decline is a long one, its seeds sown in the mid-nineteenth century. Unlike milk banks in other countries, the Irish milk banks seem to have disappeared long before the threat of HIV/AIDS in the 1980s. However, it was international campaigning that helped to re-establish milk banking in Ireland.

CONCLUSION

I developed the terms "lactation surrogate" to refer to all substitutes for direct breastfeeding, and "lactation surrogacy" to describe all attempts to harness human lactation in order to create a larger, more flexible, and holistic field of inquiry. The movement from the former to the latter requires a more systematic and clinical awareness of what is and is not a "substitute," focusing on the belief that in the case of emergency premature and low birth weight infant feeding, cows' milk is strictly speaking "no substitute" for human milk, being essentially a different product altogether.

A recent Irish dairy industry report said that the "EU is the largest milk producer, followed by the US, India, China, Russia and Brazil," with markets growing in China, India, and the Americas (More 2009: 5). This same report goes on to say that:

> In global terms, the Irish dairy industry is small, producing 5.2 million tonnes (0.94% of global production). However, the industry exports approximately 85% of annual production and is a major contributor to the national economy. The industry is also the world's largest producer of powdered infant formula (More 2009: 6). This is not however a recent phenomenon, as Irish dairy historians can attest. Seen as primarily female domestic work in the nineteenth century, by the beginning of the twentieth century the dairy industry became a male occupation (Bourke 1990). This is a not insignificant factor regarding the decline in breastfeeding throughout Ireland. The ubiquity of bovine milk as a nutritional staple for adults as well as children (and its identification as the "default setting" definition of milk itself) is a twentieth-century phenomenon that directly correlates with the "takeoff" era of Irish bottle-feeding.

Government efforts on either side of the Irish border have been made to encourage increases in breastfeeding rates that have been slowly but steadily rising, although they still remain comparatively low (EU Project on Promotion of Breastfeeding in Europe 2004).

As I have noted, milk banking can be identified as a key player in the effort to normalize human milk consumption for all infants. At the turn of the twenty-first century, in August 2000, the aforementioned U.K.'s only community-based milk bank, and the largest of the 15 currently functioning throughout these islands, began operations at the Irvinestown Health Centre, in County Fermanagh.

The Northern Ireland Human Milk Bank began in response to the needs of an infant in Erne Hospital's neonatal unit who developed NEC, and was saved through the use of donated human milk. The milk received is processed in accordance with the UK Association of Human Milk Banking (UKAMB) and the NICE Guidelines. It is then distributed to infants in need, over 700 each year since it began. The bank and its donors are clearly an exemplary representative of cross-border health co-operation (McCrea 2007).

Milk banks depend on testimony, and upon narratives of maternal trial and triumph (Condon 2006). Such narratives create a culture of empathy that sustains the recruitment and retention of donors. This paper seeks to contribute to a tradition of "public sociology" (Burawoy 2005) or "advocacy anthropology," especially in relationship to breastfeeding or breastmilk (Van Esterik 2008a; 2008b) and can therefore employ extensive use of auto-ethnographic techniques. My own personal experiences have proven crucial in eliciting information, thereby contributing to relationships of trust, and new expressions of communality, resulting in the implications of this research being disseminated beyond the traditional academy. While quantitative health research can reach the medical establishment, a reconfigured culture of lactation surrogacy demands a more qualitative approach that draws on the detailed experiences of both donor mothers and mothers of recipient babies. "Lactation surrogacy" needs stories to tell (Cassidy and El Tom 2010).

–4–

Between *"le Corps 'Maternel' et le Corps 'Érotique'"*: Exploring Women's Experiences of Breastfeeding and Expressing in the U.K. and France

Charlotte Faircloth

This chapter emerges from research involving networks of mothers in London and Paris recruited through an international breastfeeding support group. Their descriptions of breastfeeding and expressing are used here as barometers by which to explore a cross-cultural trend towards an "intensification" of mothering. This is a phenomenon identified by a range of scholars writing about parenting in contemporary Euro-American contexts (Hays 1996; Furedi 2002; Douglas and Michaels 2004; Warner 2006; Lee 2007a, 2007b; Lee and Bristow 2009), as well as beyond (Faircloth, Hoffman, and Layne 2013).

The data presented here reveal that the relationship between the dynamics of intimate relations and broader international trends is not straightforward: what is considered appropriate infant feeding practice is not cross-culturally stable. While it seems that "intensive motherhood" is being exported from the U.S. (and the U.K.) to other settings in a "global ethics of care," its reception and interpretation is far from uniform. The argument is that while the endorsement of breastfeeding by women in London is a magnification of a more generalized "intensive parenting" culture in the U.K., which encourages absorbed "sacrificial" parenting on the part of mothers, the same mothering looks very different in Paris. In a culture where maternal–infant separation and autonomy is lauded as ideal, such as France, "intensive" embodied care on the part of the mother is perceived as an impingement on female liberty, rather than a valid outlet for "identity work" (see, for example, Badinter 2010). Concordantly, the expression of breastmilk (or formula feeding) is validated as a more appropriate choice than breastfeeding. The chapter opens by providing a brief methodology of the study before presenting findings and offering a discussion of differing cultural perceptions around nature/culture, feminism, and family life by way of conclusion.[1]

METHODOLOGY

The research for this study involved long-term ethnographic fieldwork with women in *La Leche League International* (LLLI) groups, the world's foremost breastfeeding support organization. The group was founded in 1956 in the United States by a group of seven mothers to support all women who wanted to breastfeed their babies. It has now become a global organization offering breastfeeding support through publications, telephone helplines, and local meetings. While it offers support for all women who want to breastfeed, it is known among the various breastfeeding support groups to be supportive of women who breastfeed for "extended" periods, and has a significant proportion of members who practice "attachment parenting." This was a term coined by the Sears (the husband-and-wife pediatrician team) in the 1980s, and is a style of care which endorses long-term proximity between infant and care-taker (most typically, the mother). "Extended" or "full-term" breastfeeding would typically be up to the age of three or four, though ranged, in this case, between one and eight years old. Other common practices among these mothers include breastfeeding "on-cue," bed-sharing and "baby-wearing."

Feeding, arguably the most conspicuously moralized element of mothering, was the focus of the study. Because of its vital importance for the survival and healthy development of infants, feeding is a highly scrutinized domain where mothers must counter any charges of practicing unusual, harmful, or morally suspect feeding techniques (Murphy 1999). Strong feelings about feeding are derived from the fact that it operates as a "signal issue," which boxes women off into different parenting "camps" (Kukla 2005).

During 2006, and over the course of eight months in London and four months in Paris, participant observation at 18 local LLLI groups (ten in London, eight in Paris) was complemented by 39 semi-structured interviews and 48 questionnaires with individual women across the two cities. In both cases, mothers were in the vast majority white, middle-aged (on average, 34), well educated (to university level or equivalent) and married. More women in the Parisian sample than in the London sample were working full-time, as I discuss further later. Those that were identified as "full-term" breastfeeders and "attachment mothers" made up just over half of the sample in London, and just over a third in Paris.[2] Certainly not all mothers in the organization breastfeed to full term, and I would be wary of giving that impression. Where elsewhere I have focused on the accounts of attachment mothers (Faircloth 2013), here, I feature accounts from all women I encountered at the meetings—including those who were not attachment mothers—to give a more rounded picture of the cultural landscapes in which women make their decisions around infant feeding.

The WHO states that breastfeeding in developed countries should be exclusive for six months and continue "for up to two years, or beyond" in conjunction with other foods (2003). Along with other EU member states, this is endorsed by both the U.K. and French governments. Breastfeeding initiation rates at the time of research stood at 78 percent and 69 percent in Britain and France respectively,[3] with no formal statistics existing in either place for rates of breastfeeding at a year, or beyond. As I discuss below, these numbers reflect the shorter length of maternity leave women receive in France, which in turn informs (and is informed by) broader social attitudes towards women's social roles, feminism, and childcare (Randall 2000). While there were no statistics for the number of children breastfed beyond a year in the U.K., by six months 75 percent of children were totally weaned off breastmilk, and only 2 percent of women breastfed exclusively for the recommended six months (Department of Health 2005).

After Goffman (1959), I look at women's "identity work" in their infant-feeding decisions—that is, the narrative processes of self-making that mothers engage in as they raise their children. This is part of an argument that for certain middle-class parents in the U.K. (and to a lesser extent in France), the word "parent" has shifted from a noun denoting a relationship with a child (something you *are*) to a verb (something you *do*). "Parenting" is now an occupation in which adults (particularly mothers) are expected to be emotionally absorbed and become personally fulfilled; it is also a growing site of interest to policy-makers in the U.K., understood as a solution to a wide range of social ills (Lee and Bristow 2009). The "ideal" parenting promoted by these policy-makers is financially, physically, and emotionally intensive, and parents are encouraged to spend a large amount of time, energy, and money in raising their children (Hays 1996). This "intensive parenting" climate, I argue, has changed how parents experience their social role.

INTENSIVE MOTHERING

Writing about the U.K., Lee and Bristow (2009) identify two major characteristics of the contemporary "ideal" of intensive mothering: one, that mothering is defined as a practice that should be child-centered; and two, that mothers should pay attention to what is said by experts about their children. Each of these have instrumental effects with respect to knowledge and practice.

That a child's interests should be placed before the mother's is, perhaps, not to say anything remarkable—indeed, Mary Douglas has said that the "absolute morality" of motherhood is that "in all circumstances, babies take precedence over mothers" (1970: 25, in Murphy 1999: 200). But the way in which this injunction is realized is certainly novel. Hays notes that today children are not to be excluded from adult leisure time but "listened to" and "included." Weekend activities, for example, should center around maximizing children's health and well-being, and mothers are expected to act as pseudo-teachers, optimizing their children's intelligence through a range of extra-curricular activities (Hays 1996).

Indeed, the mother's role has expanded dramatically in recent years, not least because of the burgeoning interest in early infancy by psychologists in the 1950s. The interlocking "myths," as Furedi puts it (2002: 45), that experience during infancy determines the course of future development, and that parental intervention determines the future fate of a youngster, have had a profound effect on the way parents structure their relationships with their offspring. As he argues:

> By grossly underestimating the resilience of children, they intensify parental anxiety and encourage excessive interference in children's lives; by grossly exaggerating the degree of parental intervention required to ensure normal development, they make the task of parenting impossibly burdensome. (Furedi 2002: 45)

In this framing, the agency of children themselves is reduced, at the same time that the effect of peers and social climate on child development is eclipsed through this focus on parents. Accordingly, a highly interventionist approach is legitimized on their part, and the importance of the parenting role increases in congruence.

The second aspect of intensive mothering—that mothers should refer to experts when caring for their child—is also intimately tied up with the expansion of the parental role. In *Paranoid Parenting* (2002) Furedi argues that parenting is increasingly considered too important a job to be left to parents themselves to deal with. Lee (2007b) suggests that this, in turn, binds mothering to the job of risk management, at once creating and fuelling the market for a plethora of experts who "enable" mothers to avoid certain risks and optimize their children (whether that be judo teachers, osteopaths, or psychologists, to use just some of Hays' examples). This outsourcing of authority has the potential to reduce parental confidence to the extent that all parents are tinged with some degree of paranoia, Furedi argues (2002).

There are, of course, many ways of caring for children "intensively" (such as with methods which advocate strict timetabling of feeding, sleeping etc.). The philosophy of "attachment parenting," which validates attentive, embodied care for infants, offers women *one* set of norms by which to structure their "identity work" in congruence with an over-arching framework of intensive mothering. There are points of congruence and points of departure with this framework, as I explore (Faircloth 2013). Yet fashions in parenting are also best understood as barometers of wider cultural trends, which—in the U.K., at least—have recently seen a growing validation of the "natural" way of doing things in issues as diverse as what we eat, how we learn, and how we treat illness. There is an enduring conviction in this position that "nature" is a force to be trusted and respected, and with respect to parenting, deference to the "natural" bond between mother and child, which the increasingly popular "attachment" style validates (paraphrased from Bobel 2002: 11; see Faircloth 2009). Based on a "hominid blueprint" (Dettwyler 1995a), which draws on evidence of primates and "primitives" (whether in the fossil record or as represented by contemporary hunter-gatherer groups), attachment parenting is endorsed as both a traditional and "adaptive" form of care (Sears and Sears 2001). The argument is that children have evolutionary expectations (such as an extended period of breastfeeding) that must be met if they are to mature into happy, healthy adults (see Faircloth 2009 for a full discussion: women clearly do not "ape" all aspects of the hunter-gatherer lifestyle; a certain amount of cherry-picking goes on).

A CROSS-CULTURAL PERSPECTIVE: FRANCE

While numerous scholars have fruitfully used the concept of "intensive motherhood" in U.S. and U.K. contexts (Hays 1996; Furedi 2002; Douglas and Michaels 2004; Lee 2007a, 2007b; Lee and Bristow 2009) there has been less empirical work that looks at the impact of this ideology outside and across these settings.

Famously, the French government has long had a policy aimed at boosting the country's population, at the same time as increasing the amount of women in the workforce (Randall 2000). The OECD (Organisation for Economic Co-operation and Development)[4] lists the fertility rate in France as

1.94, in contrast to the U.K.'s 1.8. (These are both figures above the OECD average of 1.63.)[5] In terms of female employment, 56.7 percent of women of working age are employed in France, compared with 66.8 percent in the U.K. (The OECD average is 56.1 percent, and this includes both full- and part-time workers.)

At the time of research, in the U.K., a woman could typically expect 26 weeks (six months) of paid leave with 5 weeks additional unpaid leave if desired. (Women were not paid at full rate—it was calculated at 90 percent for the initial six weeks and then at a flat rate, approximately 33 percent of average wage, for 20 weeks).[6] In France, women could take 16 weeks of (fully) paid leave, then being eligible for longer periods of unpaid leave. Since this is generally split on a 4-week/12-week basis pre- and post-birth, women are expected to return to work when their children are between ten weeks and three months old.[7] In the U.K. this point would typically be between five and six months. (Paternity leave at the time of research in both countries was two weeks, with only 25 percent of this time paid in the U.K.)

Crucially, however, and unlike the U.K., France has a system of heavily subsidized, easily available, affordable childcare. Municipal, co-operative and parental crèches exist, able to care for infants from the age of three months at rates that are close to free through a system of pay-back from social security. From the age of three (or two, in larger cities) children can attend pre-schools (*maternelles*) for eight hours a day, for free (with the option of a means-tested after-school and holiday club, available until 6.30 p.m.). By contrast, the average cost for a full-time nursery place for one child in London in 2005 was £197/week, or nearly £10,000/annum (Daycare Trust 2005). For French mothers, the need to "juggle" careers around the demands of childcare following the end of maternity leave—practically and financially, at least—is mitigated.

So while I do not expand on it here, these data clearly chime with, or are the flip-side of the coin to, those presented by scholars working on cross-cultural variations in welfare regimes (Esping-Anderson 1999 being the classic example). Where childcare is seen as the responsibility of the family it will clearly chafe with a dual-earner family set-up, therefore precipitating the full-time breadwinner/part-time carer model, with all its usual gendered implications. In France, where the state takes more responsibility for care, it is understood as a means of protecting parents' (and particularly mothers') independence, economic and otherwise. Drawing on Pfau-Effinger's work, Edwards (2002) therefore makes the point that even for women who *do* work under the first model, such as the U.K., childcare is understood as a mother-substitute, again resonating with the anxieties propagated by an intensive mothering ideology explored here, and particularly pertinent to the infant feeding question.

INFANT FEEDING IN COMPARATIVE PERSPECTIVE

Gelling with one permutation of the "intensive" motherhood orthodoxy, new mothers in the U.K. can expect to hear a strong "breast is best" message from a range of governmental and non-governmental agencies (Lee 2007a). This message, to breastfeed exclusively for six months and "for anything up to two years or beyond" (WHO 2003b), is based on evidence from clinical studies that show benefits to infant (and maternal) health. This is largely due to the immunological character of breastmilk. Again however, while I do not elaborate on this here, it is arguable that these benefits have been overplayed by the policy and advocacy literature somewhat (Hoddinott et al. 2008; Wolf 2011; Faircloth 2013).

Current policy around infant feeding in the U.K. is best represented by UNICEF's Baby Friendly Initiative (BFI), a program drawn up in 1992 and active in the U.K. since 1994, currently endorsed as the "gold standard" of maternity care by NICE (the National Institute for Clinical Excellence) and the Department of Health. With the aim of addressing the infant feeding "problem" by increasing the numbers of women who breastfeed, maternity facilities can be accredited as "Baby Friendly" if they adopt the BFI's 10 Steps to Successful Breastfeeding. This includes having a written breastfeeding policy that is routinely communicated to all staff, informing all pregnant women about the benefits of breastfeeding, and helping women initiate breastfeeding soon after birth.[8] The 10th step of the program aims to foster collaboration between hospitals and lay support groups (such as La Leche League International).

In France, breastfeeding is not, as yet, a public policy issue in the same way as in the U.K., where it intersects with wider policy concerns such as health and social mobility. The Baby Friendly Initiative has been very slowly taken up in France, with Paris having no accredited hospitals (there were only 5 in the whole country by 2007; there were 51 in the U.K. at the same point).[9] The post of "Lactation Consultant," increasingly found in hospitals in the U.K., was not recognized in France at the time of research, and the government has only recently taken up the adoption of breastfeeding advocacy campaigns. Indeed, breastfeeding exclusively for six months, in line with the WHO guidelines, was explicitly recommended for the first time by the MS (*Ministère de la Santé*, Health Ministry) in its 2005 dossier.

Yet, in part because of EU commensuration and wider cultural shifts, it is true that breastfeeding is *beginning* to take more of a center stage in health policy, reflected (and informed) by rising rates of initiation, which increase each year—though this is, as Amelie, one of my interviewees, explains, a trend largely reserved for the educated classes:

> Amelie [32, breastfeeding her 2-month-old son, questionnaire response]
>
> Breastfeeding has become very "trendy" in the moneyed, well-educated classes, and I think that women choose it to be "good mothers"... [Yet] I live in an area with a very high amount of recent immigrants to France, and for them, the bottle is better because it is synonymous with being moneyed ("the breast is for poor people").

SAMPLE

Where in the U.K. several breastfeeding support organizations exist (such as the Association of Breastfeeding Mothers, the National Childbirth Trust and La Leche League International) LLLI is the only national breastfeeding support organization in France.[10] It therefore receives women from a more diverse range of backgrounds than in the U.K. They are largely middle-class (in the sense of being well educated), but certainly not only those with an interest in attachment parenting or long-term breastfeeding (as is more typically the case in the U.K.).

The differing policies around employment and infant feeding were also reflected in my French sample. While in my U.K. sample only one woman said that she was working full-time, and a third were working part-time, in France, a third were working full-time and a quarter part-time. So, although women were on average the same in many respects—married (around eight out of ten in each case); similarly aged (33 years old in France compared with 35 years old in the U.K.) and sharing a high level of education (with the overwhelming majority having university-level qualifications), the key difference was that *many more* women with young children were working outside of the home in the French sample.

In my responses, it was also clear that I had two fairly distinct sets of respondents in my French sample, in a more pronounced fashion than in the U.K. More women came along to meetings when their babies were under three months old in France (nine out of ten, on average) than in the U.K. (just under half), indicating an interest in breastfeeding largely within the brackets of maternity leave rather than "long" term as would be desirable according to attachment parents. As noted, just over a third of mothers answering the questionnaire fell into the "attachment mother" definition (compared with just over half in London). They constituted themselves as a marginal in relation to French society at large, framing their answers to my questions with complaints about their own marginality, in more pronounced but ways familiar to those I encountered in the U.K.

FRENCH PARENTING: NON-INTENSIVE MOTHERHOOD?

The American author Warner (2006) has written about her experience of motherhood in Paris (and for a more recent, similar take, see Druckerman 2012). She argues that unlike her in native U.S. (and, I suggest, the U.K.) motherhood was far less intensive—it was just not such a "Big Deal" in France, and certainly not something women would consider their primary source of what I term "identity work." This is corroborated by findings from this research. Just one example of this would be the differences in responses to a question in the questionnaire: where 11 out of 25 U.K. women listed their "profession" as a mother, only one in the sample of 19 women did this in France. There was far less fetishization about the role of "mother" in general; women were less effusive about the "wonders" of motherhood in their answers. This was reflected by one-word answers to, for example, "Why was it important for you to feed your child at the breast?" in contrast to long essays from the U.K. or from attachment mothers in France.

It is certainly the case that there does not (yet) exist an industry surrounding parenting as there does in the U.K. (Searching "Parenting" on the Google U.K. site generates 85,100,000 hits; *Parentage* on Google France gets just 1,660,000.)[11] "Parenting" has also not become a policy buzzword. As Warner explains, this lack of "support" for parents is double-edged, in that at the same time that it collapses choice, it also reduces anxiety and accountability:

> Guilt just wasn't in the air. It wasn't considered a natural consequence of working motherhood ... The general French conviction that one should live a "balanced" life was especially true for mothers—particularly, I would say, for stay-at-home mothers, who were otherwise considered at risk of falling into excessive child-centeredness. And that, the French believed, was wrong. Obsessive. Inappropriate. Just plain weird. (Warner 2006: 10–11)

Indeed, the argument might be that where there is less plurality about infant care (mothers in general must go back to work earlier, limiting their ability to—for example—breastfeed for several months or parent in an "attachment" fashion), less "identity work" is required about one's decisions, as a form of accountability. By the same logic, those that do, say, breastfeed to full term require even more "identity work" than their U.K. counterparts.

In her work in France, Wolfenstein (1955, with Margaret Mead) notes that for the Parisian parents she studied (in the 1950s) childhood was not about fun but about "preparation." This is, she argues, almost in direct contrast to her native America, where "childhood is a very nearly ideal time, a time for enjoyment, an end in itself" (1955: 115). In France, she says, "[c]hildhood is a period of probation, when everything is a means to an end; it is unenviable from the vantage point of adulthood" (ibid.). The child in France would not be expected to disrupt adult life, and should certainly not be the main preoccupation of adult conversation, for example (Wolfenstein 1955: 114).

This is reiterated in more recent research by Suizzo, published in *Ethos* (2004). In her article "Mother–Child Relationships in France," she uses a cultural models framework to argue for two distinctive features of the French parenting. One was that mothers wanted their children to be "*débrouillard*," a term difficult to translate into English, but which broadly means being prepared and therefore enabled to achieve one's personal goals. The second more pertinent feature was a pervasive worry about mothers being enslaved (*esclavage*) to their children who could easily become infant kings (*l'enfant-roi*). As she explains:

> [*Esclavage*] is the idea that mothers can become dependent on, even subordinate to, their children. This notion is quite different from the much more pervasive concern among parents in individualist cultures that children may become overly dependent on their mother. Mother-enslavement was described as a loss of personal freedom with very negative consequences for the mother. (Suizzo 2004: 317)

Such fear of enslavement means French parents:

> ... prefer more distal relations, maintaining separate beds and bedrooms for their infants, and engaging in less body contact, in part because they believe that separateness fosters independence in children ... French parents also avoid prolonged body contact, such as co-sleeping, holding, and carrying babies ... These findings point to a concern with fostering independence. (Suizzo 2004: 296)

Weaning would be a good example of ensuring distal relations are maintained, as Louise from my French sample (not an "attachment mother") makes plain:

Charlotte: Can you tell me what breastfeeding represents, to you?
Louise [28, just weaned her 6-month-old daughter]
... it was the "fusioned" aspect most of all, between mother and baby.
Privileging all of the senses; touch, smell. In fact, I had a lot of trouble separating
myself. So after six months it was a good moment to stop being so close to her.

There is an implication here that although breastfeeding is enjoyable (for both
the mother and the child), being "close" for too long is undesirable. Suizzo
argues that these ideas come through the ideas of the influential thinker
Rousseau, who wrote:

The first tears of children are prayers. If one is not careful, they soon become
orders. Children begin by getting themselves assisted; they end by getting
themselves served. Thus, from their own weakness, which is in the first place
the source of the feeling of their dependence, is subsequently born the idea of
empire and domination. (Rousseau 1979: 66, in Suizzo 2004: 317)

Another mother in the sample echoed the view that for the French there was
a concern about women becoming *"mères fusionelles"*:

Sandrine [28, 5 and 2-and-a-half-year-old sons, no longer breastfed]
    There is a massive misunderstanding around babies who breastfeed often,
and for a long time ... it is also difficult to breastfeed for longer than four to six
months without being seen as a *"mère fusionelle"* who is not able to separate
from her baby.

Warner notes, for example, that for mothers who do stay at home (and are
not in paid employment) it is considered important to maintain a "sense of
self" by using childcare on a regular basis for fear of becoming too tied to
one's children.

IT'S NATURAL? FEMINISM AND BREASTFEEDING IN FRANCE

To understand why the "intensive motherhood" orthodoxy (and validations
of personal liberty and/or emotionally absorbing parenting) are more or less
salient in London or Paris, a broader cultural perspective is required.
    I suggest that there is currently a more "embedded" attitude towards
the place of nature in France, in opposition to the growing fetishization of
nature as something desirable to "get back in touch with" currently prevalent
in the U.K., and so in vogue in parenting fashions (Faircloth 2009). True,

Rousseau counseled women to "look to the animals" in his campaign against wet-nursing in eighteenth-century France (Badinter 1981; Hrdy 2000). But it would be fair to argue that this injunction has been rebuked over the last two centuries with a legacy of the Enlightenment that stresses human separation from nature and, in turn, other animals. As Nicole, a La Leche League leader with whom I discussed these issues, puts it:

> *Charlotte: You said that in France there is not a "breastfeeding culture"—why?*
> Nicole [LLLI Leader]
> I think that in England there was always, at least for the last century and a half, a culture of returning to nature, proximity with nature, with one's choices, with people—there is a conscience about children that is much more ancient. In France, there was, by contrast, a "hygienist" culture, with a very strict order, "*puéri-culture*" centers [like health-visiting centers], which set the rules: "One must do it like this, and like that." It's something that's very evident ... It really harmed breastfeeding, and it's an approach that has never really been discredited. It just didn't fit with breastfeeding, where you can't be "controlled by the rod," in such a rigid way.

The 1970s "return to nature," which saw feminist movements (including LLLI) blossom in the U.K., was not replicated in France (although Badinter suggests that the same roots were present, if not as elaborated, 2010). Indeed, "being close to nature" as something desirable is a relatively new phenomenon in France, one which, I argue, is a "culture on the make" for a privileged section of society (and it's worth re-stating here that I was working in London and Paris, which, as urban capitals, cannot be said to represent Britain and France in any straightforward way. Indeed, any nostalgia for "nature" might be said to be a product of these very settings and middle-class contexts.) This was even evident in the sorts of food present, brought along by mothers to the meetings. While in the U.K. there was typically organic bread, cheese, and vegetables, in France it was normal to see packaged and processed foods, although there is a growing market for "organic" (*biologique*) food in France, which may well start to feature in much the same way as the U.K.

For many women, the idea of being "a mammal" was one reason mothers in France were put off breastfeeding, unlike in the U.S. or the U.K., where this discourse is frequently drawn upon in advocacy literature as a way of encouraging women to breastfeed:

> Sophie [25, breastfeeding her 3-month-old daughter, questionnaire response]
> Breastfeeding seems like an animal act, uncivilized.

This ambivalence about our status as mammals was seen to be part of the country's different history of both the Enlightenment, and of feminism, as Nicole expounds:

> Charlotte: *There is also the fact that people think of breastfeeding as "esclavage" …*
> Nicole [LLLI Leader]
> Yes, I agree, [French] feminism was constructed outside of and AGAINST motherhood. The battle of feminism was: equal salaries between men and women, for abortion to defend the sexual liberty of women … but not at all in favor of motherhood, absolutely not! Whereas in other countries, such as Scandinavia, feminism was constructed WITH motherhood. Moreover, the majority of French feminists didn't have children … like it was a liberty not to have children. Revenge against nature, yes, that's it, a controlling of nature. To be free was to get out of that condition.

Speaking about a friend who did not breastfeed her child, Louise explains again that her reasoning is a product of a feminist inclination which does not encourage women to adjust to the "rhythm" of their children, but rather the other way round:

> Charlotte: *Why do you think your friend didn't want to breastfeed?*
> Louise [28, just weaned her 6-month-old daughter]
> In '68 there was a big revolution, the liberation of women and all that … so in our parents' generation there weren't many feminists who breastfed. And even now there is an image of the modern woman: … she goes everywhere, does everything, she works and she is not dependent on anyone and above all not to her children. When one breastfeeds, one has another rhythm, one is obliged to adapt to the rhythm of the child …
> Charlotte: *It's interesting, the distinction between motherhood and womanhood …*
> Louise: When one looks at northern societies [such as Scandinavia], it's different; women don't get posed the same question [to breastfeed or not]: they breastfeed. If they do not breastfeed they are not considered good mothers. Whereas in France, it's the opposite, it's the woman who breastfeeds who is thought of badly, and who is thought "strange" … One must go back to work early … I took holiday, and after, I had holiday to use up … like that I was able to [breastfeed] for five months. In short, one has to fight to be able to breastfeed, you have to find combinations that work.

Many women in the French sample were therefore conscious that for mothers in France, using either formula or expressed milk, rather than feeding directly from the breast, made sense according to these cultural norms:

Diane [32, breastfeeding her 5-month-old daughter, questionnaire response]

It can appear more practical to bottle-feed [with expressed milk] as one can better manage the rhythm of the feeds; the woman is not strictly tied to her baby (for me, the idea of expressing milk with a pump is pretty distasteful, so I sometimes time where I will be with breastfeeding, not wanting to or not able to take the baby out everywhere—cinemas and theatres, etc.). The body of a woman who breastfeeds becomes totally maternal, and that can change the relationship one has with one's partner (especially if the breastfeeding is long term).

EXPRESSING MILK: THE FRENCH WAY?

So how do French women negotiate competing discourses which stress feminine liberty yet are increasingly starting to advocate breastfeeding? Since more women will go to work when their baby is only ten weeks old, there was a greater demand for information about expressing milk than in the U.K. Thus there were many more conversations about the best sort of breast pump, the storage of breastmilk, as well as questions about how to get the baby to sleep through the night, and on to solids, from as early as three months.

The expression of breastmilk (by hand or with a pump, for feeding from a cup or bottle) has been central to the infant feeding issue in the U.S. for some time, where six weeks' maternity leave is standard (Blum 1999). It is sold as offering the ultimate solution for working women, in part through the merging of the domestic and public spheres. Separating the product from the means of production means that the child benefits by receiving breastmilk even when it is unable to extract it itself, or when the mother is absent. The mother is therefore able to invest her energies in other labors (such as employment). A woman doesn't have to expose her breast in public; a third party can engage in the feeding process (meaning that "bonding" can be shared) and parents can see exactly how much the child is eating.

Yet critics of the "pump-culture" claim that children (and mothers) greatly miss out by not actually being in skin-to-skin contact for feeding, since jaw and eye development is hindered, the supply–demand relationship of milk production put out of kilter, and the production of antibodies specific to the maternal–infant environment disrupted. To many breastfeeding advocates, any sort of separation, in the form of a bottle or teat, is seen as damaging for the child. There was concern among some of the "attachment mothers" that something essential to the mothering relationship—the bonding—was missing, when mediated by a bottle or pump.[12]

Expressing was therefore understood to be less than ideal by many LLLI leaders, though there was pragmatism about women's ability to delay their return to work in France, which was near impossible. While in the U.K. women were sometimes asked, either by other LLLI members or leaders "Could you possibly afford not to work?", this was rarely asked in France—instead tips on combining breastfeeding and working would be proffered.

Furthermore, although French women generally considered themselves to be less prudish than their British counterparts about nudity, they found a contradiction between *"le corps 'maternel' et le corps* 'érotique'" to be more problematic than the majority of my British respondents. (Certainly, intensive [attachment] parenting can intersect with couple relationships in a problematic way, which Layne [2013] observes in her recent case study of a single-mother-by-choice.) Interestingly, there was a difference in how British and French women narrated this contradiction: French informants seemed to prioritize descriptions of their bodies in their accounts of breastfeeding. Where women in France would talk about "my breasts," for example, women in Britain spoke of "the breast." Bobel notes that this latter term is a form of objectification, which at once resists and accepts cultural prescriptions about breasts, put to the service of another (Bobel 2001: 136), though I also remember one woman in the French maternity hospital saying "my breasts are for my husband" when asked why she had chosen to formula feed.

"The Body" has been the focus of much discussion in the social sciences, particularly since the arrival of technologies of modification. It is notable that breasts—in both the U.K. and France—are probably the greatest site of female bodily modification in the form of plastic surgery (which often precludes breastfeeding). In contradistinction to the typical emphasis in social science on the commodification and objectification of bodies, McDonald and Lambert, in their recent volume *Social Bodies*, aim to consider the extent to which "bodies and their elements are themselves 'social'" (McDonald and Lambert 2009: 2). To this extent, breasts can be considered as a site of women's identity work, albeit with different emphases in Britain and France, with respect to the transition between the maternal and erotic bodies. McDonald and Lambert note that the transformation of bodies is "never confined solely to the biologically functional in their effects but inevitably entail[s] the reformulation, reconstruction or re-establishment of social relations between persons and between human groups" (McDonald and Lambert 2009: 5). We might say that the moral relations of accountability (to the child, or to the partner) are made corporeal by women through their breasts.

Thus, when in the U.K. group attachment mothers mentioned co-sleeping as having an effect on their relationship with their husband, it would usually be in a dismissive tone. Generally, less "intimacy time" with a partner would be considered a reasonable sacrifice for a "family bed" philosophy:

> Judy [39, breastfeeding her 2- and 4-year-old daughters, questionnaire response]
> Yes, our children have access to our bed and we do not exclude them from our evening time. Overall—bar a few bad colds and a few restless nights—we sleep very well, and are a very close family. I see it as a reflection of the commitment we have to the wellbeing of our girls and believe it has strengthened the relationship I have with my husband. The extra evening time our children have had, especially with their father, has been very important.

By contrast, Nayanika, in the Parisian Anglophone group, also practicing attachment parenting, gave this story about her relationship with her (French) husband and her breastfeeding daughter:

> Nayanika [28, breastfeeding her 1-year-old daughter]
> My husband was having his breakfast, and she started fussing. I was in the middle of making coffee and I just undid my bra. Then he said "I suppose that's why a lot of women don't breastfeed, because men stop feeling sexual afterwards. I've just grown to accept that they're [her breasts] not mine anymore." I don't feel sexual about my breasts any more as they're so nutritive and practical. It's not the same as before.

The non-attachment French LLLI members I spoke with seemed more concerned about the effects of this, speaking less about the "bonding" of children with the father than with the effect of their parenting practices on their intimacy as a couple:

> Diane [35, breastfeeding her 3-month-old daughter, questionnaire response]
> Effectively, to be able to breastfeed during the night, I moved her into our bed, which had a positive side, for being able to nurse whilst sleeping, but also had negative effects:
> 1. She wakes up more often, three times a night, whereas when she slept alone in her cradle she wouldn't wake up more than twice—I am more tired because my sleep is broken.
> 2. The intimacy with my partner has been really limited, and I think that to put her back into her own bed would be nearly impossible. (But at the same time I wonder how and when? When will she sleep through?)

Overall, then, we can say that for my French informants there was an association between feminism and the work of de Beauvoir (unlike the

U.K. responses, which drew on cultural feminist trends, as Nicole explains above). Her work *The Second Sex* describes how female physiology renders women subservient to the requirement of the species to procreate, in ways vastly more costly than those accrued to men. Her view of breastfeeding was indeed as some sort of enslavement. As Layne and Aengst note, "[s]he celebrates human society which exerts mastery over nature: '[h]uman society is an antiphysis – in a sense it is against nature; it does not passively submit to the presence of nature but rather takes over the control of nature on its own behalf' (1989: 53)" (Layne and Aengst 2010: 73). So, breastfeeding *at all* is seen to be against the ethic of "French" feminism. Breastfeeding "to full term" makes one even more marginal.

There was therefore a difference in the ease with which French women consider themselves able to "sell" attachment parenting to their partners when compared with their British counterparts. I cite the following conversation between myself and two members of the Anglophone group in Paris, both practicing "full-term" breastfeeding, to show how women negotiate these multiple accountabilities—in this case to their French husbands (who would prefer their wives to socialize more), and to their children (who, cared for according to attachment parenting guidelines, prevent them from doing so):

Charlotte: Do you work?
    Vicky [34, breastfeeding her 1-year-old daughter]
    I did, but … I want to stay with her as much as I can and I want to have another baby as well. I like the idea of having more kids.
    Nayanika [28, breastfeeding her 1-year-old daughter]
    I like the idea as well—but three years of breastfeeding, times [multiplied by] however many children. I'm not sure my husband can take it! My husband definitely wants to stop at two. He loves it but I don't think he can do this life of staying-in. You have to stay in all the time. She won't go to bed with anyone but me.
    Vicky: Life is so different when you breastfeed this way. I see other mums who stopped breastfeeding much earlier and they go out to dinner once a week with their husbands. Their life is almost back to pre-baby social.
    Nayanika: But I didn't have a baby to get back to pre-baby as quickly as possible. That's my logic. That's not entirely my husband's logic and I have to respect the fact that there are two people in this marriage and family. It's fair enough. I really wanted to get pregnant and he was less ready to have a baby.
    Vicky: I often hear talking about people putting their baby to bed early, getting them to sleep from an early hour. But I don't want my evening back. I put her to bed early for her, but I would rather have her up with my husband and me. Though, of course, I am tired.

Nayanika: I don't want to go and sit in a restaurant when I can be with her. [The time] is so precious and it goes by so quickly.

Vicky: I don't have the desire to go and sit in a restaurant.

Nayanika: I think from my husband it comes from the people around him. The fact that a lot of people have found having children so difficult. We really are freaks [compared to how the rest of our friends do it].

Vicky: I have other people who I'm in touch with who are like us, but we don't see our friends very often. We don't have people over for dinner, the husbands don't see each other any more. He's very different from his friends that he talks to, and to the people at work.

Charlotte: Not going out for dinner, and not meeting friends for a drink, I think that's something I would miss ...

Nayanika: I do miss it, but only from a social perspective. Rather than go out, we have had people over for dinner, but it's a circus. My husband ends up entertaining them a lot more than I do, and I go and put her to sleep, which takes an hour.

Vicky: If I had my friends over for dinner, it would be [my husband] entertaining our friends and I would be in the bedroom with her.

Nayanika: It has spoilt some of my friendships. I know that [my daughter's] godmother is slightly disappointed that I've stopped working and I'm staying at home. She has a really high-flying job. She's surprised at me, and I see a lot less of her. She's found this whole side to me that she can't quite deal with. On the other hand I have some friends with whom I've got in touch with again, and some who think what I'm doing is really wonderful—and all the new people at LLL.

SHIFTING ORTHODOXIES

Yet there are counter-currents to the "typically French" parenting these mothers describe. Recently, Badinter, the author and philosopher, has argued that the traditional French model of motherhood is under threat from a rising orthodoxy of "Good Motherhood"' (of the kind familiar to many British women), which champions "natural" practices such as (long-term) breastfeeding, using washable nappies, and cooking organic food, and impels women to take a considerable periods of time off work to look after children (2010). Indeed, an article appearing in *Elle* magazine entitled "The End of Feminism? What Happens when Super-woman Returns to the House" featured two of my informants, describing their feminism in a language reminiscent of "attachment mothers" in London:[13]

Stephanie [34 years old, in a couple, 1 child]
I never "found" myself in feminism. There are fundamental differences between men and women. Motherhood is an essential one. I intend to be a mother as much as a woman. I have the chance to work at home, so my son, who is nearly three years old, has never been looked after [by anyone else]. There is a rhythm with the rest of the world. I breastfed him for a long time, and until the age of one he was always by my side, in a scarf next to me. Yet, I have an active life; I am a journalist and a translator and I work in public associations. But to work should not be synonymous with separation from one's child. I do not want to impose that on him. Moreover, I did not register him at school: I like the idea of him being free in his activities.

Like attachment parents elsewhere, and in line with an "intensive motherhood" orthodoxy, women practicing attachment parenting in France speak about being emotionally absorbed and personally fulfilled through their parenting practices, which in turn form the basis of their "identity work." Yet their approach to parenting, which relies heavily on a validation of nature as opposed to culture, is not, in general, endorsed in broader French culture (or philosophers such as Badinter), which validates the Enlightenment legacy of humanism and domination over nature. They are therefore not seen to be helping the traditional feminist cause—quite the reverse.

Yet like in the U.K., attachment mothers in France considered themselves to be "beacons" who were "spreading the light" about attachment parenting, in distinction to mainstream patterns of care. Indeed, women who practice attachment parenting in France have a commitment to the cause that was even stronger than those I met in the U.K., perhaps as a result of their exacerbated non-conventionality. Typically, and to a greater extent than in the U.K., they spoke of their marginalization. This mother (who was French, but living in London) noted:

Audrey [35, breastfeeding her newborn son]
My friends in Paris think I am totally mad for not wanting an epidural during the birth, and for breastfeeding for five months—if only they knew I might do it for five years! They say to me that I pick him up too much when he cries and that "*il faut frustrer le bébé*"—I don't know how you would translate that, but it basically means I am making a rod for my own back by making a clingy baby, or "you must frustrate the baby."

CONCLUSION

What is interesting in this discussion is how the experiences of French and British women who practice attachment parenting challenge the prevailing norms in each country. We see that the length of maternity leave routinely given to women, the importance of work outside of the home for self-realization, and notions of individual autonomy combine to have a substantial impact on how women go about narrating their experiences of parenting. Where in the U.K. breastfeeding (and indeed attachment mothering) might be said to slot into the prevailing climate of "intensive motherhood" (a prevailing climate for the middle classes, at least), in France breastfeeding (and certainly attachment mothering) goes against this grain. Indeed, in a culture where maternal–infant separation and autonomy is lauded as ideal, intensive, embodied care on the part of the mother is perceived as an impingement on female liberty, rather than as a valid outlet for her "identity work." Yet—as evidenced by the rapid growth of mothering boutiques, magazines, and clubs, many of my "attachment" informants frequented—it seems that the climate in France is on the cusp of a change, in which case women there will start to face a similar but exacerbated cultural contradiction between their working and domestic lives.

Badinter's analysis of shifting orthodoxies around motherhood is useful, although it does not highlight the struggle of many French women who would like to spend more time with their children in the early months—attachment parents or otherwise—and who resent the social pressure to return to work. What she does show, however, is how this "struggle" is itself a result of these very shifts, which, I suggest, appear to be turning towards a validation of intensive, "natural" mothering. How each group of women negotiate these shifts—one with a generous system of childcare (in France), the other with a long length of maternity leave (in the U.K.)—and its implications on infant feeding patterns will undoubtedly be a source of feminist interest for some time to come. As she says, "The majority of French women reconcile maternity with professional life. Many of them work full-time when they have a child. They are resisting the model of the perfect mother, but for how long?"[14]

–5–

The Naturalist Discourse Surrounding Breastfeeding among French Mothers

Gervaise Debucquet and Valérie Adt[1]

In the order of nature, breastfeeding necessarily succeeds birth as it delivers the nutrients that are vital to a newborn's growth and development, establishing and facilitating the emotional and psychological bond that unites the mother with her infant. However, in other respects, breastfeeding is a practice that borders "nature" (as opposed to culture). Its methods, its exclusive or non-exclusive nature, and the path toward weaning are almost invariably defined by culture. Through breastfeeding practices are staged the question of the relationship between the sexes (Héritier 1996), the connections between parents (Lévi-Strauss 1949), and the changing roles of "mother" and "woman" (Maher 1992; Badinter 2010). In other words, mothers do not have any real freedom of choice when it comes to matters of breastfeeding (Jodelet 1987; Jodelet and Ohana 2000). The renewed discussions of both naturalists and ecologists in Europe (most particularly in France) demonstrate that this boundary between nature and culture is never decisively fixed and that it continues to elicit debate such as that highlighted in a recent publication by Badinter (2010). In effect, Badinter poses the question of choice between breastfeeding and bottle-feeding, a choice she considers "doubly constrained" under the pressure of particularly active associations promoting breastfeeding and the medicalized highlighting of the nutritional value of breastmilk. In some ways, this is a reversal of the biomedical stand of the 1960s and 1970s. Furthermore, according to Badinter, the conjunction of medical and naturalist discourses surrounding breastfeeding tends to present it as an ideal model for the mother and the child, while at the same time helping to generate a sense of guilt among mothers who use formula milk. In fact, the rise of breastfeeding in France, particularly among women from higher social strata, is a phenomenon without precedent, since the rate of breastfeeding at hospital discharge increased from 52.5 percent to 62.5 percent between 1998 and 2003, according to data from INSERM. The weight of the naturalist, medical, and familial arguments in the discourse of mothers and maternity is to be described, taking into account mothers' social origin. We must also ask about the "rationales" for all those who feed their babies with formula milk.

This chapter proposes to answer these questions by analyzing the conceptions French mothers have regarding the issue of perinatal nutrition for children. Indeed, feeding the newborn addresses a number of nutritional, psychological, social, and cultural issues. The educational concerns occupy a place sometimes as important as the strictly nutritional concerns (Antier 2003) and we will see in what follows that the question of education, in particular food education, holds a very important place in French mothers' discussions. For French mothers, feeding an infant or young child is simultaneously not only feeding but also teaching him/her to "eat in the French style." This involves the transmission of a certain culture of taste, the promotion of a natural and balanced diet, as well as ensuring the absorption of a number of rules, such as eating at regular times (Poulain 2002a; Fischler and Masson 2008). We will show that the choice of breastmilk versus formula goes beyond the discussion of nutritional differences (real or imagined), and turns out to be the choice of a "method" to transmit these standards and cultural norms. The analysis of the arguments of the "artificial milk" mothers shows that they see the bottle as an effective way to create a rhythm and regulate food intake, which thus allows the infant to quickly internalize the rules and family eating habits. "Breastmilk" mothers, however, value breastfeeding on demand and rely heavily on naturalist arguments to prove the superiority of breastfeeding, including in matters of food education. This leads us to relativize the diffusionist view (Boltanski 1969), since "breastmilk" mothers (who are viewed as more educated) tend to relegate to second place the scientific and medical arguments promoting breastfeeding.

After having presented the methodology and the context of the research, we will present the results by comparing "breastfeeding" versus "bottle-feeding" mothers, looking at (1) the nutritional virtues ascribed to breastmilk and artificial milk in connection with the conceptions of the body, and (2) the representations of the advantages and disadvantages of each type of feeding in terms of transmission of taste, of balanced diet, and of regulation of food intake. Finally, we will discuss our results by considering how the naturalist discourse around breastfeeding connects with the current concerns of French mothers about food and how it leads one to reconsider the question of receiving medical or dietary recommendations in the perinatal period.

RESEARCH CONTEXT

Our thinking is part of a broader research program (NUPEM[2] 2007–10), co-ordinated by the CHRN (Centre for Human Nutrition Research in Nantes), to better understand the impact of diet in the perinatal period (pregnancy and the first year of life) on the future health of adults. A too-low birth weight and a too-high growth rate in the first year of life may increase the risk of obesity and cardiovascular disease in adults. The recent concept of a *nutritional footprint* tends to account for the persistent exposure to certain nutrients, in particular omega-3, oligosaccharides, and proteins or their deficiencies during a key period of perinatal life, hence the need for certain optimization of the nutrition of mothers and children to prevent diseases later in adults. Breastmilk may have many advantages over various artificial milks currently available on the market, but this research has a twofold purpose: (1) assessing the impact of an enrichment of the mothers' diet in terms of certain nutrients during pregnancy and lactation; and (2) optimizing the ingredients for infant formula. These works, therefore, are of interest to both feeding choices but they raise an important issue—that of the reception of a new scientific argument around perinatal feeding by mothers—and this in a context in which the naturalist discourse discovered numerous shifts of emphasis and direction. It is this concern expressed by some representatives of the medical profession that led us, along with researchers from various disciplines (neonatologists, obstetricians, metaboliciens, chemists, and psychologists), to shed light on the sociocultural determinants of the acceptance or rejection of medical recommendations or prescriptions by the mothers. But to answer this very specific question, we could not do without, as we said in the introduction, a wider reflection on how the nutritional concerns are articulated with the educational questions, indeed cultural identity issues, inherent to perinatal feeding.

METHODOLOGY

The methodological approach we have chosen is exclusively qualitative and is based on semi-structured interviews with a total of 33 women, 19 of whom were interviewed once, and 14 of whom were followed from the end of their pregnancy to the first months of the life of their child. Recruitment was done through the offices of gynecology, midwives, pediatric nurses, delivery preparation offices, or the La Leche League association. Additional people were monitored, via an internet discussion forum. The criteria that were selected for the formation of the sample are the number of children (multiparous/ primiparous), gestational weight gain (less than 10 kg, 10–15 kg, over 15 kg), the weight of the child at birth (small, medium, and heavy weight), the socio-professional family profile (higher class, intermediate, and lower), and finally the type of feeding (breastmilk, formula, or mixed). The interviews were conducted partly in the Pays de la Loire, Paris, and across eastern France to take into account the regional variability in the choice of perinatal feeding; the west of France recording the lowest rates of breastfeeding and the Paris region the highest rates (55 percent vs. 74 percent according to INSERM 2003).

The interviews were structured around four main topics: (1) the determinants of the choice of breastfeeding versus formula, noting the role of knowledge, representations, and identification of familial continuities and discontinuities; (2) the practices of perinatal feeding, noting maternal nutrition, details of feeding, and weaning; (3) the nutritional knowledge and beliefs as well as perceived benefits/risks of breastmilk versus formula; and finally (4) the relationship between perinatal feeding and food education (Table 1). It is important to note that the interviews were conducted in the mothers' homes and all were punctuated by either breastfeeding or bottle-feeding, thus allowing observation of actual practices.

RESULTS

The in-depth interviews that were conducted indicate that, in reality, the opposing views about breastfeeding versus formula feeding conceal a variety of influential representations foreshadowing practices in perinatal feeding, almost invariably resulting in a set of physiological, psychological, social, cultural, and even medical as well as economic constraints. Our purpose is not to reflect the entire spectrum of practices but to compare the discourse of two ideal types (Weber 1956): first, mothers with strong convictions in favor of breastfeeding, and second, mothers who favor artificial feeding.[3] In other words, we choose to present those practices that evidence strongly anchored representations, and whose discourse demonstrates consistency and coherence. Without ignoring the use of formula as a default choice, it should be noted that "artificial milk" mothers could not escape the temptation to justify their choice in response to what is perceived as a naturalist offensive, of a kind that Badinter specifically denounces (Badinter 2010). For "artificial milk mothers," it is therefore necessary to take into account the discourse of destigmatization and whether or not it was spontaneous.

Table 1: Structure of the interview guide

Themes	Main questions
Determinants of choice (breastmilk / formula milk) (identification of familial continuities / discontinuities)	• Tell me about the way babies have been fed in your family (mother, grandmother, mother-in-law, sisters). • When did you decide about the kind of feeding? Why? • And for your other babies? • What does a "beautiful baby" mean to you? – What is "good milk"/"bad milk" for you?
Practices	• Tell me about your food during the pregnancy and after child's birth. What has changed? Why? • Did you take nutritional supplements for you? • "Breastfeeding" one's baby—what does it mean for you? • Describe, in your own words, a baby fed with breastmilk and a baby fed with formula milk. • Breastmilk versus formula milk: what are the differences? • How do you imagine the feeding of your baby during the first year? And then what? • What difficulties have you come up against?
Nutritional beliefs	• When breastfeeding, is it possible to have "bad milk"? • And "bad" formula milk? • What "goes through" breastmilk? Positive and negative things? What happens between mother's body and baby's body? • Advantages/disadvantages of maternal milk versus animal milk?
Educational stakes	• What does "succeeding or failing" mean for you regarding the management of your baby's food? • In the end, what is expected? • "Learning to eat to one's baby"—what does this mean for you? • From this point of view, is there a difference between a baby fed with breastmilk and a baby fed with formula milk?

These spontaneous discourses will be the focus of what follows and we will compare discourses of "breastmilk" mothers in order to highlight diametrically opposed conceptions of body, health, contamination, and finally, food education. These comparisons are based on representations, beliefs, and knowledge that we analyzed. The socio-demographics of the two ideal types are presented in detail elsewhere (Table 2), but are in line with Gojard (2000).

REPRESENTATIONS OF THE NUTRITIONAL BENEFITS OF BREASTMILK VERSUS ARTIFICIAL MILK: SYMBIOTIC BODY AND PERFORMATIVE BODY

Breastfeeding, as a natural consequence of pregnancy and childbirth, constitutes a theme that questions the body, its representations, and the beliefs

Table 2: Characteristics of the ideal-types

	Mothers in favor of breastfeeding	Mothers open to breastfeeding	Mothers in favor of formula feeding
Socio-demographics	· Upper social classes · In parental vacation or breastfeeding carried on after going back to work · Often multiparas · First successful experience of breastfeeding	· Middle social classes · Break of breast-feeding before or when going back to work · A first baby rarely breastfed	· Middle and lower social classes · No breastfeeding at the maternity hospital · No child breastfed
Relation to social and medical norms	· Mothers "free" from familial practices · Distance from scientific and medical views (including food diversification)	· Distance from familial practices in progress · Confidence in medical and pediatric views (including food diversification)	· Continuity of familial practices (including diversification) · Critical attitude towards scientific and medical view (its changes and contradictions) · Confidence in science for formula milk
Arguments	· Pleasure and personal blooming · Relationship between mother–baby · Nature as moral argument · Educative issues of breastfeeding at least as important as nutritional issues	· Affective re-appropriation of the baby · Confidence in nature but lower in their body · Nutritional issues more important than educative issues	· Good balance between the roles of woman, mother, and wife · Share of roles in the couple (significant role of fathers in infant food) · Low confidence in nature and their body · Negative perception of breastfeeding (modesty, suffering, aesthetic) · Educative issues of feeding bottle at least as important as nutritional issues

associated with it. From this point of view the two ideal types reveal two opposite conceptions of the body without knowing to what extent concrete experience of breastfeeding, familial practices, adherence to values, or nutritional knowledge in general have helped shape them.

In "breastmilk mothers," the body is, in terms of its representation, a body that "knows" what the child needs and provides milk that is suitable for all stages of growth; that is to say, a body fully symbiotic (Lecourt 2003) with the child. These mothers then offer us the image of the self-sacrificing mother who gives herself entirely to her infant, paying special attention to her/his own lifestyle and diet, on which milk quality is supposed to depend. Here one finds an echo of the French representations of "eating well" since these mothers talk about the rigor with which they vary and balance their meals and choose the most natural foods possible (that is to say, food labeled "organic" or simply food from their own garden). Research elsewhere has indicated that among some other Western nations, the French value a balanced meal, pay attention to the origin of food ingredients and that what is natural for them is what originates close to home: i.e. from the garden or from small domestic producers (Merdji and Debucquet 2008). Even when talking about the enrichment of formula milk, its value is heavily pervaded with environmentalist and naturalist ideas:

> I eat everything balanced and varied vegetables from my garden, I do not see why we must supplement. The iron fed to the baby … it is not easily assimilated, not as much as that which passes through breastmilk. Same problem with formula! [...] Formula doesn't have everything, not the same vitamins, even though the manufacturers say they do. For example, Vitamin D is not as assimilated in formula because there are also plenty of other vitamins in formula. It's better to breastfeed than to put vitamin D in the yoghurt!
> *And whenever the added vitamin D would be natural, for example from fish oil?*
> Yes … but it's not as good as when it passes through the body. It's not natural. The body is designed to receive small doses of vitamins, not in large doses unless there are deficiencies! So normally it's not worth giving more things to the baby! The same thing with all these added vitamins. I fear that my baby will become dependent on these substances.

We see here through the distinction that is made between "natural" vitamins progressively "distilled" and "added" vitamins (sometimes in excess) that the body (or rather the passage through the mother's body) constitutes a symbolic guarantee of the value of the nutrients. Even when discussing the issue of nutritional supplements for mothers during pregnancy or lactation, most of these mothers refuse, considering them "useless," "ineffective," or "against nature." Elsewhere, we have observed that most French people are very much opposed to nutrient enrichment of food for these same reasons, but they accept more easily natural enhancements (for example, through animal feeding for milk cow) than industrially prepared enrichments (for example, milk with added nutrients) (see Merdji, Debucquet, Fischler, and Masson, 2008 Research Program ALLEGNUTRI, publication pending).

As for "artificial milk mothers," a totally opposite concept of the body has been found since it is a performative body that is to be seen in the discussions. Even if these mothers belong more to the middle and lower classes, some of them, particularly from the middle and upper middle classes (Gojard 2000), could have an ideological relationship with the cutting edge of science which, as Habermas says, leads to a certain "rationalization" of the effects of scientific progress, in this instance those who have served as points of support to the emergence of a functional food. This concept of performative body is also echoed in the work of Le Breton (1998) which shows how an anatomical–physiological knowledge has gradually established itself in the minds of lay people, even if they do not comprehend more than a small fraction of it. But this knowledge has contributed to a mechanistic view of the body, which is reduced to a machine that can optimize its operation. However, when considering the first expressions of "artificial milk mothers," we detect recurring themes that refer to a lack of confidence in their bodies and in the ability of the latter to produce "good milk." In this regard, a recent article shows how the image of one's own body plays an important role in the management of breastfeeding. Among obese women (BMI > 30), initiation rates of breastfeeding in hospital and extended breastfeeding beyond one month and three months are lower than in normal-weight women (18.5 < BMI < 25). Moreover, they feel a greater discomfort with breastfeeding in public (Mok et al. 2008).

It is unclear whether this particular relationship to the body evokes a certain psychological profile or derives from a more and less conscious construction because of the existence of substantial continuity of family practices (bottle-feeding for the last two generations and/or the failure of breastfeeding) in popular circles. Whatever it may be, this sentiment predisposes these mothers to a greater trust in formula. Unlike the "breastmilk mothers," those mothers adhere to dietary supplements during pregnancy that can "enhance their bodies," deemed by expectant mothers as "incapable" of providing necessary nutrients to the babies. And almost all these mothers occasionally or regularly took vitamins, iron, or other minerals during their pregnancy and see the choice of artificial feeding as a logical extension of these practices.

BREASTMILK AND FORMULA: THE NATURAL VERSUS THE NORMALIZED

The answers to the question asked at the beginning of the interviews—"According to you, what is a 'good' milk for your baby? What are its characteristics?"—confirmed the two opposing visions described above. For "breastmilk" mothers, breastmilk is best because it is intrinsically adaptive and changing:

> There are alternatives, such as formula milk ... but we cannot manufacture milk as good, it is alive, it changes all the time, during feeding, over time, at 3 months, at 6 months. We cannot imitate it ... it is what it is at any given time. Living with antibodies, more or less rich in water, fat, sugar; water is the starter, the rest is the main dish! It's the baby who chooses. The other milk which is formula is inert. Milk is not only a collection of nutrients, there are also antibodies in it, and so it is well designed to be assimilated, it contains iron and the enzyme which goes together for digestion ... this is the living part.

In contrast, formula can be summarized in terms of a fixed quantity of nutrients, "such as a powder that you can never completely dissolve in water." What such a statement brings to light is the opposition made between breastmilk and formula milk, the singular versus the standardized and the living versus the inert. More broadly, the fundamental opposition is between the natural and the artificial. These representations allow us to understand why these mothers refuse any somatic explanation that can be given to "bad" milk—some of them evoking the intergenerational conflicts they may have about this with their mothers or mothers-in-law, who, as a general rule, did not breastfeed and who pressure their daughters and/or daughters-in-law to resort to biological analysis to assess the quality of their own milk.

The worldview of the "artificial milk mothers" is completely different and steeped in "science." Their vision is to be able to "optimize" the nutritional quality of milk and produce a milk "rich enough and in large quantities." Thus, the nutritional supplement and enrichment are perceived as "normal" because it is needed, according to their statements, "to correct what nature does." This confidence in scientific research was fully expressed when we directed the attention of the mothers during the interviews toward the table with the nutritional composition of the infant formula cans they used. Indeed, most of them were unaware that the formula milk was made from animal milk; formula milk is, in their minds, a fully synthetic milk.

"Breastmilk" mothers and "artificial milk" mothers differ markedly in terms of the schema they use to think about the quality of both types of milk and which gives each of their discussions a remarkable coherence. We will give another example in what follows through their conceptions of contamination.

THE TWO CONCEPTIONS OF CONTAMINATION

First, it is important to note that we found in our two ideal types of mothers a number of beliefs described as "permanent" by the many researchers who are interested in the issue of breastfeeding. The theme of the contamination of milk by the bodily fluids—in particular semen and blood—(Verdier, 1979; Speltini and Molivari 1998; D'Onofrio 2004) is, in fact, invariably present in the discourse of "breastmilk mothers." Hence the idea of milk being altered upon the return of one's period or avoidance of intercourse during lactation, in addition to the refusal of oral contraceptives, which some mothers regarded as potentially dangerous. They believe sex hormones can be absorbed by the baby, just like alcohol, tobacco, or drugs. This absorption is morally unacceptable for many and hence these mothers feel the need to devote themselves entirely to their feeding function. This last point resonates with a number of requirements concerning lifestyle (physical hygiene and food but also customs and moral life) made for nursing mothers by various doctors of the 1900s, notably Dr. Vallembert, but is found to be still partially believed today. The 1930s French family booklets echoed these views, many of which prevailed and were repeated to us during our research. The permanence for what, in part, falls within the scope of beliefs, attests to the symbolic equivalence that is established between the physical and moral qualities of the maternal body and milk quality (Merdji 2006).

Regarding other considerations, representations of contamination, or, more precisely, pre-representations associated with "undesirable components" of milk, show that the differences we have discussed previously in relation to the body, nature, or science still actualize themselves here in the responses of "breastmilk" mothers versus "artificial milk" mothers. In a nutshell, the debate so far raises an important question: Is it milk that can contain negative attributes? If the answer is "yes," then where does that view come from? We will limit ourselves to the case of "chemical" contamination that we have addressed through the case of dioxin, a problem largely ignored by all interviewed mothers, none of whom mentioned this spontaneously.

The evocation of the possible contamination of breastmilk by dioxins provoked strong reactions in "breastmilk" mothers as shown in this excerpt from an interview:

Dioxin? I had never thought ... If you eat things with dioxin in them ... But, I think the formula made with cows' milk ... they also have dioxin! So there is more benefit to eating organic but to continue breastfeeding.

You mean that if you eat organic food it is less likely to absorb the dioxin?

Yes ... and that mothers' milk will always be less contaminated than powdered milk.

The words of this mother are another illustration of the weight of the naturalist argument within the mechanisms of lay, uninformed reassurance, thereby actualizing the representations associated with breastmilk, that is to say those of "symbiotic" milk produced by—and through—the mother's body and thereby ensuring its purity. This in turn leads to the symmetrical representation of formula milk as being tainted by the mere fact that it is "artificial":

In breastmilk, certain negative things can pass through [if consumed in excess]: smoke, alcohol, pesticides ... But in the end it is less detrimental than formula even if it is very controlled ... because this milk is artificial: it's powdered milk with lots of things added into it.

For "artificial milk" mothers, the reasoning is reversed in all respects, because in their view it is precisely the existence of "scientific control" that gives formula milk its purity, while at the same time contributing to reify it:

I'm more reassured with powdered milk because everything is controlled from start to finish in the manufacturing plants, while breastmilk will always be milk from a woman who may be more or less [not] clean ...

Breastmilk is perceived as dirty precisely because it remains symbolically attached to the body where it originates and therefore, in the minds of these mothers, is directly dependent on the hygiene and lifestyle of nursing mothers. Thus we find, through these two opposing visions, a validation of the anthropological theory of the impure and dirty (Douglas 1967). But dirty and clean are never absolute concepts, but relative to all pre-existing representations and to the network of ordered correspondences they constitute.

Thus, the knowledge associated with nutritional benefits or risks of perinatal nutrition have a representational part, including, as we suggested earlier, among the most educated mothers or the most scientifically trained. The comparison of our two ideal types of mothers helps to identify two distinct approaches to ensure consistency of the discourses.

If the nutritional dimension of perinatal feeding appears to be essential in the discourse of mothers, its educational function is at the heart of maternal concerns. Thus, what we will be precisely analyzing hereafter is a complex question, strongly concerned with "identity" within the transmission of food culture, which rests in our two ideal types, with their symmetrically and diametrically opposed views.

TRANSMISSION OF FOOD CULTURE AND THE CHALLENGE OF PERINATAL FEEDING EDUCATION

Before returning to our detailed analysis of educational practices related to perinatal feeding, it is important to consider the schools of thought that have always marked and influenced family perceptions of infant feeding. In effect, the history of medical, psychological, or childcare prescriptions surrounding perinatal feeding shows that transmission of social rules in early childhood has always figured prominently in debates, and has always confronted two major conceptions of education (De Singly 2009). On the one hand, we see the educational model formalized by Durkheim in his *Treatise on Moral Education* (1884), but which had already been promoted as early as 1840 by a series of doctors, particularly Dr. Alfred (head of the clinic at the University of Paris). The "reformist doctors of the 1900 generation" had in some way contributed to relaying this model (Boltanski 1969), based on the experience of frustration regarding the earliest possible transmission of social rules. Hence arose the need to address infant feeding at fixed times, a rule invoked originally to fight against gastroenteritis, thought at the time to be caused by prolonged breastfeeding. Very quickly, this assumption metamorphosed into a moral argument: "do not give infants immediate pleasure, nor rock them when they cry." As Durkheim (1884) stated, only reason can overcome the singularity of each individual. Therefore, we must restrain children from an early age so that they become "reasonable" through education, distancing them from their feelings or impulses. Today we find an extension of this vision in those of the pediatrician Naouri (2004), who opposes any "justification" of a command or an order and strongly advises against breastfeeding on demand.

At the other extreme of this educational model, we find a very different concept of education, one that is communicated from early childhood according to diametrically opposed principles and practices. It is based on a full rehabilitation of the individual and his/her distinctive identity, a thesis developed by the sociologist Simmel (1917) almost at the same time as

Durkheim, but whose major ideas had already been proposed by Jean-Jacques Rousseau (in *Emile* 1762). Spurred on by Rousseau, the second part of the eighteenth century became devoted to breastfeeding, which was elevated into an unprecedented cult based on the idea that feeding on demand met infant needs and did not contradict nature. It is to be noted that it was mainly the cultivated and privileged classes who were concerned with and participated in this debate (Palmonari and Speltini 2008). These ideas were echoed centuries later by the pediatrician Antier (2003) and through the network of the La Leche League, and also by the pediatrician and psychoanalyst Dolto (1977), who emphasized psychological development. The latter states: "Every child has his nature; a happy child is one who has been able to develop with their particularities that are respected" (Dolto 1977). What is central to this model is not the transmission of external rules to the infant but the meeting of conditions permitting the self- expression of the infant and his/her needs.

On another level, what also plays into these two concepts of education is the question of the child's autonomy, in the first case, precocious and constrained, and, in the second case, delayed and spontaneous. We will see in what follows that these two educational models emerge clearly from mothers' discourse and can be opposed into our two ideal types. However, we will focus on how mothers more or less consciously summon these two educational models within their discourses to explain how they transmit French food culture in early childhood. As we will see later, the decision to feed one's baby with formula milk or breastmilk goes beyond a nutritional choice, becoming a choice of "method" to sustain food identity.

BREASTFEEDING AND REGULATION OF FOOD INTAKE

In "breastfeeding" mothers, we find Rousseau's previously developed argument, since the value of breastfeeding in their eyes sometimes goes beyond the purely nutritional considerations to embracing the possibility of better satisfying the infant's needs for as long as he/she demands. However, what is particularly interesting here is the link that mothers very explicitly make between feedings at will with the future regulation of food intake and the prevention of obesity. Here is an example of how they oppose formula milk:

> The advantage to breastfeeding your baby is that they digest very well and they cannot ingest too much; they won't become ill and they know when they are hungry, without being frustrated. In contrast it's totally different with the bottle:

> The baby gulps it down very quickly, so they don't have their dose of suckling ... the mother makes more bottles when they cry out, and so follows obesity! When they grow older they don't know the difference between being actually hungry and the need for suckling. I believe they don't know "when they are really hungry or not" and "when to stop eating."

What this excerpt from the interviews brings to light is the idea that the lack of listening to infants and their needs leads to a kind of "forced feeding," thus denying them the possibility of self-regulating their food intake. The image that these mothers gave us of the bottle-fed baby is that of "a chubby, plump, overweight" baby who develops in this way as an expression of disrespect for the child's uniqueness:

> Bottle-fed babies are more at risk than others, they are forced to finish the bottle, there are small eaters and large eaters, therefore, each eats according to their own needs. But some will be force fed to respect the rhythm of the bottle ... at any price. There is the problem of weight curves/differences, and the fear of the bottom line! With the bottle, as mothers see what they are giving, they are always comparing it to the norm, to the little brother, the neighbor ... and then they end up constantly saying "finish your bowl" and require them to swallow the entire quantity! How horrible!

Moreover, one of the points on which these mothers insist is the internalization of the rules around meals, i.e. having meals at fixed times, to which the French are attached (Fischler and Masson 2008). Almost paradoxically, they are convinced that feeding on demand allows the child all "alone" to learn to eat at mealtimes. Everything happens as if eating meals at fixed times (which is a cultural practice) was supposed to come "naturally" to young eaters. That shows the scope of social and cultural representations in the conduct of food, including in infancy.

Among "bottle feeding" mothers, it is a largely Durkheimian concept of education that is expressed. The bottle is the device that allows effective and early imposition of healthy rhythms upon the child. These mothers do not believe in the ability of infants to regulate their own food intake, rather it is breastfeeding on demand which in their minds leads to being overweight and obese:

> If the child feeds all day, they will inevitably become fat ... while with powdered milk, if you give it to them every four hours, they will quickly learn the rules ... In France we eat at specific times. And since powdered milk is perfectly balanced, even if the baby drinks too much, they will never become fat!

In sum, this transcript reveals the moral dimension related to the question of food intake. What is specifically challenged here is a kind of food liberalism "necessarily" leading, in their minds, to obesity; references to the dietary practices of Americans "who eat whatever they want at any time of the day" are also common. It is very striking that the question of controlling intake quantity, weight, and size of babies plays an important role in the discussions of these "bottle-feeding" mothers:

> I wonder, moreover, how one can control what the baby intakes by breastfeeding! ... I write everything in a notebook, hours, quantities, and the weight of the baby every day. And when my daughter is sick or doesn't finish her bottle I ask myself a ton of questions!

These remarks on formula milk reveal the importance of mothers' belief in science as well as its ability to rationalize/streamline feeding, since "optimized formula" of these milks symbolically is perceived to erase the risk of obesity. These views take us back to the issues of the research program NUPEM cited above and which aims to analyze the impact of levels of nutrients, either too high or too low, in formula milk on the risk of obesity in young children and future adults. This point is not unrelated to a recently made observation regarding the levels of consumption of nutritional food in adults who are reported as having a tendency to overeat things just because they are reported by the industry as being "good for your health" (Provencher et al. 2009).

In the light of comparison of our two ideal types, we can ponder the fact that the relationship between perinatal feeding and obesity is primarily moral and inscribed in the system of representations for each ideal type.

BREASTFEEDING AND FORMATION OF TASTE

The question of the transmission of taste is also a major issue of perinatal feeding and the strategies used by French mothers to expand the sensory experience of the newborn are numerous. In particular, "breastmilk mothers" consider, from this point of view, that breastmilk has no equivalent:

> When you breastfeed, from an early age the child is already "at the family table." They taste everything the mother eats. The milk never tastes the same ... and in addition I drink herbal tea with thyme, fennel, cumin, etc. ... Initially it is to have more milk, but I use it mainly for taste [...] It is also because of this problem

of taste that I prefer to diversify as late as possible., My baby will taste more through my milk than if he was eating by himself so young.

The misappropriation of use evidenced here by herbal tea is extremely interesting, as are other "techniques," such as putting a tiny piece of cheese (such as Roquefort) on the tip of a baby's tongue "in order to accustom them to eating strong cheese." This explains why these mothers quite logically delay the time that other foods/flavors are introduced and expect it to be dictated by the baby. In their eyes, the transmission of food culture begins *in utero*, the mother's body providing more than one biological function since it is the link through which food preferences are perpetuated. Comments on formula milk are, incidentally, from this point of view particularly emblematic.

> Formula milk has nothing additional! There is no difference in taste between all the formula milks ... even if we have added lots of, or different flavors. It's not at all the same! It doesn't pass through the mother's body, which serves as a filter; it will know what is right to give to the child.

Beyond these real or imagined differences in taste, it is clear that taste is a social and cultural construction. If formula does not have the same status as that of breastmilk, it is because the "real" taste is that of "natural" milk, that is to say that which is transmitted from one generation to another by "passing" through the mother's body. All others are then artificial in these mothers' minds.

For "formula" mothers, the question of the education of taste doesn't arise in the same terms. The "artificial" flavors of infant formulas are expected to fulfill an educative function and early diversification is the necessary condition for infants "to learn to eat as quickly as adults." We observe these mothers, who belong to lower social classes, distancing themselves from medical discourses; early diversification of food is highly valued because, in their view, it allows them to initiate the infant more quickly to family habits:

> It's very important to diversify early enough for the infant to eat everything quickly, meat, fish, and lots of vegetables because it's good for their health. My mother did the same with me and I love everything now! [...] Our tastes develop early when we give other foods before 4 months! From this perspective, breastmilk has no more taste/flavor than formula milk. It has no advantage in this plan!'

In sum, for these mothers, a sense of taste cannot be made only through milk, but above all through the early introduction of varied and solid food. During the interviews, we saw the importance that the mothers from the lowest social classes (many of these women were "bottle" mothers) placed on the early consumption of meat. When they discuss this, it is not only in terms of nutritional value or taste, but also because meat can teach the infant "to not be difficult and strengthen his/her stomach, making it accustomed to take in the most diverse foods," as already stated by Boltanski (1969: 124). On another level, the stated order of the foods introduced was first meat, then fish and vegetables, as observed in several interviews. The report illustrates the particular link the lowest social classes have with their bodies and with satiation regarding their attachments to meats and *charcuterie*-valued foods because they "nourish and support better than vegetables" and sooth the infant, making him/her sleep more easily (Boltanski 1971; Poulain 2002b). Following the comparison between the practices of "bottle-feeding mothers" and those of "breastfeeding mothers," it is confirmed that the conduct of perinatal nutrition and nutritional diversification responds not only to medical or paramedical injunctions, but reaffirms, on the contrary, the role of this premium diet in food education, sensory education, and also in the learning of social and cultural norms.

CONCLUSION

Our analysis of the knowledge, beliefs, and representations associated with perinatal feeding in its nutritional and educational dimension has shown extreme coherence of discussions both in "breastmilk mothers" and "artificial milk mothers." We are particularly committed to restore the correspondences that are established, usually unconsciously, between the biological body, the sociological body, and what might be called the symbolic body, in the words of Douglas (1967). The first one refers to the physiological and psychological dimensions, the second one pertains to a social and cultural collective sense, and the latter is an expression of the link between the image of nature and its equilibrium and that of the body. According to most of the women interviewed, breastfeeding is well endowed with a very strong symbolic valence and, as already shown by Heritier (1996) and Lévi-Strauss (1949), it is much more than just a natural reflex. We have shown that, for French mothers, breastfeeding is a practice charged with serious meaning, since breastmilk is the first "vector" for transmission of taste and rules governing the procedures of meals, That is, in short, the issue of transmission of food identity "à la française."

Among mothers in favor of "formula," we have shown that they have found, through the bottle, another "method" to ensure the continuity of food culture and use distinct explanatory schemas to justify choices. The analysis of discourses and declared practices related to perinatal feeding involving both mother and infant has revealed a weakening of what we have called the "symbolic body" as a result of certain relaxation of relationships held with nature, its images, and its real or imagined equilibrium. How is this phenomenon to be explained? Rather than give an unequivocal explanation, we investigated the predisposing factors, which connect triply, as we have already stated, to a lack of family experiences relating to successful breastfeeding, to a more negative maternal body image, and finally to a greater propensity to trust science. In fact, it is among "formula milk mothers" that we found substantial "traces" of scientific discourse—mostly referring to (but without fully understanding) the meaning of lipids, carbohydrates, or antibodies, all of which formula is, in essence, supposed to contain. Yet these mothers are recruited mainly among the middle and lower classes, while "breastmilk" mothers are largely from the upper classes. This observation leads us to relativize Boltanski's points (1969: 101–2) on the discursive categories used by mothers to talk about perinatal nutrition. According to him, it is mainly women from ordinary backgrounds who use the naturalist argument to describe the properties of these milks, preferring breastmilk as "more natural" than powdered milk or rejecting the industry-prepared jars as "less natural" than "homemade" purées, these categories themselves being self-sufficient principles of explanation. According to Boltanski, for the lower classes, the concept of "natural" is a universal self-sufficient principle that fails to acknowledge more scientific concepts. It is very interesting, four decades later, to discover directly opposite findings, since it is mothers specifically from the upper classes who use the naturalist argument to discuss their practices, and this well before evoking more scientific arguments concerning antibodies, nutrients, digestibility, etc. The scope of natural symbolism is measured in terms of the exaltation of breastfeeding, including its educational dimension. This phenomenon is sustained, according to our studies, as a result of the combined effects of, first, the promotion of breastfeeding over the past 20 years, and second, the return of "the natural" in French nutrition, born partly out of suspicion surrounding the food industry in response to food crises, but equally to the strength of the French food identity. In France, especially among those from higher social classes, evocations of the current imperative to "eat well" also carry along with it all the positive values associated with "natural" and "real taste," both of which are seen to be embedded in land and farming, moreover associated with ideas of conviviality and sociability (Merdji and Debucquet 2008). We found all the traces of these representational worlds in "breastmilk" mothers and we understand why the problem of transmission of this cultural model occupies a place at least as important as nutritional issues.

To conclude, our reflections lead us to extend the thinking of Gojard (2000) on the limits of the diffusionist theory—according to which knowledge is always transmitted from top to bottom and faster when "social" distance is smaller—in order to analyze the dispersion methods of the childcare standards or, in this chapter, of nutritional standards. Indeed, as noted in this article's introduction, our research is part of a broader reflection, which concerns the reception of the latest scientific knowledge on the optimization of perinatal nutrition. From this perspective, our research findings lead us to two observations. The first is that the issue of the appropriation of "learned" standards cannot be reduced to a problem of social distance. In higher social circles, the rehabilitation of naturalism, referred to above, and some older practices specific to popular categories, such as sleeping with parents, show that practices related to food and education are constantly changing and never designate a definitive mark of social class. We have also observed that more educated mothers are not more likely to rehearse the scientific argument, and they even tend to value certain practices with the single motive of "self-evident" to ensure the continuity of food culture. The theme of the transmission of food culture is also reflected in the discourses of mothers from lower social classes who instead opt for artificial feeding. Their choice of this "educational method" is sanctioned by a greater confidence in science, which does not prevent some of them from overcoming a number of recommendations on further diversification under the influence of family practices. Finally, this means that adherence to medical or nutritional recommendations depends not only on the level of education or the scientific knowledge of mothers, but also the worlds of representations that they associate with breastfeeding. This involves their relationship with medical knowledge and with science in general as well as the values they are attached to at a given period. If certain values are found to be specific to a given social class, we found that others seem to transcend the social divide, for example, the sentiment of belonging to the same food culture, which must be transmitted in early childhood.

This brings us to our second remark on the interest of the anthropological approach to identify all the meanings that are attached to the body during the very specific perinatal period. Furthermore, it outlines the challenge the medical profession has to face to disseminate a "new" nutritional discourse among mothers. In fact, anatomical and physiological knowledge of the body today is relayed through the notion of *nutritional footprint*, but emphasizes, along with the growing naturalist discourse, the phenomenon of the symbolic break previously analyzed by Le Breton (1998). A rupture between the body and the cosmos is perceived, which is reflected here in the relaxation of the link between images of nature, both its balances and those of the mother's body, leading to a greater individuation of the latter. The anthropological perspective has shown, however, the importance of considering the social and cultural stakes in the premium diet to understand the body in all its dimensions and connections that link the biological, the social, and the symbolic. It remains to be seen how the medical sphere can integrate all these dimensions to better convey the idea of "nutritional optimization" of perinatal nutrition among mothers.

"Who Knows if One Day, in the Future, They Will Get Married …?": Breastmilk, Migration, and Milk Banking in Italy

Rossella Cevese

The spread of milk banks in the (Western) world can be viewed as a way to cope with the need for fresh human milk to feed newborn babies when their own mother's milk is not available (Golden 1996b). According to the WHO, breastmilk is the best food for newborn children, and it is particularly important for premature and sick babies (SIN 2006). The practice of milk banking in a multicultural society opens a range of problems related to different ways of thinking about and using human milk. This essay is based on my doctoral fieldwork followed by subsequent research with a group of Moroccan women in Verona in northern Italy. It delves deeper into two issues: first, the impact of milk banking on ideas about kinship, and particularly on the Islamic institution of milk kinship; second, the fuzzy and changing meaning of breastmilk in a multicultural context.

As a matter of fact, Italy is becoming an increasingly multicultural country. In January 2010, there were 4,235,059 resident immigrants, forming 7 percent of the total population (ISTAT 2010), and of whom 32 percent were Muslims (Caritas 2010). In Verona the migrant population exceeds 11 percent. In 2009, there were 17,256 immigrants from north African countries in Verona, constituting 17.92 percent of total immigrants (for details see Cestim 2011). Islamic women in Verona come mostly from north Africa (Morocco, Tunis, Algeria, and Egypt) and the Middle East (Saudi Arabia, Lebanon, Iran, Turkey); a few people come from Albania, Senegal, Pakistan, and Bangladesh.

MILK KINSHIP: "FAR FROM A DEAD LETTER!"

In her paper about modernity of milk kinship, Morgan Clarke states that:

> Despite an undoubted decline, milk kinship is far from a dead letter. [...] Milk kinship is an elaborate and enduring Islamic legal institution, that finds varied expressions in the lives of Muslims [in the Middle East]. (Clarke 2007: 291, 294)

An important dimension embedded in the statement "Milk kinship: far from a dead letter" was raised by Fatema, a Moroccan woman I met during my Ph.D. research. Fatema is a 25-year-old from Marrakech; she arrived in Verona in 2004, and in 2008 she gave birth to Layla. She reports:

> At birth Layla had a hematologic problem, and had to be hospitalized in the Newborn Intensive Care Unit for several weeks. I had a lot of milk, but Layla was very weak and she ate very little. As I had some milk left, a nurse proposed me to donate it to the milk bank. This request astonished me, and I refused ... I have to know the baby who would suck my milk, because he would become my "milk son" and Layla's "milk brother." Who knows if one day in the future they will get married ...! [Fatema, 23, housewife, Verona, June 2009]

So, Fatema preferred throwing her surplus milk away rather than donating it to an unknown baby. Fatema's position seems to support Clarke's words. Islamic law, in fact, acknowledges at least three kinds of kinship ties: the "*nasab*," the relation of lineage (agnatic and uterine); the "*musahrah*," the relation by marriage, and the "*riḍā*, رضا" the relation by breastfeeding. To that, popular Islam adds further kinship bond created by mixing of blood of two individuals following incisions made for the purpose (personal communication with Abdullahi El Tom). While heritage rules are different, all these relations limit marriages. In the case of milk kinship, the marriage prohibition involves milk brothers and other relatives, but the debate about which relatives is open (Clarke 2007).

Beginning with the pioneering work of Soraya Altorki (1980), milk kinship has attracted large anthropological attention, and encouraged a very dynamic debate. Indeed, although milk kinship is acknowledged throughout the Arabic world, there are several differences in individual Islamic schools and social practices (Clarke 2007). The interest of scholars focused on the structure, social meaning, and practical use of milk kinship in different Islamic countries (Khatib-Chahidi 1992; Heritier 1994; Long 2001; Parkes 2001; Clarke 2007). In short, scholars underline the social use of milk kinship in order to limit marriage, create and strengthen domestic and clientage relations, respond to practical needs of baby's feeding, create social kinship, and promote social mobility (Ensel 1999).

Notwithstanding the importance of milk kinship in the Arabic world, many authors underline a progressive decline of practices of milk sharing (Altorki 1980; Khatib-Chahidi 1992; Parkes 2001; Clarke 2007). Scholars link this decline to the transformation of some living patterns, such as higher mobility of people, the choice of a nuclear pattern of family, and the introduction of formula milk.

Recently, the topic has attracted the interest of the branch of "new kinship studies," which approaches the implications of new reproductive technologies in kinship (Carsten 2000; Conte 2000b; Parkes 2005; Clarke 2006). The implementation of technologies that provide substitutes for bodily parts and secretions like milk, blood, ovaries, and organs challenges the traditional rules of kinship. Milk banking, in particular, affects the institution of milk kinship and opens interesting questions linked to the meaning and power of breastmilk.

MILK KINSHIP AND THE HUMAN MILK BANK

The human milk bank is a "place" where mothers who produce a large amount of breastmilk can donate it. The term "place" refers to a virtual presence but domiciled in a fridge in a hospital. The first human milk bank in Italy was created in 1971 in a Florence hospital, but the development of a network of human milk banks started in the 2000s (www.aiblud). Due to the controversial history of breastfeeding in Italy (Pizzini 1981; Pancino 1984; Balsamo, De Mari, Maher, and Serini 1992; Sbisà 1992), milk banking is still something new in this country and with limited proliferation. Italy counts 23 milk banks, organized in a network and referring to international guidelines (www.aiblud). According to these guidelines, the milk bank takes care of the collection, screening, elaboration, preservation, and distribution of human milk. All these processes allow this bodily substance to become available and movable (Aria 2008; Dei 2008; Lepore 2009; Boyer 2010).

The bank's milk is used for premature babies hospitalized in newborn intensive care units (< 32 week) and babies with particular illnesses, when their own mother's milk is not available. These illnesses include chronic renal failure, metabolic problems, allergies, and complications associated with feeding after surgical operations. The bank removes any personal relationship between donor and receiver. After the donation, in fact, the name of the mother disappears and milk is classified by a number. Then, milk is analyzed, pasteurized, and frozen, and it becomes the "bank's" milk, ready to be sent to the neonatology center that applies for it. Moreover, the amount of milk to use for the baby-in-need is composed by mixing milks from different donors.

All these processes can be interpreted as a way to purify the breastmilk by removing any subjective and corporeal connotation. As Mary Douglas (1975) suggests, indeed, bio-substances outside the body are considered potentially dangerous and contaminant, and need a transformation to be used in a public sphere.

Moving from Appadurai's reflection on social life of things (Appadurai 1986), the historian Janet Golden analyzes the history of breastmilk in the U.S. (Golden 1996b). The author highlights how, during the twentieth century, the status of breastmilk has changed, shifting from commodification to sacralization. In the early twentieth century, in fact, selling milk to hospitals was a common practice for wet nurses, who did it as a job. Beginning in the 1960s, this practice was gradually replaced by milk donation, and breastmilk was gradually sacralized. Golden's reflections are very relevant to the discussion presented in this paper. As with other kinds of donated bodily substances, in fact, once outside the body, breastmilk takes an "ontological" status and becomes a "public entity" (Appadurai 1986). In the public space of the institution, a bank's milk is considered as a sacred substance with therapeutic powers, extremely precious for babies' survival.

Milk donation can be conceptualized in the debate about blood and organ donation. In this regard, Dei proposes a comprehensive analysis of the main works about blood donation, deepening the aspects of gift, social networks, imagination, and social use of blood donation (Dei 2008). Unlike blood, however, breastmilk doesn't need medical procedures to cross body boundaries and circulate, and can be shared using informal and not institutional networks. In fact, milk sharing and wet-nursing are documented in diverse societies, either along formal or informal networks (Cavallo 1983; Golden 1996a; Parkes 2004). A milk bank makes the difference because it institutionalizes milk donations and keeps lactation practices out of the provider's control.

As donated blood, a bank's milk embeds peculiar characteristics: it is anonymous, movable, mixable, and, above all, it is totally detached from the provider. These characteristics are the core of the social and legal debate about milk banking in societies of Islamic background (Ghaly 2010). Indeed, milk banking makes the identification of donor/receiver impossible. On the other hand, the debate about the amount of milk and the method of ingestion required to create a milk kinship is open for social and legal debate. Issues that are far from settled include the quantity of milk to be ingested to create a kinship tie, the method of ingestion whether breast or bottle, the duration of breastfeeding, and the number of relatives concerned by marriage prohibition (Khatib-Chahidi 1992: 124; Clarke 2007: 295).

The position of the Islamic authorities on milk banking is ambiguous. Clarke reports that in 1985 the Organization of Islamic Conference (OIC) declared that "milk banks lead to confusion [*ikhtilat*] and doubt [*ribah*]," and prohibited "the spread of such institutions in the Islamic world, and the use of milk from them" (Clarke 2007: 295). In a recent writing, Ghaly analyzes a fatwa issued in 1983 by the Egyptian scholar Yusuf al-Qaradawi, who saw no religious problem in establishing or using these banks. As Ghaly narrates, the fatwa was interpreted both in Egypt and in Western countries where Muslims live. However, the same fatwa led to opposite recommendations: milk banking was prohibited in Egypt and allowed in the diaspora countries (Ghaly 2010; www.Islamset). In general, the OIC's opinion seems to be widely accepted in the Sunni Muslim world. Fatema's position, therefore, finds social and legal support.

Moreover, the topic of milk kinship in Islamic culture seems to be known by Italian medical professionals (midwives, gynecologists, nurses) who work in the field of breastfeeding, and it is specifically addressed in the Italian milk banks' "guidelines":

> Concerning the informed consent by the legal tutor of the receiver, doctors that prescribe the milk should give correct and complete information about the use of donated milk and should accept a possible refusal. The informed consent becomes basic if parents are Muslims [...] Differences between breast feeding and bank milk-feeding must be explained. Bank's milk, indeed, is pasteurized and so it is a therapeutic device and cannot be considered as wet nurse's milk. (BLUD Guidelines 2007: 52)

The hospital in Verona, where Fatema's story takes place, provides a milk bank; the service is managed by Dr. C., a professional midwife.

> I started taking care of Verona's milk bank three years ago. Until now, I have never met a Moroccan donor ... We had a few migrant donors, mostly Albanian ... but never an Islamic one [...] They are not accustomed to donating their milk because of milk kinship. After many refusals, I gave up advising them. [Dr. C., midwife, June 2010]

Fatema explains that breastmilk cannot be shared with everyone, and this is why she refused to donate. Milk kinship is not created by chance, but it is managed by important social rules. Fatema's refusal must be related to the impossibility of knowing who will drink the milk, and to the desire of avoiding a situation of "kinship confusion" (Clarke 2007: 295) and unwitting forbidden marriage.

THE "ESSENCE" OF THE MOTHER: EMOTIONAL INVESTMENT IN THE BREASTMILK

The topic of milk donation raises interesting issues over the range of meanings that those involved give to this bodily substance. Unlike Moroccans, Italian mothers seem to be very keen to become milk donors. While in the 1970s and 1980s breastfeeding was not widely supported in Italy, in the twenty-first century a new "culture of breastfeeding" was promoted and encouraged by Italian doctors and society; nevertheless, not all Italian women breastfeed their babies. Those who do may also limit it to a few months. For example, it has been reported that in 2000, 81.1 percent of Italian women breastfed their babies for an average of seven months (USTAT 2000; cf. www.allattare).

Mothers who decide to become donors are usually very motivated and experience easy breastfeeding. Donation is a voluntary act, but becoming a donor is not for everyone; like other kinds of donors, mothers must cope with some physical and "moral" requirement: good health, a healthy lifestyle, and good milk (see Dei 2008). Furthermore, a milk donor should donate during the first six months of her child's life. When a mother decides to become a milk donor, she is interviewed and screened for infection; if she passes all the tests, she's registered in the donor book.

Dr. C. points out that the milk bank in Verona has an increasing number of (Italian) donors. She explains that informal networks are very important for the recruitment of donors; indeed, mothers who have abundant milk tend to find a way to use rather than waste it. This attitude is also confirmed by Dr. P., a gynecologist from the public consulting room who follows pregnant women—both Italians and foreigners—from pregnancy to puerperium. She has spent many years working in the field of breastfeeding, and she states:

> Italian women put a big personal investment in their milk ... donors or not, when there is milk left, they tend to store and preserve it. [Dr. P., gynecologist, August 2010]

Italian women seem to consider breastmilk as a precious and nourishing substance, directly connected to the "quality" of the mother. Marisa, a 42-year-old woman, points out:

I had a lot of milk. In my family, all women had natural births and breastfed the baby until one year of age. My son ate and grew as an animal. He had an abnormal growing curve. I felt like a real woman [...] I had milk left and I wanted to donate it, but it was too difficult. At that time (12 years ago), you had to go to the hospital and to pump your milk there. Pumping milk is not easy; it's painful and takes a lot of time [...] And more, my milk, so thick, good and nourishing, would become another thing. It's sterilized, pasteurized and mixed with others' milks. There is nothing left of me [...] so I threw my extra milk away; it was a pity for me ... [Marisa, 42, beautician, Verona, June 2010]

Marisa is very proud of her milk. She traces a sort of familiar mythology, where breastfeeding is seen as a "rite of passage" to becoming a "real woman." For her, the nourishing value of the milk is composed partly by bodily substances, and partly by the essence of the mother. Dr. P. adds an interesting reflection in this regard. She splits the Italian women into those who simply breastfeed and those who do it thinkingly, or "with the mind" (*allattano di testa*). In her reflections, the latter category experience difficulties breastfeeding, because they "think a lot, they have inherited and embody a medical logic based on quantity, so they are very stressed."

Milk banking eliminates this individual value, transforming Marisa's milk into bank milk. This passage, basic for the logic of banking, demotivated Marisa to donate. Consequently, donating milk can be viewed as a way to cope with the need for not wasting the mother's essence: the breastmilk.

Nevertheless, milk banks are not the only way to share; mothers tend to freeze any extra milk in order to create a supply, and show a good attitude about sharing this with other babies. Although further research is required, it is our impression that milk sharing among Italian women outside the medical gaze is not uncommon. Silvana, a 33-year-old mother, remembers:

I had enough milk for Elena and more. I wanted to donate my left milk, but the hospital nurse told me that it was difficult, because Bologna hospital doesn't have a milk bank. So, I threw my extra milk away ... I was very sorry ... Once, I went to see a friend complaining because of lack of milk. I saw her baby so hungry and agitated ... and I offered to breastfeed him ... but she refused. [Silvana, 33, agronomist, Verona, July 2010]

Silvana's words suggest ambiguous facets about breastmilk; breastfeeding, indeed, either creates networks of self-help and solidarity, or engenders feelings of competition and mortification (Sbisà 1992; Boyer 2010: 16).

Like Silvana, Italian women I spoke to showed a positive attitude about donating or sharing their milk, considering it as precious nourishment.

Moroccans, instead, seem to be more worried about the consequences of the donation, as Fatema's experience suggests.

Even if milk sharing is less common nowadays in Morocco, Moroccan women I spoke to counted several milk relatives; for these women, milk kinship remains an important part of social relations, and it plays an outstanding role in their lactation practices, both as donors and as recipients. Concerning this, Ibtisan, a Moroccan woman in Italy since 2007, reports:

> Kamal was born by an emergency Caesarian. He spent his first three days in the intensive care unit. My milk hadn't yet arrived, and I don't know how he was fed. I didn't ask and nobody told me ... I noticed small bottles of milk in the fridge of the hospital, and I assumed it was human milk. In that moment there were other Italian and Romanian women hospitalized, so I imagine that Kamal could have Italian or Romanian milk brothers ... [Ibtisan, 32, housewife, Verona, April 2010]

Ibtisan's words reflect Fatema's concern of a possible "kinship confusion" created by the milk of an unknown donor.

The feeling of uncertainty that permeates Ibtisan's story often characterizes Morocco's health narrative (Beneduce 1998; De Micco 2002; Sayad 2002) and raises a core question about the relationship of power between doctors and migrant patients.

Milk kinship, and its consequences, does not matter in Italian culture nor for Italian doctors. Despite Italian milk bank guidelines recommending that doctors inform parents about the use of this milk, in praxis this recommendation is not always followed. As Dr. C. states, if the baby is in need (and human milk is available), doctors do what is best for the baby and use the bank milk without informing parents, in order to avoid a possible refusal.

> When we decided to give bank milk to a very premature baby, Moroccan or Tunisian ... we never told mothers ... I know very well that, due to their culture, mothers tend to refuse it ... they refuse to donate or receive it, because they consider babies as milk brothers ... [Dr. C., midwife, June 2010]

Thus, parents (foreigners as well as Italians) are often excluded from this decision. The attitude of Dr. C. above seems to be very common, though should not be taken for granted. As a consequence of effective politics of cultural mediation, some hospitals are particularly careful to deliver proper information for donors and receivers. On the other hand, Islamic women's choice of not donating milk can also be read as an "endogamy strategy" (personal communication with Vanessa Maher). In a multicultural context, not spreading the milk helps prevent a situation of "kinship confusion" by lowering the probability of future forbidden marriage (above all if the partner is also Muslim).

As many scholars underline, milk kinship can be viewed as a strategy of managing social relations by limiting or creating milk ties. The strategic use of milk kinship seems to be particularly tense in a context of immigration, where social relations are weak, fuzzy, and provisional. However, milk kinship can also be used deliberately to strengthen and make a friendship bond enduring. Concerning this, Fatema reports the case of Hanan and Meryam.

> Here in Verona, an Algerian woman I know [Meryam] created a milk kinship with the Imam's wife [Hanan], who is Yemeni. They met at the Islamic center and they became very close. Both women were in Italy temporarily; before going back to their countries, they decided to create a milk kinship between their daughters. So, Meryam breastfed Hanan's daughter and vice versa. [Fatema, June 2010]

Fatema stresses that Meryam and Hanan used the milk kinship to strengthen their friendship, and to create an enduring bond for them and their daughters, in spite of the distance. Fatema also added that she would not do this in Italy, because she did not feel like having any such relationship. This view is also confirmed by other Italian Moroccan women, citing unwillingness to create kinship ties that cannot be honored.

The experience of Meryam and Hanan shows how, in the context of migration, milk kinship is still used to create or strengthen alliances and affective bonds (Long, cited in Parkes 2005: 23). Similar experiences seem to be not uncommon between Islamic women in Italy, and should be investigated more deeply.

Majda, a cultural mediator, reports:

> Sometimes women do it … they swap children in order to create a milk kinship and strengthen their relation[ship]. I know few cases [here in Italy] … I think that this is a matter [for] women and they don't share this practice with men. [Majda, cultural mediator, January 2010]

Majda suggests an interesting hypothesis that should be compared with the field: the use of milk sharing to perform women's agency.

CONCLUSION

In this chapter I have suggested some considerations about the donation of breastmilk in a multicultural context, where different meanings of milk intersect and confront each other.

The experiences discussed support Clarke's idea that milk kinship is "far from a dead letter." This idea seems to be effective also in the context of migration, where living conditions are often ambiguous and social relations can be breakable and fragile, while also being very close and intense (Salih 2003). As the experiences I reported highlight, milk kinship remains an important aspect of the lactation practices of Moroccan women in Italy. Moreover, practices of milk sharing are used tactically to control social relations, by creating or avoiding social bonds, in order to prevent situations of "kinship confusion" (Clarke 2007: 293).

The importance of milk kinship has emerged in milk donation; milk banking, in fact, challenges the rules of milk kinship, because it breaks and nullifies the personal link between donor and receiver. For Moroccan women, the connecting power of breastmilk is still great, but it is impossible for them to control the "milk relation" (*riḍā*), so, they refuse to donate their milk to the bank.

Moreover, milk banking projects breastfeeding on to a public space and allows milk to take an ontological status (Boyer 2010: 5). In his analysis of blood donation, Titmuss (1970, in Dei 2008) identifies three groups of "actors" involved in the process: donors, receivers, and intermediaries (nurses, doctors, organizers ...). This pattern can be used to analyze milk donation as well. Once outside the body of the woman, breastmilk takes the status of a "public entity"; it ceases to be a private matter between mother and son or daughter, and becomes a public matter, managed by intermediaries.

Milk banks are places of power that respond to the logic of the institution (the hospital); the actors involved in the process, however, share a different degree of agency, and are not equals in the decision-making process, as Ibtisan's experience shows.

Talking about the mobility of breastmilk, the geographer Kate Boyer states: "I suggest that this case [of milk donation] provides an example of how mobile biosubstances are increasingly travelling in hybrid forms that reflect elements of both gift-exchange and commodity-exchange" (Boyer 2010: 6). According to Boyer, bank milk embodies features of both gift and commodity. Indeed, like blood, milk is donated spontaneously and for free, without a material counterpart except a moral acknowledgment (Titmuss in Dei 2008;

Golden 1996b). On the other hand, bank milk is mobile and potentially exchangeable with money (Golden 1996b; Boyer 2010).

As situations presented in this paper show, breastmilk takes on different meanings for different "actors." Donors and receivers have a large emotional investment on this substance. In particular, Italian women stress a "moral connotation" of the breastmilk; they see it as a nourishing and precious substance to be shared and preserved. Moroccan women, instead, emphasize the connecting power of breastmilk and consider it an effective substance that creates ties. Intermediaries, finally, separate the milk from any personal and moral qualities and consider it as a "public entity" and powerful medicine, to use to save sick babies. So, milk banking involves polyphonic meanings of breastmilk, especially in a multicultural context. I suggest that this complexity should be considered in the politics of public health in order to avoid situations of disparity and quarrel.

Religion, Wet-nursing, and Laying the Ground for Breastmilk Banking in Darfur, Sudan

Abdullahi Osman El Tom

The Berti live in the state of Northern Darfur, Sudan. They are sedentary farmers who combine agriculture with animal husbandry. The Berti are followers of the Maliki School of Islam. For several generations, they have spoken Arabic only, and are now reasonably grounded into the Arab Islamic culture (for more details see Holy 1974; El Tom 1989). In the current Darfur war, the Berti fall within the so-called African divide that pits them against their nomadic Arab neighbors. As such, they are primarily supporters of the rebels, while most of the Arabs are sympathetic to the government of Khartoum (for more on the Darfur conflict see El Tom 2005; Flint and De Waal 2005; Daly 2007).

EL TOM'S PERSONAL TESTIMONY

I was born sometime in the mid-1950s in Broosh, a small town in North Darfur. At the time of my birth, Broosh had no medical facilities, and the nearest clinic was a day's journey on a donkey or a camel. Passing trucks were rare and unscheduled and most people did not rely on them for urgent journeys. A couple of traditional birth attendants helped with childbirth, as a trained midwife did not appear in the town until about 15 years later.

I had many friends in my early childhood, but I was closest to Mohamed. My family shared my affection for Mohamed and always treated him almost as a family member. Mohamed lived only two houses away from us. His family's house was identical to ours and both of our fathers had their shops attached to their respective homes. Whenever Mohamed was around during mealtimes, my late mother always had a share of the meal for him. Mohamed's mother was among the first to show up in our house when extra hands were needed. My father was a well-connected man and often had to host some visitors who passed through the town. Mohamed's mother was always there to help with cooking. There were no hotels or restaurants at the time and visitors to the town had to be hosted and fed by the locals.

I might have been around 11 or 12 when I first realized that Mohamed was more than a friend, and that his special relationship with my family had its justification. In a casual talk that I overheard, a woman said to my mother: "Mohamed is a wonderful boy, it is such a shame that he cannot marry one of your daughters in the future." The remark that intrigued me was of a passing interest to my mother and her companion, who proceeded to talk about something else. What interested my mother's companion most was that my mother had an abundance of milk, perhaps so much that it had to be expressed away in order to ease breast pain she often had after each delivery.

It was not until a few days later that I learnt of Mohamed's mysterious relationship with my family. As it transpired, Mohamed and I were born almost at the same time, but his birth came close to a disaster. Both Mohamed and his mother were lucky to survive. Mohamed's mother had a difficult labor, lost so much blood, and was very sick for a while. As a result, she was not able to breastfeed for quite some time. Luckily, my mother was there to lend a helping hand, thus transforming Mohamed into our milk brother.

I cannot recall whether Mohamed realized his relationship with my mother at the same time as I did, but he certainly acted as a second child to my mother. Mohamed and I attended the same educational establishments until we went up to university. Later, we went to work for different organizations away from Broosh. Every two or three years, we visited Broosh, sometimes together but often separately. In his visits home, Mohamed always went to my mother with gifts, and was treated as a returning child. I responded to Mohamed's kindness to my mother by treating his in a similar fashion, even though she is not my milk mother.

BREASTFEEDING

Berti customs are influenced by Arab–Islamic traditions. Family law among the Berti is an approximation of Islamic law. This arises from the times of pre-British colonialism, in which family relations were derived from Islam, with only minor local variations. Family law runs parallel to other laws that have either a national or local basis, and are often at odds with Islamic principles.

Traditionally speaking, mother's milk is regarded as the best for a baby, and it is the ideal to continue breastfeeding for two entire years. Obviously, this ideal cannot always be adhered to. Breastfeeding for two years requires collaboration of senior female relatives as well as the husband. This is reminiscent of the WHO "doula" system, recommended by this body. The Berti commission a senior female relative to advise young mothers on how to breastfeed, while other relatives take over routine daily housework. If the mother experiences some difficulty at first, the breast is massaged with sesame oil, and she is encouraged to continue trying until milk flow is secured. Early milk (colostrum) is particularly regarded as crucial for healthy progress of the baby and is often fortified by butter made from goat or cow milk. This butter is the only external feeding given to the baby in the first five to six months of life. Modern medical personnel in the area now advise against use of butter, but are rarely listened to. The use of butter at this early stage is similar to the practice of giving dates to a newborn, a custom reported in central Sudan but unknown to the Berti (El Tom 1996). As soon as a baby is born in central Sudan the Traditional Birth Attendant (TBA) chews a small piece of date and then deposits it in the mouth of the baby. Dates were regarded as the Prophet's favorite fruit and are hence intended to be the first food the baby tastes in his/her life.

The commitment of the father is important for maintaining the ideal of breastfeeding for the duration of two years. Parents of the breast-fed baby are expected to abstain from having sex for the entire duration of breastfeeding. This is to ensure the avoidance of pregnancy, which is believed to spoil the milk of the lactating mother. The local view asserts that as soon as the mother gets pregnant, her milk is no longer suitable for breastfeeding. In their words, the milk then belongs to "the baby inside the womb rather than the one outside." In fact, the breast-fed baby will be harmed either by being weaned prematurely or being fed on defective milk. Such milk is seen to be a common cause of particular types of diarrhea, which can be tested and verified. The test consists of pressing a thumb on the forehead of the sickly child and observing how the skin bounces back into position. If the skin is too slow when bouncing back, the diarrhea is certainly caused by defective milk due to pregnancy. Modern medics take this as a likely sign of malnutrition. The Berti agree, but see the cause differently, giving it a moral twist. In their culture, this is indicative of callous parents who are irresponsible enough to sacrifice their baby for their own pleasure. Hasty and damaging methods are then used to get the baby off the breast. Methods of abrupt weaning may include sending the baby to a relative in a different village, smearing the breast with salt, or even chili pepper, or simply attaching frightening objects, like feathers and cotton wool, to it.

The Berti live in the female circumcision zone in the Sudan.[1] The rate of female circumcision among the Berti as a percentage is the same as it is among all the ethnic groups that live around them. Not surprisingly, the Berti experience a high rate of maternal mortality at birth. Much more recently, the adjusted rate of maternal mortality in the Sudan for the year 2000 was estimated to run at 590 per 100,000 (UNDP 2006). While the Berti do not attribute their high maternal mortality directly to female circumcision, they clearly recognize that giving birth is a cause of death of many mothers and newborns (for more on circumcision see El Tom 1998). This is clearly evident from traditional greetings used in addressing expectant mothers as well as in congratulatory terms for new mothers. In their exegesis, the pregnant woman is earmarked for death by God, and her grave remains open until she is out of the danger zone, indicated by the 40 days' confinement period that Berti women adopt. Successful delivery is followed by 40 days' confinement to the house, where the mother and her newborn are kept away from evil onlookers and other malicious forces. It is during this period that the immediate community is mobilized to help and give the mother a good rest while also allowing delivery wounds to heal and the mother to establish a successful breastfeeding relationship with the newborn.

Among the greetings used for expectant mothers are:

May Allah release you or unfasten you—from the death post—with good health.

Successful delivery greetings include:

Praise be to Allah who has unfastened you—saved you from death—and with good health.

Or:

May Allah complete your recovery and that of your child and give you more siblings for your baby.

The high significance attached to breastfeeding for two years among the Berti is unmistakably of Islamic origin. Islam has survived for more than 1,400 years in a geographical span from south-east Asia to the Atlantic at Morocco only because of its ability to accommodate diverse and numerous cultures. The flexibility of Islam also enabled it to survive infinite changes through the centuries. Whether credit goes to Islam or to the accommodative nature of these diverse cultures remains a debate for a different space. What is important for us here is that in their accommodation of Islam, different cultures indigenized Islam and adapted it to their own culture. The Berti are no exception in this regard. Due to a high rate of illiteracy among the Berti, indicated by school enrolment that is as low as 30 percent, adults have to rely on collective memory for Islamic justification of their acts. However, religious leaders are able to read the Qur'an and other Islamic sources for backup when necessary.

Islamic jurisprudence stipulates three major sources of religious rules and in a strict order of importance: the Qur'an, the *hadith* (Prophetic speeches and descriptions of his actions), and deliberations of Islamic scholars and theologians. The Qur'an is quite explicit on the rule regarding length of breastfeeding. Reference to breastfeeding and its derivatives occur 14 times in seven chapters and eight verses in the Qur'an (see the note for all Qur'anic verses). Below are Qur'an verses that refer in particular to the length of breastfeeding:

> The mothers shall give suck
> For two whole years,
> If the father desires
> To complete the term.
> But shall bear the cost
> Of their food and clothing
> On equitable terms.
> (Ali 1983: 93; chapter 2, verse 233)

> And We have enjoined on man
> (To be good) to his parents:
> In travail upon travail
> Did his mother bear him.
> And in years twain
> Was his weaning: (hear
> The Command), "Show gratitude
> To Me and to thy parents:
> To Me is (thy final) Goal."
> (Ali 1983: 1083; chapter 31, verse 14)

> We have enjoined on man
> Kindness to his parents:
> In pain did his mother
> Bear him, and in pain
> Did she give him birth.
> The carrying of the (child)

To his weaning is
(A period of) thirty months.
(Ali 1983: 1370; chapter 46, verse 15)

Sources other than the Qur'an also give the same advice regarding the two years' code. However, they seem to have come in the context of interpreting or justifying the Qur'anic verses above, and hence there is no need to repeat them. Theologians interpret the 30 months referred to in the last Qur'anic verse as including a pregnancy of six months. Thus, according to a theological source:

> As narrated by Ibn Abbas, the baby stays in the womb for six months. If it lasts for seven months, then it shall be breast-fed for 23 months; and if it remains in womb for 9 months, then it shall be breast-fed for 21 months. (Elqutubi chapter 3: 108)

While this precise computation is available to local theologians, the average Berti is neither aware of it nor ready to indulge in it. What is significant for them is the recommended duration of 24 months for breastfeeding. They also recognize that this recommendation may remain inspirational and is often disrupted by one factor or another.

WET-NURSING

It must be noted that the Berti make little fuss about wet-nursing. Chances are that it is much more prevalent than it is talked about. As my own biography illustrates, people recognize the relationship, but they do not boast about it. This reticence perhaps resides in the fact that wet-nursing is a gift that one gives without expecting any direct gratification and that its very essence is undermined by boasting. The value of children in the society, and the centrality of that to motherhood and hence femininity, colludes in its disguise. Few women would want to admit to their inability to breastfeed their babies and their surrogate mothers may prefer not to expose them as unfortunate mothers who have had difficulty in asserting their motherhood. Moreover, wet-nursing mothers may find it denigrating to reduce their service to a simple, commercialized good that can be paid for. Indeed the altruistic value embedded in wet-nursing defies boasting about it, as this reduces it to an individual enterprise. However, long-term as it may be, personal gain accrued from wet-nursing cannot be underestimated. In a society where children and grandchildren constitute the only old age insurance, it makes little sense to forgo a milk-adopted child for temporal commercial gain. It is within these premises that we should see the relationship between Mohamed and my mother. Although my mother did not need to rely on Mohamed for her old age support, it would have been difficult for him not to help her, should she have needed it.

Given the relative marginality of the Berti to the Arab–Islamic culture, it would perhaps be safe to say that adoption of wet-nursing is either inspired and/or augmented by Islam. It is common knowledge for the Berti that Prophet Mohamed himself was wet-nursed. Schoolchildren across Muslim Sudan can even name Halima Alssadiya as the Prophet's wet nurse. However, details of Islamic theological debate on wet-nursing have not filtered into the Berti's collective memory of Islam. Such knowledge is, nonetheless, available to local religious leaders. References to wet-nursing in the Qur'an are as follows:

> No mother shall be
> Treated unfairly
> On account of the child.
> Nor father
> On account of the child,
> An heir shall be chargeable
> In the same way.
> If they both decide
> On weaning,
> By mutual consent,
> And after due consultation,
> There is no blame on them.
> If they decide
> On a foster mother
> For your offspring,
> There is no blame on you,
> Provided ye pay (the mother)
> What ye offered,
> On equitable terms.
> But fear God and know
> That God sees well what ye do.
> (Ali 1983: 93; chapter 2, verse 233)

> Prohibited to you
> (For Marriage) are
> Your mothers, daughters,

Sisters; father's sisters,
Mother's sisters; brother's daughters,
Sister's daughters; foster-mothers
(Who gave you suck), foster-sisters;
Your wives' mothers;
Your step-daughters under your
Guardianship, born of your wives
To whom ye have gone in,
No prohibition if ye have not gone in;
(Those who have been)
Wives of your sons proceeding
From you loins;
And two sisters in wedlock
At one and the same time,
Except for what is past;
For God is Oft-forgiving,
Most Merciful.
(Ali 1983: 186; chapter 4, verse 23)

Style as ye live,
According to your means:
Annoy them not, so as
To restrict them.
And if they carry (life
In their wombs), then
Spend (your substance) on them
Until they deliver
Their burden; and if
They suckle your (offspring)
Give them their recompense:
And take mutual counsel
Together, according to
What is just and reasonable.
And if ye find yourselves
In difficulties, let another
Woman suckle (the child)
On the father's behalf.'
(Ali 1983: 1564–5; chapter 65, verse 6)

The Qur'an is quite categorical about the legitimacy of wet-nursing. The same is supported by ample narratives of the Prophet Mohamed as well as by Islamic theologians.

What is striking is the right of the mother to abstain from breastfeeding and her entitlement to support in case of divorce at the time of breast-feeding. Moreover, Islamic edicts oblige the "father" and not the mother to shoulder the cost of breastfeeding. At the same time, Islam instructs that the mother should be allowed to breastfeed her child even if the father of the baby is divorced. An interpretive text in this regard reads:

> Whether she is divorced or in marriage, a mother is entitled to breastfeed her baby, if she chooses to, and nobody is entitled to deprive her of that right. (Source unknown to the author)

As far as the Berti are concerned, children of both sexes remain with their divorced mother for their early childhood. As such, the possibility of separation does not occur, unless the mother proves incapable of taking care of the babies.

The Qur'an is also quite explicit on its edict that a wet nurse be paid for her service. That also applies to the mother who is divorced at the time of breastfeeding. It is here that the Berti offer a different interpretation. Among the Berti, wet-nursing belongs to the so-called "gift economy" domain. It is done for altruistic reasons and for enhancing community relations. This, of course, does not preclude the wet nurse receiving personal gifts in return. It might be strange to contemplate how the early Arabs had commercialized wet-nursing in the seventh century while the Berti have not done so in the twenty-first century. The Berti are certainly not new to a commodity economy. Nonetheless, they opted not to apply a commodity economy to wet-nursing. We must caution that this fact can only be labored on up to a point. After all, most societies, including modern ones, combine both commodity and gift economies in their cultures. For example, blood banks as well as milk banks in the Western world operate under gift rather than commodity economies.

At a different level, the Berti are careful regarding the selection of a wet nurse. In their culture, certain women do not make good wet nurses. They are likely to transmit diseases to the breast-fed baby and/or convey undesirable characteristics. Some diseases like TB, epilepsy, mental illness, and leprosy are believed to run in certain families and might be transmitted through wet-nursing. Peculiarly, the Berti also think certain ethnic groups have a tendency to turn into haunting ghosts after death. This feature, too, is likely to be transmitted through breastfeeding. As far as possible, women of bad moral character are equally to be avoided as possible wet nurses. Interestingly, little differentiation is made between learnt characteristics and attributes that are of a biological nature. Some of these perceptions can be found in early Islamic exegeses. Thus, Imam Ali Ibn Abi Talib is quoted as having said:

> Discriminate in the choice of wet nurses, as you do in marriage; for breast-feeding affects characters of your offsprings. (Al Mustadrak)

The Prophet Mohamed too had left a similar note:

> Do not commission wet-nursing of the idiot and the bleary ('amshaa') for breast milk transmits diseases. (www.theindependentbd.com)

Or in the context of transmission of positive characters, the Prophet said:

> I am the most articulate among all Arabs. I am from Quraish ethnic group but my tongue is that of Bani Saad Bin Bakr. (www.theindependentbd.com)

It is to be noted that Bani Saad were regarded as the best Arabic speakers at the time and it was they who provided Halima Assaidya (of the Bani Saad ethnic group), who wet-nursed the Prophet.

Wet-nursing is also restricted by consanguinial relationship of the baby to the potential nurse. Those who are prohibited in marriage—all of which are referred to in the following Qur'anic verses—cannot act as nurses:

> Prohibited to you
> (For Marriage) are
> Your mothers, daughters,
> Sisters; father's sisters,
> Mother's sisters; brother's daughters,
> Sister's daughters; foster-mothers
> (Who gave you suck), foster-sisters;
> Your wives' mothers;
> Your step-daughters under your
> Guardianship, born of your wives ...
> (Ali 1983: 186; chapter 4, verse 23)

A prophetic speech also comes in line with the above Qur'anic verse:

> Whoever is forbidden in marriage is also forbidden in breastfeeding.

Or differently expressed in another prophetic speech:

Breastfeeding is forbidden in accordance with what is forbidden in procreation.

The Berti are aware of future marriage restrictions imposed by wet-nursing. As their culture lays preference for marriage within the group (endogamy), wet-nursing within the group is only reluctantly pursued. Furthermore, the Berti do not have to worry about any unknown breach of the marriage code related to wet-nursing. Wet nurses come from the community and they and their children are known to all.

DISCUSSION

The complexity of wet-nursing and milk sharing should be understood within its power—with wide ramifications—to transform social relationship into kinship bond among milk sharers. In Islamic societies, kinship (*qarabah*) is created through procreative blood that includes uterine or agnatic (*nasab*), affinity (*musahara*), and breastfeeding (*riḍā*). Hence we have blood, affinity, and milk kinships (see Altorki 1980; Clarke 2007, 1994). Modern biomedical reproduction techniques such as in vitro fertilization, egg donation, surrogacy, and organ transplant might produce new forms of Islamic kinship yet to be explored (see Clarke 2007). The relatively well-developed Islamic jurisprudence in milk sharing will undoubtedly provide a blueprint for dealing with these new forms of kinship in Muslim societies (ibid.). These issues have not yet surfaced in Broosh.

In the case of milk sharing discussed herein, we must recall again the divide between popular and orthodox or theological Islam, for which most of the illiterate Berti have no aptitude. As far as Mohamed is concerned, his milk sharing fortune transforms him from a near-stranger to a kin of my family, replete with its specific marriage rules. By being breast-fed by my mother, Mohamed is placed exactly in my position regarding marriage prohibitions. In line with Berti Islam, Mohamed therefore acquires a whole set of milk (foster) relatives whom he cannot marry. His new foster relatives and who come under marriage prohibitions include:

milk mother
milk mother's sisters
milk mother's lineal ascendants and descendants
milk/foster father's sisters
milk/foster father's lineal ascendants and descendants.

In the Berti version of Islam, the marriage prohibitions faced by Mohamed are restricted to him and do not exclude his siblings, who are free to marry children of his milk mother. Likewise, children of Mohamed's milk mother are free to marry among siblings of the former, as they are not involved in the sharing of milk. It is to be noted that these rules are far from uniform in different Islamic societies and may not satisfy some conservative theologians (for an extended list see Altorki 1980; Clarke 2007).

While the Berti confer kinship relationship between a milk child and the husband of his/her milk mother, as implied above, they do not see the father as involved in the production of milk as such. This is the case in some societies that conceive of the husband as instrumental in the production of milk through impregnation and its hormonal effect on the lactating mother. Through the concept of "stallion's milk" ("*laban al fahal*"), a direct link is established between a foster child and his/her foster father (Altorki 1980: 233).

Kinship relationship ushered in through breastfeeding is not only confined to marriage prohibition. It equally introduced new forms of gender relationship, particularly in the field of modesty and veiling rules that are significant for some societies. It is here that the apt concept of "tactical use" of milk kinship bonding rises to prominence. Kinship bonds created through milk sharing could be tactically and deliberated used in at least two distinctive ways for specific motives, although neither of them is corroborated by my research or personal biography.

The first strategy is to override oppressive parallel or cross-cousin marriage that is hegemonic in some Islamic societies. Parents who for one reason or another do not want their children to conform to cousin marriage can entice their sisters-in-law to breastfeed their children, thus rendering them unmarriageable to their cousins in the future. Through this strategy, a family opts out of obligations to meet undesired cousin-marriage bids in the future.

The second form of tactical use of milk sharing is employed to ease gender relationships among certain individuals. In particular, this pertains to societies bound with rigid modesty rules in which men cannot come into domestic contact with women unless they are *muhram*, i.e., forbidden to marry. This dilemma is bolstered by a unique experience in the biography of Prophet Mohamed but still resonates with current conservative Muslim societies in the Middle East. A rather controversial narrative of Prophet Mohamed is stated below, and I report it in full and in its unconventional style:

A'isha (Allah be pleased with her) reported that Salim, the freed slave of Abu Hudhaifa, lived with him and his family in their house. She (i.e. the daughter of Suhail) came to Allah's Apostle (may peace be upon him) and said: Salim has attained (puberty) as men attain, and he understands what they understand, and he enters our house freely, I, however, perceive that something (rankles) in the heart of Abu Hudhaifa, whereupon Allah's Apostle (may peace be upon him) said to her: Suckle him and you would become unlawful for him, and (the rankling) which Abu Hudhaifa feels in his heart will disappear. She returned and said: So I suckled him, and what (was there) in the heart of Abu Hudhaifa disappeared. (Sahih Muslim, Book 8, Number 3425; www.daruliftaa)

This *hadith* has recently come into the spotlight, triggering hot debate in Saudi Arabia, Egypt, and among some Muslims in the diaspora. Not surprisingly the *hadith* raised the question whether adult breastfeeding can be used to circumvent modesty rules regarding the presence of unmarried couples in a secluded public space such as an office. The mere suggestion of this abhorred official theologians as well as others. Sheikh Muhamed ibn Adam of Daruliftaa argued that the *hadith* provided only a mere "personal dispensation governed by its specific circumstances" and cannot be applied to others. He further indicated that breastfeeding was not direct and was in fact provided via expression of milk in a cup, a narrative challenged by other reporters. The source outlaws sucking by adult altogether (www.Daruliftaa). While intricacy of theological debate lies beyond the interest and scope of this essay, I hasten to add that the debate reflects a huge margin of opinions and openness to pragmatism in Muslim societies. Such a feature should be noted by those interested in the introduction of milk banking in Muslim societies.

Supporters of milk banking in particular and wet-nursing in general in the context of Muslim societies have another thing to celebrate in the above *hadith*. Clearly, breastmilk does not have to be ingested through suckling. It can be expressed or pumped and later procured from a receptacle. A further ruling on the side of milk banking pertains to the quality of milk that can create a kinship bond. According to at least some Islamic schools, ingested breastmilk must be pure in order to create milk bonding (Shah 1994: 4). As milk banking involves mixing a woman's milk with other milk or other substances, it is possible to argue that it fails to create kinship relations with any particular donor. Fortunately, the Berti approach gender modesty with relative ease, and most of them would see this as an unwarranted theological debate and a luxury unworthy of further pursuit.

Turning back to the Berti, there can be no doubt that their culture is fully supportive of breastfeeding and that it is equally accommodating for wet-nursing. While the influence of Arab–Islamic culture is evident, survival of strong breastfeeding culture among the Berti is a function of their poor exposure to modernity. Invariably, breastfeeding has declined in all Muslim societies that have shifted to the modern way of life. Sadly, this will also be the future of Berti society, and the time is ripe to counter such influence. In this regard, efforts must be made to preserve the current preference for extended breastfeeding in the area.

As far as wet-nursing is concerned, we can be assured of its groundedness in Berti culture. Nonetheless, wet-nursing in this culture is community-based, a situation that may not be sustainable in the future. As the society becomes more individualistic and urban-oriented, wet-nursing will face a formidable challenge. In the current wet-nursing arrangement, the possibility of a person unknowingly marrying a milk sibling is beyond contemplation. This situation will not remain the same if milk of unknown donors is used.

Modern milk banking systems in the Berti's rural setting may be both unnecessary and unpractical. This is due to poor infrastructure, as the entire area lacks transport, communication networks, electricity, and reliable health amenities. To this, one may add sparse population distribution in the area. Luckily, the current community-based wet-nursing can be enhanced, and there is ample room for that. Restrictions based on traditional health beliefs can be tapped upon here. Exclusion of potential wet nurses on the bases of beliefs in ghosts or transmission of disease must be negotiated.

Prospects for the introduction of milk banking are far better in the urban areas where modern facilities are already in place. Moreover, community-based wet-nursing is unlikely to be sustained in urban zones. Hence, milk banking could serve as backup if not as an alternative to community-based wet-nursing.

While wet-nursing remains the focus of this essay, we must not lose sight of our ultimate objective: better health and higher survival rate for newborn babies and their mothers. If that is the case, then wet-nursing must be seen as a component of a series of measures towards that objective. Issues like nutrition, antenatal care, female circumcision, infectious diseases, diseases of poverty, etc., must all be part of our strategy.

Between Proscription and Control of Breastfeeding in West Africa: Women's Strategies Regarding Prevention of HIV Transmission

Alice Desclaux and Chiara Alfieri

When the first data about cases of HIV transmission through breastfeeding were published in 1985 (Ziegler 1985; Dunn et al. 1992), the abandonment of breastfeeding was rapidly adopted as a medical recommendation for women living with HIV in developed countries. They were told to formula-feed their infants, and that formula would be provided to them through social insurance systems or social programs. The number of infants born from HIV-positive women was limited, and formula feeding appeared an easy strategy. It was already available, known to be acceptable, and was quite efficient, since it would fully eliminate the risk of HIV transmission.

In developing countries, the history of prevention of HIV transmission through breastfeeding was complex. A number of factors hindered the scaling up of the abandonment of breastfeeding as a preventive strategy regarding HIV risk. The main risks related to formula feeding in settings where the sanitation level was low and drinking or potable water was scarce; where access to fuel or electricity for heating and refrigerating formula-based milk was not generally avaliable; where literacy rates among women were limited; and where the epidemiological environment made diarrhea common and malnutrition a leading cause of infant mortality. Meanwhile, a number of scientists underestimated the impact of the AIDS epidemic at a time when it had not reached its peak in all African sub-regions, and doubted the necessity of setting up specific policies (Jelliffe and Jelliffe 1988: 142).

When formula feeding was considered in developed countries as the only means to avoid HIV risk, it was understood in developing settings as an "option" with various infectious and nutritional attached risks. Its feasibility, accessibility, and acceptability were not guaranteed and proscription of breastfeeding was to be considered among other feeding options, with the aim of balancing and reducing a significant number of risks, rather than only eliminating the risk of HIV.

From 1998, the WHO and other United Nations agencies set up policies for the reduction of HIV transmission through breastfeeding based on the selection of low-risk feeding options defined in relation to the sanitary environment (UNAIDS et al. 1997). Between 2000 and 2009, in many developing countries the main preventive feeding options promoted at national level were twofold: on one hand, proscription of breastfeeding and use of formula; on the other hand, control of breastfeeding through the limitation of its duration to three to six months and through its exclusiveness, since some publications had shown that mixed feeding might increase the rate of HIV transmission through breastmilk (WHO et al. 2003). This general policy slightly changed when antiretrovirals provided to the mother and to the infant showed their efficacy for "preventive coverage" of breastmilk; in 2009, WHO recommended choosing only one feeding option as a strategy at national level (WHO 2009a). Then, when developed countries still recommended formula feeding combined with antiretrovirals to eradicate HIV risk, developing countries mostly opted for breastfeeding "protected" by antiretrovirals. In 2010, the divide observed during the early period of the HIV epidemic returned: different preventive strategies were promoted in developed and in developing countries. However, owing to the efficacy of antiretrovirals, the "virtual elimination" of mother-to-child HIV transmission is expected in 2015 (UNICEF et al. 2010).

Over almost a decade, some West African countries implemented national programs for the Prevention of Mother-to-Child Transmission (PMTCT) that permitted HIV-positive women to decrease or eliminate the risk of HIV transmission and avoid extra infectious and nutritional risks by providing them with information, counseling, guidance, and support for prevention, as well as formula, under certain conditions. Besides its content of human experience and suffering, the "2000–2009 window" illustrates an interesting period from a social science point of view, since international policies giving similar recommendations for all world countries allowed comparative studies of local interpretations for the same preventive propositions and their effects.

The issue is important for public health. When international organizations started providing estimates, in 2000, figures of 200,000 to 500,000 infants infected annually by HIV through mother-to-child transmission were mentioned; breastfeeding was responsible for a third to a half of these transmissions (WHO et al. 2003). In 2009, more than 1.3 million HIV-positive women were pregnant in Sub-Saharan Africa. About 700,000 were involved in PMTCT programs and received antiretroviral treatment (WHO et al. 2010); they had to face the issue of infant feeding. In spite of the achievements of PMTCT programs, the estimated number of children newly infected by HIV was 330,000 (190,000–460,000) in this region (when fewer than 100 children were similarly infected in Western Europe). About a third are supposed to have been infected through breastfeeding. Ninety percent of all HIV-positive children in the world live in Sub-Saharan Africa (as well as 80 percent of all HIV-positive women). These differences in scale of the populations concerned between developed and developing countries—particularly in Sub-Saharan Africa—make it relevant to carry out an in-depth analysis of attitudes when breastfeeding is loaded with risk.

Have women who participated in PMTCT programs in West African countries widely adopted the proscription of breastfeeding, as in developed settings? Why did some women use other feeding options? Were these experiences determined by material and environmental contexts? Or were they more influenced by the social and cultural contexts regarding infant feeding?

From a larger perspective, what do HIV-positive women's practices and experiences reveal about breastfeeding in contemporary West Africa? Do they show changes in perceptions due to the AIDS epidemic, as has been discussed elsewhere (Liamputtong 2010)? Do these experiences reveal some trends related to local issues, or do HIV-positive women living in West Africa share more general concerns with women who also must discontinue breastfeeding in other regions?

Burkina Faso is a country where such issues may be studied fruitfully, as its situation gathers several characteristics common to many West African countries. Ranked 183 for Human Development Index (UNDP 2013), it is considered a "Least Developed Country." Its 17.5 million inhabitants in 2012 (UNDP 2013) mainly live from agriculture in rural areas, while its population is now gravitating towards Ouagadougou, the capital city (with 2 million inhabitants) and Bobo-Dioulasso, the second main city (with 400,000 inhabitants). The HIV epidemic is "generalized," according to the WHO definition, which means that more than 1 percent of the adult population of Burkina Faso is HIV-positive and all social groups and geographical areas are concerned. The peak of the epidemic occurred in the late 1990s, reaching about 8 percent; the prevalence rate slowly decreased to 1 percent in 2012 among the general population aged 15 to 49 (UNAIDS 2013); the estimated number of persons living with HIV is 110,000. The country may be considered as having been strongly affected by the HIV pandemic, and the majority of families have suffered from the loss of members. About 40,000 persons took antiretroviral medications in 2014, which called for huge improvements in the health system organization and efficiency. With the involvement of many local social organizations from all sectors (from "civil society" to public services) and the financial support of the Global Fund for AIDS, Tuberculosis and Malaria (GFATM), the public health situation is in a phase of "normalization": HIV infection is more and more considered as a chronic ailment and prevention has been scaled up beyond health services all over the country.

From a social and cultural point of view, AIDS has not become a "commonplace disease." The moralizing context that was related to HIV contamination during the first decade, owing to perceptions of the infection as due to extramarital sexual relationships and sex workers, and the load of misfortune attached to a deadly disease, have not faded away. Though antiretroviral treatments are successful in providing health to many adults and children, stigma is still attached to HIV infection, and people avoid any action or discourse in public spaces that might evoke a connection to HIV.

METHOD

Between 2003 and 2007 we conducted a research program on social and cultural aspects of the prevention of HIV transmission in Burkina Faso, in a comparative approach with four other resource-poor countries (Cameroon, Cambodia, Kenya, Ivory Coast).[1] Research used ethnographic methods combining non-structured data collection by immersion in health services and associations supporting people living with HIV, 84 structured interviews with 45 HIV-positive mothers (with infants aged between one and three months, then again between six and nine months), interviews with seven health and social workers or NGOs members, focus group discussions with the same populations, and month-long observation and recording of individual and collective counseling sessions. Data collection was implemented in Ouagadougou and Bobo-Dioulasso in public health services applying national programs. In some of them a PMTCT program was supported by an NGO, an association, or a clinical trial, while others only could provide the average national standard of care. Data collection was done by Chiara Alfieri, with the help of a translator for interviews, and by a team of research assistants for the recording of some counseling sessions. Interviews were recorded, translated from Mooré, Dioula, and Fulfuldé into French when necessary, and transcriptions were processed using Word for textual analysis. The analysis was based on the explication of emic categories and social and cultural logics, not on a normative approach that would identify compliance or resistance to medical recommendations. The results were compared with the results of previous research into infant feeding perceptions, stakeholders, and practices in Burkina Faso and Ivory Coast before the AIDS epidemic, in 1998–9 (Desclaux and Taverne 2000). This enabled us to identify the main trends in perceptions and practices, the changes over a five- to eight-year time span, and variations between pilot sites hosting PMTCT programs held with external support, and "ordinary" sites from the national program. It also enabled us to identify common situations across countries and local cultural particularities regarding counseling for the selection of infant feeding modes and maternal choices (Desclaux and Alfieri 2009), interactions between mothers and health-workers (Desclaux et al. 2006), the dynamics of social constraints (Desclaux and Alfieri, 2008), and the way mothers deal with contradictory influences and discourses regarding preventive strategies (Desclaux and Alfieri 2010). This chapter will focus on women's feeding practices to identify patterns, and will analyze the social logic underlying women's strategies.

CASE STUDIES: FOUR WOMEN, FOUR INFANT FEEDING PRACTICES

The situations observed among Burkinabè women generally followed four patterns. These women applied: (a) proscription of breastfeeding, replaced by formula feeding; (b) control of breastfeeding through exclusive breast-feeding limited to a duration less than six months; (c) limited control over infant feeding completed by lay preventive practices; (d) successive control and proscription through "sequential feeding." Four case studies will allow us to understand women's experiences and situations as well as the logic underlying these practices.

1 Fatou: Proscription of breastfeeding

Fatou is 35 and her infant is 45 days old when we meet her for the first interview. She is married to a polygamous man who works either as a traveling salesman or as a peasant farmer; they have four children. They live in an extended household belonging to her husband's mother; she has a co-spouse who lives in the same household. Fatou is a hairdresser (doing braids), and when she can work, she earns about 300 FCFA a day (0.6 USD), which allows her to prepare food for her family. She has completed primary school. She is a Protestant.

When she and her co-spouse were ill three years earlier, she got tested, and she and her last child were diagnosed HIV-positive, but her husband and her co-spouse refused to take an HIV test. She did not tell him her HIV status, but she thinks he knows it. As she was still breastfeeding her 13-month-old child when she got her test result. She weaned him immediately. She was encouraged by the doctor and health worker team, who provide follow-up care for persons living with HIV. At a health center supported by an international NGO. They provided her with formula. As her baby was already grown, it was not very difficult to give him formula, though she needed an excuse for this "early" (according to local standards) weaning:

> I looked for a way to say it, and I said that as I was ill myself, strengthless, with little blood, and the doctors allowed me to wean my infant and said I will have more strength for myself. They [family and neighbors] would not try to look further on the subject, they did not think it might be THE disease.

Then, she started ART (antiretroviral therapy) and she regained enough weight to feel much better: her weight was 65 kg after decreasing from 72 to 47 kg when she was ill. At that time, her husband requested her to come back to their household, though he had previously told her to return to live with her own family when she was ill. Then she had a new pregnancy.

> Q: Then, what led you to choose formula?
> A: As I already knew that breastmilk is poison, I did not feel like breastfeeding my baby. I also knew that if I chose formula I would not have to pay for it. That's why I said I will formula feed this baby to prevent him from getting ill as the previous one.

> Q: What did your co-spouse say?
> A: She asked why [I did not breastfeed him] and I said it is because of ulcers I was requested to avoid breastfeeding.

> Q: And what did your parents say about formula?
> A: Ah, they often say I should also breastfeed him to make him fat, because "the whiteman's milk" (formula) cannot make him fat quickly. Then I say that usually when I have a baby I do not have much milk, then as they [the health team] help me [by providing formula] I am not going to look for something else.
> [Ouagadougou, 2006]

In Burkina Faso, nearly all women breastfeed their infants, as did Fatou when she was diagnosed HIV-positive: 84 percent of infants are still breastfed at the age of 18 to 23 months (INSD and ICF 2012). Using formula is uncommon out of a PMTCT program, if not for women who work in the paid employment since the legal duration of work leave after giving birth is limited to two months, and women are seldom permitted to bring their child with them to their workplace. Women using formula belong to a minority, usually living in urban areas, and are better off than the general population: 44.6 percent Burkinabè live on less than 1.25 USD per day (UNDP 2013). In semi-urban and rural areas, most women are seen with an infant on their back, as the fertility rate is 6.5, which means that on average they spend more than 18 years of their lifespan being pregnant or "holding their infants." The infants held on their mothers' backs during daytime may be breastfed on demand until they can walk, and usually are breastfed long after they get teeth.

However, the majority of women we interviewed said they had chosen between proscription and control-selected formula feeding, as Fatou did. All these women said that they preferred it because it totally avoids HIV risk. Though formula feeding holds different infectious and nutritional risks that have been explained to women during antenatal counseling, those are seldom considered as important compared to HIV transmission, a risk that no mother tolerates. Nearly all women mentioned that if they could choose without constraints they would choose formula, i.e. zero risk of HIV transmission.

Most women who were able to make a choice accessed a PMTCT program in a health service supported by a "project"—either a research project held by an international institution or a support project held by a non-governmental international organization. As these "projects" would reinforce teams, material means, and professionals' skills in health services, these women were able to get counseling for infant feeding in the context of HIV during antenatal and postnatal visits, to get nutritional support through follow-up postnatal care, and provision of formula, sometimes along with utensils for the preparation of formula. Projects allowing women with limited means to access formula illustrates these women's capacity to manage formula safely in environments of scarcity—even, in some cases, when there is no tap water or electricity in the house.

Some women might also choose formula in "ordinary" mother and child services if they lived in a social situations or had a professional employment that permitted them to meet extra expenses. All women considered seriously the social risk of being stigmatized as a "bad mother" because they were using formula, but they were able to devise strategies to overcome that risk. In "project sites" or in "ordinary" services, the women that formula-fed their infants often have a social profile, a higher education level, a position in the household, or are of an age that allows them some autonomy: Fatou, for instance, is 35 and already had four children, which protects her from criticism about her ability to care for a child, and she knew how to deal with gossip. As she said:

If my neighbors ask about it, I say that I have not enough milk, and as I am getting support [i.e. I am provided formula] I have no need to look further when I already get help. I say it like this, briefly [in order to avoid further questions].

In Fatou's case, the fact that she already had a successful experience with breastfeeding discontinuation and use of formula made it easier to choose this feeding mode. Moreover, she had stopped breastfeeding her previous child very late according to international standards—if not by local ones—when milk was only a part of his daily intake. As this child had started eating diverse food, his health was not affected by the change, and Fatou would not consider that any intercurrent disease might be due to the interruption of breastfeeding, which might have an impact on her perceptions.

As the "tree" of economic exclusion is solved by support organizations or projects, the "forest" of other determinants of feeding strategies comes into view. Fatou's case makes apparent the main factors that lead women to choose proscription of breastfeeding: a strong will to avoid any HIV risk for their infant; some autonomy towards "significant others," such as the head of the household or its influent members—usually the husband, mother-in-law or co-spouses; the capacity to face and avoid criticism and a previous experience of early weaning or formula feeding.

2 Rokia: Control over breastfeeding

Rokia is 27, and she has been living in Bobo-Dioulasso for two years when we meet her. She was born in Mopti, Mali, where she was married at the age of 13 as the fourth wife of an Islamic priest and had two children. Her husband migrated to Côte d'Ivoire and left her without resources. She went to Bobo-Dioulasso and married a man who said he was an ambulant salesman. When we met her, she lived with her husband, a ten-year-old girl from her first marriage, and the baby. She has a co-spouse who lives in another neighborhood. Her husband's goods were recently confiscated by the police and since then the family has had no resources. She says that "eating is a problem," since they do not have enough money, and they survive on the food that their neighbors give them. However, they have access to tap water.

Rokia was diagnosed HIV-positive during her last pregnancy in Bobo-Dioulasso because she was ill, and antiretroviral treatment was prescribed to her for PMTCT. Her husband discovered the medicines, went to his doctor to get an explanation, and had a fight with her back home. Rokia mainly relies on help from a community-based organization: she is given some food and medicines; she also attends community meals organized there. But she doesn't like to go there because she doesn't want to be seen by her neighbor who works there. She explains her infant feeding choice as follows:

> I chose to breastfeed him because nowadays if you do not breastfeed people think that you have THE disease. I thought that if I start with formula they will have their idea. But I breastfed him and he was not comfortable. After 26 days he was complaining about his belly and he got bad diarrhea.
>
> Q: And why do you think he had diarrhea?
> A: Because the disease is in my body. Thus as my infant drinks from my breast he may get the disease. Then I thought I should stop breastfeeding him.
>
> Q: You thought he was getting the disease?
> A: Yes, that's why he had diarrhea [...]
>
> Q: And what did you do to avoid people being suspicious?
> A: The way I did it ... [they wouldn't]. First the baby had diarrhea. Then when they started asking why I was stopping breastfeeding I said that my right breast hurts and the milk from left breast is not sufficient. And also my breast was swollen, they would not understand [that she turned to formula to prevent HIV: they would think she was using it because of her swollen breast].

Rokia applied a transitional feeding mode over the course of four days, as advised by a social worker. This time span was necessary to get utensils to prepare formula, meet the doctor and "get his authorization," learn how to prepare formula with the social worker and to have a home visit by the PMTCT counselor. During that time she put ice on her breast to stop lactation. People stopped enquiring after this. Rokia gives long and detailed explanations about the way she prepares formula milk.

When asked about her baby's health, Rokia answers that he is well, owing to formula and herbal teas. But before, she had to "fight" to avoid extra water: because the baby was crying from his first day of life, her neighbors and other women—especially one who works at a pharmacy—told her the baby was thirsty and wanted to give him water.

According to Rokia, the disease is conveyed not through milk but through blood only. She thinks that the manner of breastfeeding is even more important than breastmilk itself. Rokia can talk about some positions for breastfeeding that have been taught to her during information sessions during antenatal visits, which are necessary to avoid sores on the nipples, leading to blood sucking by the baby. She explains that she avoids bringing milk to the baby's mouth through pressure on the breast in order to avoid blood emission, believing that mastitis may have the same consequences.

Rokia talks about the importance of support that she finds in community-based organizations and in the project that reinforces the mother-and-child health service she attends:

> My heart cried from anxiety but owing to counseling and medicines, they give us advice, they encourage us, they give us money for transportation, even more, and if you feel weak they come to your home to support you, to help solve your problems and anguish. I really found peace there. It is like if God knew what I was feeling. I was sitting thinking that I had no more milk. That day if he [my baby] drunk milk there would be no more left for the day, then I would have to go get some more. And I had no more money for transportation.

Rokia's story—and particularly the time span when she was breastfeeding her infant—shows that she was able to "control" breastfeeding, which contributed toward allowing her infant to stay HIV-negative. However, in defiance of predictions of some Burkinabè health professionals who say that breastfeeding is "natural" and exclusive breastfeeding should not be too difficult (Desclaux and Taverne 2000), there are many social consequences associated with early weaning of exclusive breastfeeding.

In Burkina Faso, besides the long breastfeeding durations mentioned earlier, only 25 percent of infants under six months are breastfed exclusively (INSD and ICF 2012); 52 percent are breastfed and receive complementary food when six to nine months old. Exclusive breastfeeding is thus uncommon, as breastmilk is complemented by liquids for most infants. Local culture pertaining to infant feeding also tends to add water in many contexts: during the first days to replace colostrum, which is thrown away as unclean; to pacify a crying baby when the mother is not available for breastfeeding; when the weather is hot and dry, or the baby must stay out of the shade and may be thirsty; when the baby's body is "hot"—which, according to emic perceptions, means that he has got a fever, or that he has been exposed to symbolic heat in sites where some rituals were performed, or through contact with a body heated by strong emotions (including sexual relationships). Moreover, water is also given to a baby without the purpose of hydration: as a welcome gift ("*eau de bienvenue*"), water is usually offered to a woman coming for a visit in a household, and some water is also given to the baby. One more reason for the provision of water by somebody besides the mother involves hygiene and infant care. Infant cleaning requires that the baby is given a daily bath, with an enema in the first days of life, using water in which some herbs have been soaked. The techniques of bathing include gestures to force the infant to drink some water used for the bath, which helps cleaning the guts and is considered as a preventive practice.

During the last ten years, the national program for promotion of breast-feeding and the UNICEF program "Baby-friendly Hospitals," held in pediatric wards, have spread messages in favor of exclusive breastfeeding for all mothers in mother and child health services and in the media. These campaigns helped reduce the feature of exceptionalism linked to this practice. Unlike the HIV/AIDS prevention information messages that aimed at popularizing the notion that breastfeeding may transmit HIV, these recent messages were useful for avoiding the attachment of HIV-related stigmatization to exclusive breastfeeding. However, the risk that suspicions about HIV infection might be attached either to the practice of exclusive breastfeeding or to formula feeding (as about any uncommon feeding mode) is still relevant and provokes the fears of HIV-positive mothers.

Since giving water to an infant is so common, applying exclusive breast-feeding requires that a mother avoid social situations with her infant. Some women say that they no longer want to attend meetings and ceremonials such as baptisms, where they know they will find other women who may give water to their infant. They also may go there before or after the liveliest stage of the gathering in order to meet fewer people. In their own household, they do not leave the infant under the supervision of an elder child or a young girl cousin or housemaid, which is common for other infants.

The narrative of Rokia's management of weaning shows not only the set-up of a new feeding technique, but also her efforts to control its interpretations by significant others, or by any person in a position of enquiring or giving comments about her feeding practices. Through exposing a partly fictive etiology that cannot be easily checked by somebody else (pain in the right breast and insufficient milk in the left one) and relying on a visible symptom, she builds a "cover" medical explanation, consistent with lay perceptions of breast ailments, as an excuse for applying early weaning.

Rokia's case illustrates the many dimensions of control that HIV-positive women apply to breastfeeding in order to reduce the risk of HIV transmission while maintaining their role of caring mothers. They control: (1) the techniques of breastfeeding, including gesture, position, and time of feeding; (2) the provision of any other feeding to the infant, including water; (3) their participation in social activities outside the household to avoid complementary feedings; (4) the sharing of the childrearing role in the household; (5) the time and duration of weaning, to reduce it as much as possible; (6) their comments on infant health to avoid raising suspicion and defuse any comment that might result in a breach in confidentiality about their HIV status; (7) their anxiety over the transmission of HIV to their infant while feeding, a psychological burden mainly relieved through support by community-based organizations.

3 Leila: Infant feeding out of control

Leila is 26 years old when we meet her, with her child, a two-year-old boy. She lives with her mother and her six brothers and sisters, but without the child's father, who abandoned her when he knew she was pregnant. She has an exceptionally high education level, since she obtained a university degree in international trade. However, she has no work position, and depends on the household head for her resources; she prepares and sells cakes as an informal part-time job, but earns little money this way.

Leila got an HIV test after she suffered from a zona. She says that she has no idea how she was infected. She told her HIV status to her mother, who reacted badly, and has reproached her since for spending too much money on treatment for her and her child. Leila's mother is not pleased about her daughter's informal activity, and she refuses to give her any money.

When she was counseled about infant feeding, Leila preferred to breastfeed her child. When he was three months old, she started giving him some gruel since she wanted to wean him at four months. Her mother did not want this, and she went to see a cousin gynecologist, who was not informed about her HIV status, to ask him to tell Leila that she should go on breastfeeding her baby. As for exclusive breastfeeding, Leila could not practice it, since her mother told her:

> We [me and my generation] have given you water when you were born. I gave water to you and you grew up healthy. Everybody needs water to live, so does a baby.

Leila started giving other food besides breastmilk when her son was three months old and finally weaned him when he was 14 months old.[2] Unfortunately, he was infected by HIV. Since he was an infant, Leila had also used folk remedies that were taught to her by "*les vieilles*"[3]—elder women of her mother's generation:

> You give them a "canari"[4] and then a "vieille" puts some leaves in it, I don't know which ones. These leaves do well against HIV and pain due to teething. An

old traditional healer and a "vieille" ask about the color and consistency of the stools, about vomiting and spitting, or fever at night, to select the right leaves.[5] As long as the leaves look good the medicine is OK. You may buy some for 200 FCFA or 100 FCFA [0.4 or 0.2 USD].

I give this medicine continuously, and when I don't have money the old woman gives it free. Even in the hospital we put that in a bottle and I gave it as water. The doctors do not approve it, but mothers think that doctors and traditional healers may collaborate together for people's sake.

Knowing her education level, one would expect that Leila would apply the preventive measures advised by health services. However, she mostly adopted the lay child feeding and care mode that is usual for infants who are not exposed to HIV. Her infant was breastfed during 14 months and was given water and early complementary feedings. Some herbal teas were used for prevention and care, their traditional applications for pediatric ailments being extended to HIV infection. Leila combined traditional and biomedical treatments, which is common among the mothers we interviewed.

These feeding practices were decided by Leila's mother, following the usual distribution of roles in families. Elder women ("les vieilles") play an important role in childcare and rearing in the household, in particular for a mother's first offspring. Usually, in most ethnic groups in Burkina Faso, women live in their husband's extended family household—when the household is not nuclear— and childcare practices are governed by the father's mother. When the mother does not live with the child's father, as in Leila's case, her own mother holds the power to make such decisions, or drive her daughter's.

Leila received some information from a community-based association, but this was not before she had to take a decision about infant feeding options. Though this interview collected little in terms of personal feelings, Leila's words on feeding, care, and HIV topics suggest that she was informed about risk and prevention, but her absence of control over the feeding mode adopted for her infant resulted from a lack of autonomy in the household, lack of acknowledgment by her mother, and lack of early support by a community-based organization.

Leila's case illustrates failures in applying proscription or control of breast-feeding for the prevention of HIV tranmission, mainly due to social reasons. Though she knows about preventive feeding patterns, Leila cannot apply them because of a lack of autonomy and social legitimacy in front of her mother, who has the cumulative authority of a "vieille" and of a household head. Leila's story shows the micro-social dimension of practices, which go beyond the relationship between mother and child, the social frame usually considered in biomedical culture and services. To be implemented, unusual practices of proscription or control of breastfeeding must also have a social substratum, such as approval by a supportive household, follow-up and support by a community-based organization, regular care by a health team, or regular exchanges in a self-help group.

4 Madina: Sequential control and proscription

Madina is 26 and her baby is 44 days old at the time of the first interview. She lives with her husband, a bus driver, in Ouagadougou. She is his only wife in the household, but he also has another partner with a six-year-old child, living somewhere else. She is a Protestant. She never went to school and cannot read. Madina has a six-year-old child, plus the infant who is the subject of the interview reported here. She had another child who died when seven months old, two years before this interview. Two younger brothers of her husband, who is the head of the family, also live in her household, as do the wife and small child of one of them. Madina mostly looks after the household and prepares food, with the very limited amount of money that her husband gives her (about 500 FCFA = 1 USD per day for 14 people). Sometimes she sells small goods.

Madina discovered her HIV status during her last pregnancy. Only her husband knows her HIV status, but he refused to undergo a test himself and never spoke to her about his status. She sometimes gets some help or support from her husband's brother's wife, but the support she really appreciates comes from associative members of a support community-based organization who visit her. She also goes to the organization's center when she feels the need to be encouraged.

Since she had an abscess when breastfeeding the infant who died, two years ago, she did not want to breastfeed her next infant.

> I was shown how to care for my infant after delivery. I was asked whether I was going to breastfeed him or to use formula. I said I was going to formula-feed him, but my husband did not want me to do so, because his mother was going to come from the village. And if she found that the baby was formula-fed she was certainly going to make troubles. Thus my husband told me to breastfeed him and later we would formula-feed him ...
>
> I wanted to do so [to mention her previous abscess as a reason to avoid breastfeeding], but as the vieilles had not seen the sores I had before, they would say I must breastfeed. If I had said I had no milk they would also check.

When compelled to breastfeed, she fought to avoid extra feedings, especially water. At the time of delivery her mother-in-law was in their household; before Madina had milk, the woman wanted to give some tap water to the baby. Madina knew that giving water was wrong, but she could not prevent it, thus she had bought some mineral water and the mother-in-law used that. The infant had water on his first day, then he was breastfed.

During the second interview we could find out more about Madina's baby's feeding history. At the medical center, her decision to wean her baby very early was supported, and she was offered an appointment for three months later, to be given formula. She went on breastfeeding the child until he was three-and-a-half months old, then formula-fed him. The baby was growing well, but he died of reported neurologic troubles when he was six months old.

Madina's case illustrates a strategy that was chosen by many women we interviewed. According to the biomedical categorization of infant-feeding patterns for the prevention of HIV mother-to-child transmission, this should be labeled "exclusive and early weaning," since this categorization is focused on the first months of the baby's life and on the choice of an option, rather than on the feeding itinerary for the two-and-half-years' time span of infant life when he or she may be breastfed. Though the medical categorization is based on an opposition between breastfeeding and formula feeding, the mothers who opt for breastfeeding use formula when weaning; in a social context where prolonged breastfeeding is the main practice, this may be interpreted as temporary proscription of breastfeeding.

Unlike other mothers who started exclusive breastfeeding without planning the situation at weaning and had to face stigma, lack of food for their infant, or criticism for not feeding properly, Madina planned this weaning, eliciting support from her husband, from the community-based organization team, and the medical team from the health center.

Madina also had to face conflicting influences: for instance, the feeding mode she adopted first was not her choice. However, for each meaningful event regarding her infant feeding, her interventions seem to be the result of a weighing—a "balance"—between social and biological risks: the social risk of being considered a bad mother or as an opponent to the authority of the "*vieilles*," between the risk of being labeled as HIV-positive on one hand, and the biological risk of HIV transmission to her infant on the other hand. Her mode of dealing with risks follows a risk-reduction model rather than a "zero risk" one. When she cannot avoid risk, she tries to limit its extent and reduce its consequences. Without any formal education, and with a social status that does not give her much autonomy, Madina applies a contextual rationality and negotiates with all these elements, which makes the succession of control and proscription of breastfeeding the most relevant strategy in her case.

OVERALL STRATEGIES AND UNDERLYING LOGICS

Among the rich information brought by this set of women's narratives, we will discuss three aspects, in order to answer the initial questions.

The social substratum of preventive feeding practices

Unlike women in developed countries, the women we interviewed in Bobo-Dioulasso did not "apply a medical recommendation" regarding infant feeding, since they had to select between two options. It was not only a matter of "choice," since all of them said that they preferred formula feeding as the only method that fully eliminated the risk of HIV transmission. Apart from the economic factors, their feeding decisions were the result of a matrix of tensions between contradictory perceptions of antagonistic risks and benefits regarding formula and breastfeeding, the eventuality of social support and stigma, as well as diverse discourses or opportunities about feasibility.

Whatever feeding option they selected, the women we met faced difficulties in applying it, since none of these feeding practices is common in the lay culture of infant feeding in the 2000s (Desclaux and Taverne 2000). Either complete proscription of breastfeeding or other liquids, or reduced duration of breastfeeding, may be criticized by co-spouses, neighbors, friends, and elder women, particularly the infant father's mother, in a patrilinear society where a woman remains a stranger with few rights in her husband's lineage and where elder women are considered as experts in infant care. Women are thus confronting a situation rather different from the one described by health professionals, who consider formula feeding as rarely possible, and breastfeeding as a "default option" easily feasible if the mother is convinced of its utility.

Besides, women's narratives show that both preventive feeding practices are possible if a mother has enough autonomy and gets social support—either from a husband, significant others, a community-based organization, NGO, or a health team. Feeding practices are only secondarily influenced by their material and environmental context regarding water and hygiene. Contrary to the approach developed in health services, which is focused on access to tap water and electricity, perceptions on the one hand and relational and social aspects on the other hand seem to be at the forefront of facilitating factors or obstacles for applying control or proscription.

The perceptions of breastfeeding

The study of perceptions of breastfeeding and breastmilk shows their evolution over the last 20 years, due to biomedical communication on this subject that started before the set-up of the national program for breast-feeding promotion and the rise of the HIV pandemic. When 20 years ago, every classified mother might have regularly breastfed a baby, and a woman would easily feed a baby crying in the absence of his mother, health professionals have advised that an infant should be fed exclusively by his biological mother, or by a surrogate. The benefits of breastfeeding are regularly taught during information sessions, and notions of "bad milk" due to heat have faded slightly.

While building on overall highly positive representations of breastfeeding through erasing prior lay reluctance, medical discourse has also introduced the notion of HIV transmission; as a result, breastmilk is presently the object of ambivalent perceptions. The highly positive value attributed to breastmilk may explain to some extent the fact that, as with Rokia, some women think that HIV transmission through breastfeeding is due to blood. This positive value may also be seen in the words of mothers of infants that were infected by HIV while undergoing the PMTCT program, who attributed transmission to mistakes in feeding on their part rather than to breastmilk as a vector of residual risk (Desclaux and Alfieri 2008). The very particular discourse that presented exclusive breastfeeding as a preventive method when breastfeeding was considered as a mode of transmission might also have participated in the building of ambivalent perceptions. Among all the women interviewed, few had positive perceptions of formula. The only quality mentioned was its completeness and scientifically fixed composition: for some women who do not have access to enough food for themselves, this feature makes formula more suitable than their own breastmilk.

Infant feeding practice and the intimate household history of HIV

Most women who opted for proscription of breastmilk took this feeding decision alone, whether or not they informed their husbands. When husbands are not concerned about the payment for formula, they have less power over decisions. However, the autonomy shown by some women on this matter is rather unusual. Fatou and Leila's cases show, in very different ways, how women's personal autonomy regarding feeding decisions and practices is framed by the history of HIV in the household.

In Fatou's case, her husband was suspected of having transmitted HIV to her and her co-spouse, which weakened his symbolic capital and authority as the head of the household: in local gender values, a man is accountable for the prosperity and protection of his household members (Bila 2011). Had she needed support, Fatou might have found it easily among health workers who would criticize him for having ignored the possibilities of getting an HIV test earlier and protecting his spouses and children. Tacitly acknowledged as a "victim" of HIV transmission in her household, Fatou had enough legitimacy for acting as she wanted, following medical recommendations regarding her infant, or taking decisions on other matters.

Unlike Fatou, Leila was not considered a victim in her household. Her pregnancy "without a father," then her HIV infection, fully disqualified her in her mother's perceptions. When she shattered her mother's expectations about a bright future following her university studies, she was no more seen as able to make an appropriate decision, either for earning a living or for caring for her child. Considered "guilty" for her HIV infection and social failure, she was compelled to apply her mother's decisions regarding infant feeding and care, which might have caused her son's HIV infection.

Other women like Madina took their decision after discussion as a couple, or, like Rokia, started a process of communication about HIV. Several histories show that the father may himself be aware of his HIV status and shared with his wife a concern for the infant's health without always speaking explicitly about it; other fathers are supportive, as described in Côte d'Ivoire (Tijou et al. 2009). In some cases, suspicion and resentment toward the infant's father seem also to have an incentive effect on women's affirmation of their own agency, as if they felt disengaged from their obligation of mutual support by their husband's prior defection from his responsibility to protect the couple from HIV.

CONCLUSION

The women living with HIV in Burkina Faso, the majority of whom discovered their HIV status during their last pregnancy, could, in health services supported by international projects and community-based organizations, choose between proscription and control of breastfeeding. When all preferred formula for its capacity to avoid HIV transmission, their feeding decisions were the result of complex arbitrations resulting from the diverse discourses and social tensions usually constraining women, as in other matters within a patriarchal society.

More than applying medical recommendations, women would set up strategies built on lay understanding of risk reduction that in some cases were relevant from an epidemiological understanding, though they were not fully acknowledged in medical discourse. As for sequential proscription and control, or the use of bottled water when extra feedings cannot be avoided, these strategies may be considered as the result of an indigenization of WHO recommendations that contribute to the building of a local lay knowledge in HIV prevention regarding children.

Women's experiences and discourses show that information about HIV did not, as feared by health experts, engender a loss of confidence in breast-feeding, nor a "spillover" in the use of formula, which is not accessible to the general population for economic reasons. Rather than erasing the value of breastfeeding, the notion of HIV transmission seems to be associated—under an additive process—with overall perceptions which, following increasing medicalization, tend to value breastfeeding and breastmilk more and more positively. In the end, HIV-positive women have a very ambivalent perception of breastfeeding, which makes infant feeding even more sensitive at a psychological level, an aspect that has also been shown in East Africa (Blystad and Moland 2009). This ambivalence to breastfeeding related to the polarization of discourses may endanger the communication about other risks that challenge breastfeeding, such as the toxic risks of nicotine or dioxines, which have an increasing importance in developing countries.

A particularity of the ongoing social construction of the HIV pandemic is the moralities at stake. The categorization of women as "guilty" or as "victims" regarding HIV infection, as a result of intimate stories of HIV transmission in the micro-social context of households, determines women's agency, including their ability to apply preventive infant feeding patterns. This study shows that the social and cultural dimensions that shape decisions of proscription or control of breastfeeding and women's practices in Burkina Faso have a complexity underscored when only economic and environmental explanations are given for differences in practices between developed and less advanced countries.

Acknowledgments

We acknowledge all of the women and health teams who kindly participated in this study. We also acknowledge Sharon Calandra for her linguistic
correction of a draft version of the chapter.

–9–

"Impersonal Perspectives" on Public Health Guidelines on Infant Feeding and HIV in Malawi

Anne Matthews

> An action can be judged as the right one if it gets the best overall result from an impersonal perspective. (Beauchamp and Childress 2001: 340)

Public health guidelines, such as those of the World Health Organization (WHO 2006, 2009a, 2010) on infant feeding and HIV aim for best "overall result." These guidelines and their recommendations draw on quality-graded evidence to calculate the relative risks of breastfeeding and its alternatives for women, taking HIV into account. The evolution of these guidelines will be explored. There are considerable sociocultural and ethical issues arising from the implementation of these guidelines in resource-poor settings where there is high prevalence of HIV infection, such as in Malawi. Therefore a guiding question of this chapter is whether impersonal perspectives on topics such as infant feeding and survival are, in fact, possible or desirable.

HEALTH AND SOCIAL CONDITIONS IN MALAWI

Malawi is a land-locked country in south-eastern Africa, with a population of over 15 million (15,381 million in 2011). It is ranked 170 from 186 countries in the United Nations Human Development Index (HDI), which is a composite measure of three components of wellbeing: health, education, and income (UNDP 2013). HIV prevalence rates are estimated at 10.8 percent among adults aged 15–49 years and 1.1 million people were estimated to be living with HIV/AIDS in 2012, of whom 560,000 were women aged 15 years and upwards (UNAIDS 2014).

Life expectancy in 2011 was 58 for both sexes in Malawi (WHO 2014). Maternal mortality is very high, at 680 per 100,000 live births, for 2010

(Countdown to 2015, 2013). These maternal deaths are avoidable, either preventable or treatable, being due mainly to uterine rupture caused by obstructed labor or to infection or hemorrhage (Leigh et al. 2008). With very high rates of infant and child mortality, diarrhea is the stated cause of 11 percent of deaths of children under five for 2008 (WHO 2010a). There are serious difficulties in implementing maternal and child health services in Malawi. Although there has been investment in healthcare facilities especially at local health center level, many facilities lack basic drugs, equipment, and, critically, healthcare workers (Maliwichi-Nyirenda and Maliwichi 2009). Severe shortages of healthcare staff persist.

HIV AND CULTURE IN MALAWI

HIV probably began to affect the Malawian population in 1977 (Lwanda 2005) and people with its effects became in need of health services in the 1980s. Specific factors led to its high rate of spread: the involvement of the Malawian army in the Mozambican war, the displacement of Mozambican refugees into Malawi, as well as the movement of Malawian migrant workers to South Africa. In his Ph.D. research entitled *Politics, Culture and Medicine in Malawi: Historical Continuities and Ruptures with Special Reference to HIV/ AIDS*, Lwanda (2005) explores the effects of history and politics on how AIDS was understood and responded to in Malawi. British colonialism and the postcolonial "dictatorship" of the Hastings Banda regime and its reluctant response to HIV interacted with traditional, cultural religious beliefs and practices. Reactions to HIV/AIDS were based on beliefs about witchcraft (*ufiti*) and were in particular related to sexual taboos. Reviewing Lwanda's work, Fonseca (2007) notes how the perceived distance of AIDS versus the economic threat of hardship and starvation meant the rational choice was to choose survival and unsafe sexual practice. She also highlights Lwanda's stress on how decades of repression have produced "a cultural alibi," whereby Malawians could abdicate their responsibility for HIV prevention. Lwanda (2005: 115) describes how "Banda's stance against western immorality and decadence" placed the blame for AIDS elsewhere, and that AIDS was described as an American disease, or an American family planning plot. Cultural practices embodied *ufiti* witchcraft rituals and in particular sexual taboos and practices were often in conflict with biomedical scientific explanations of disease causality, including HIV/AIDS.

Lwanda (2005: 118, 199) describes the term "EDZI" as an onomatopoeic "meaningless" Chewa version of the term AIDS. He claims that this weakened an opportunity to communicate something of the nature of the infection and its means of transmission in its title. He suggests that this would have been the case with "*chiwerewere*," which is Chichewa for "promiscuity," and which did continue in minority use. He also refers to the term "*magawagawa*," which means "something shared" in Chichewa, as being more indicative of the meaning of the virus. Lwanda describes that the HIV virus was known as the small AIDS beast, so that the idea of removing the beast (germ) implied that a cure was plausible. Muula (2005) describes the ongoing reluctance of health professionals to name HIV/AIDS on medical notes for fear of stigmatization and discrimination by others and emphasizes that while these efforts may be well-meaning it may be more fruitful to tackle these issues head-on rather than by using euphemisms. He outlines the lay terms associated with HIV/AIDS, including *matenda aboma* (the government's disease), *matenda amasiku ano* (the disease of these times), *kaliwondewonde* (slim disease), *zomwezi* ("these things") and *ntengano* (the disease that leads to both wife and husband dying together or one after the other) (Muula 2005: 187). In their study of university students' perceptions about those who have AIDS, malaria, schistosomiasis, and a cold, MacLachlan and Namamgale (1997) conclude that "AIDS was the most easily distinguished from the other three by being seen as the least easily cured, having the most gradual onset and being the most contagious. Moreover, people with AIDS were seen as being 'the most to blame for their illness and the most likely to die soon'" (MacLachlan and Namamgale 1997: 212). Women's multiple burdens in particular were highlighted in a qualitative study by Rankin et al. (2005), leading to risk-taking behaviors. These religious and gendered attitudes especially about sexuality interact and compound women's positions and constitute their "donkey work."

THE WHO GUIDELINES ON HIV AND INFANT FEEDING

Primarily, two sets of WHO guidelines on HIV and infant feeding (and related sources WHO 2003a/b/c) will be highlighted and compared:

1 The 2006 HIV and infant feeding update (based on 2000 and 2006 technical consultations)
2 The 2009 HIV and infant feeding revised principles and recommendations RAPID advice (also included in the 2010 guidelines on HIV and infant feeding report).

The core recommendation of the 2006 guidelines states that:

> The most appropriate infant feeding option for an HIV-infected mother *depends on her individual circumstances*, including her health status and the local situation. The health services available and the counselling she is likely to receive should be considered. (emphasis added)

and that:

> The WHO recommends HIV-infected women breastfeed their infants exclusively for the first six months of life, unless replacement feeding is *acceptable, feasible, affordable, sustainable and safe* (AFASS) for them and their infants before that time. When *those conditions* are met, WHO recommends avoidance of all breastfeeding by HIV-infected women. (emphasis added)

The 2009 guidelines were introduced based on "significant programmatic experience and research evidence regarding HIV and infant feeding" that had been accumulated since the 2006 update (WHO 2006: 1). This mostly relates to the effectiveness of antiretroviral Therapy (ART) in preventing mother-to-child transmission of HIV, described in the report as "transformational" (WHO 2006: 8). The 2009 recommendations are stated to be either strong where benefits outweigh risks or weak and conditional where benefits probably outweighed risks whereby "the majority of well-informed individuals would want the interventions but an appreciable proportion might not" (WHO 2006: 3). The quality of evidence is judged to be high, moderate, low, or very low, according to the criteria based on the work of the Grading of Recommendations Assessment, Development, and Evaluation Group (GRADE). Both sets of guidelines were developed taking account of the risk of the oral transmission of HIV virus in breastmilk. Research is ongoing and challenging this premise, for example, Fouda et al. (2013). If breastmilk is in fact confirmed to be protective against oral HIV transmission, this would confirm the current approach of recommending exclusive breastfeeding for six months. The dangers of mixed feeding may endure in that case, so guidelines may remain as they are.

The core recommendation in the 2009 guidelines is that national or sub-national authorities should principally promote and support one approach and the recommended approach is *breastfeeding and ART interventions*, to give infants born to mothers known to be HIV-infected the greatest chance of HIV-free survival. Within the recommended strategy, WHO states it "will work with partners to secure access to ART for all HIV-infected mothers," and when ART is not available, the recommendations in the 2006 HIV and infant feeding update "still provide useful guidance for mothers and health workers" (WHO 2006: 8) that is based on individual circumstances and not breastfeeding if AFASS conditions are met. Certain conditions required for formula feeding are again restated in the 2009 guidelines, though the widely used acronym "AFASS" from the 2006 guidelines has been rephrased as six points covering safe water and sanitation, access to formula, preparation, family support, and access to health services (WHO 2009a: 19).

There are eight key principles outlined in the 2009 report, which are stated to "reflect a set of values that should contextualise the provision of care in programmatic settings" (WHO 2009a: 4). It is stated that they cannot be subjected to formal research but represent public health approaches and preferences. These are:

- balancing HIV prevention with protection from other causes of child mortality
- integrating HIV interventions into maternal and child health services
- setting national or sub-national recommendations for infant feeding in the context of HIV
- informing mothers known to be HIV-positive about infant feeding alternatives
- providing services to specifically support mothers to appropriately feed their infants
- avoiding harm to infant feeding practices in the general population
- advising mothers who are HIV-uninfected or whose HIV status is unknown
- investing in improvements in infant feeding practices in the context of HIV (WHO 2009a).

These principles underpinning the recommendations are explained. The first principle, "balancing HIV prevention with protection from other causes of child mortality," highlights the higher risk of mortality and morbidity for children who are not breastfed than the risk of acquiring HIV through breastmilk, where resources and access to water and sanitation are not guaranteed. Access to clean water and sanitation were stated to be prerequisites for formula feeding, according to the AFASS criteria.

"An unhygienic and unsafe environment is the main contributor to child deaths worldwide" (Engebretsen et al. 2007: 2). The key factors associated with HIV-free infant survival identified in a South African prospective cohort study examining the effectiveness of the implementation of the 2006 guidelines were piped water, electricity or gas or paraffin for fuel, and disclosure of HIV status (Doherty et al. 2007). Coutsoudis et al. (2008) highlighted the dangers of piecemeal interventions, such as providing formula milk based on the 2006 guidelines, to families in severe and persistent poverty; their call for more fundamental steps to alleviate poverty remains unanswered.

Principle 6 underpinning the 2009 guidelines, "avoiding harm to infant feeding practices in the general population," focuses on any weakening of the promotion of the "universal breastfeeding" public health message. The guidelines state that HIV has caused great confusion among health workers in relation to their promotion of breastfeeding. In particular, confusion is sharper for those who are HIV-positive and for whom breastfeeding may be safer than formula feeding even without antiretroviral drugs (ARVs), but also the "spillover effect" to those who are HIV-negative or unaware of their HIV status. As it became known, formula companies exploited that confusion. For example, Greiner describes the baby food companies' actions as those of the "heroin dealer," knowing the dependency-creating power of offering a free sample when substitute solutions were being tested (Greiner 1999: 6). Early media and scientific reports about the transmission of HIV through breastmilk had serious consequences from the 1980s (Greiner 1999), with one scientific source publishing a headline in 1998 that said: "UN says no to breastfeeding" (Greiner 1999). In a WHO Bulletin in 1999, a call was made to provide universal replacement feeding methods and support their safe use for women who are HIV-positive, plus those untested for HIV (Berer 1999). Berer also then highlighted the limited capacity of antenatal and delivery services to implement optimal programs in resource-poor countries such as Malawi, and where these limits persist, particularly in relation to human resource capacity.

THE IMPLEMENTATION OF THE 2009 RECOMMENDATIONS

The success of the implementation of the "breastfeeding and ART" strategy recommended in the 2009 guidelines depends on at least three critical factors:

- women knowing their HIV status, based on access to and uptake of reliable and ethical HIV testing
- reliable access to antiretroviral therapy (ART) for those who are HIV-positive *and*
- exclusive breastfeeding practice, up to six months.

These factors will be considered in relation to their implementation in resource-poor country settings.

Exclusive breastfeeding

Mixed feeding is associated with the highest rates of mother-to-child trans-mission, which are higher than exclusive breastfeeding (WHO 2007). Therefore promoting exclusive breastfeeding for six months (and thereafter weaning) is a very real concern. Data for Malawi for 2010 shows 71 percent of infants are exclusively breastfed to six months (Countdown to 2015, 2013). In an earlier cross-sectional study of infant feeding practices in Balaka district in Malawi, almost half the mothers surveyed and who reported breastfeeding had given non-nutritive substances such as water to babies (n=179) before four months of age, as well as breastmilk (Hotz and Gibson 2001). Studies in South Africa show that, while recommended in the context of high HIV prevalence, exclusive breastfeeding is not always practiced. Perceived milk insufficiency meant that supplements were given to 46 percent of infants (n=134) in one longitudinal study (Bland et al. 2002). While 43 percent of women self-determined their feeding choice, other influences were health staff (22 percent) and grandmothers (16 percent), stressing the need for wide communication and support. The authors concluded that mixed feeding is the socially and culturally accepted mode of feeding in township and rural areas studied and that in fact most infants were not being exclusively breastfed by two weeks. A later cohort study by the same group found that lay counseling visits were strongly associated with exclusive breastfeeding at four months (Bland et al. 2008).

Mataya et al. (2013) in a qualitative study in southern Malawi suggested that women who were HIV-positive understood why exclusive breastfeeding for six months was recommended, but stigma, lack of social support, and poverty—meaning lack of access to weaning foods—make it difficult for them to stop breastfeeding after six months. An earlier qualitative study in Malawi (Ostergaarrd and Bula 2010) had found similar problems with stigma and lack of support. Explicitly studying the implications of the guidelines in contexts of abject poverty, Chinkonde et al. (2012) highlight the feeding dilemmas women face, caught between medical and social expectations. Stigma about HIV-positive status and the indications of this through infant feeding practices is at the root of the difficulties women face, found in all of these studies. Chinkonde et al.'s article title, "HIV and infant feeding in Malawi: public health simplicity in complex social and cultural contexts," captures the tension well. Mixed feeding, in particular prelacteal feeding, was also found to be the norm in Uganda, where under-5s mortality rate ranges between 81/1,000 and 140/1,000 infants (Engebretsen et al. 2007), though high education and formal marriage were protective factors against mixed feeding. Two-thirds of women in the study areas had access only to dirty water; 57 percent of the rural population in Malawi were using improved sanitation in 2008 (from 41 percent in 1990) and 77 percent of rural people were using improved water source in the same year (up from 33 percent in 1990) (WHO 2010a). Health professionals also widely practice routine and unnecessary prelacteal feeding, as was found in a study of 1,100 health workers in Nigeria (Akuse and Obinya 2002), though this is discouraged by the WHO.

HIV testing and treatment

The percentage of women who undertook voluntary antenatal HIV testing in Malawi was recorded as 8 percent in 2004, and 50 percent in 2007, rising to 68 percent in 2008 (WHO 2009c). Other sources record 52 percent in 2009 and 66 percent in 2010 (WHO 2014). Fifty-three percent of eligible women who were HIV-positive received ART for PMTCT in 2011 (Countdown to 2015, 2013). The introduction of the Option B+ of the WHO recommendations on PMTCT in 2011 will hopefully mean this rises, if ARV supply is supported. Option B+ involves commencement of ARV treatment for all HIV-positive women (regardless of CD4 count) in pregnancy, intra-partum, and postnatally, with lifelong ARV treatment subsequently. Place of delivery may also affect adherence to preventive MTCT strategies; Kasenga et al. (2007) show how delivering outside the hospital was associated with lower adherence to prophylactic treatment, especially for infants. In 2010 71.4 percent of women giving birth had skilled attendance at birth (up from 54 percent in 2006) (WHO 2014). This suggest a likelihood for greater ART coverage, where appropriate, though with over one quarter of women giving birth doing so without a skilled attendant (therefore outside the formal health system).

Beauchamp and Childress (2001: 66–7) acknowledge that "HIV testing carries psychological and social risks" in their discussions of autonomy, privacy, and mandatory testing. The approach that is most respectful of autonomy and privacy is to offer and allow access to voluntary testing, and this is in place in Malawi. In a study of women's perceptions of maternal health in Mchinji district in Malawi involving participation by 3,171 women, the most common causes of maternal deaths were accurately identified, although HIV/AIDS was ranked low as a priority (Rosato et al. 2006). The authors concluded that the taboo surrounding HIV/AIDS persists and makes discussion difficult. This is linked with low uptake of testing. The authors state that only 15 percent of pregnant women in Mchinji had gone for counseling and voluntary testing, though the dates of data collection are not specified by Rosato et al. (2006). At this time, MTCT prevention was only available in two of the 14 Mchinji district health facilities. The authors acknowledged that perceptions that "AIDS was untreatable" are explained by these factors at the time.

Ethical implications of the guidelines

The WHO guidelines raise many significant ethical challenges. Preventing mother-to-child transmission while also protecting infants from the other causes of death in the absence of breastfeeding were described as "the most pressing public health dilemmas" facing policy-makers, professional, researchers, and HIV-infected women, especially in developing countries (WHO 2007: 1). As Bland et al. state, HIV has "complicated" breastfeeding advice (Bland et al. 2002). It is acknowledged that "recommending any breastfeeding has been perceived by some as a double standard compared to the standard of care expected in well-resourced settings" (WHO 2009a: 16). The option for mothers who know they are HIV-positive in developed countries is to avoid all breastfeeding, and it can even be forbidden or outlawed, as in Sweden in 1987 (Greiner 1999), whereby breastfeeding is seen as abuse or neglect, even if ART is available and taken by the mother (WHO 2009a: 7). However, avoidance of breastfeeding in settings where safe and sustainable formula feeding is very difficult is just not a safe option (Bland et al. 2002). Those who do work in a service job in Malawi could earn maybe 200 Malawi Kwacha (€1) per day. A tin of infant formula cost 4,000MK, which amounted to three weeks' salary in 2010.

The earlier guidelines espouse respect for autonomy of women in their own decisions about feeding, usually laudable by ethical norms.

Beauchamp and Childress define autonomy as: "self-rule that is free from both controlling interference by others and from limitations, such as inadequate understanding that prevents meaningful choice" (2001: 57). This is a complex definition. There is little meaningful choice in the context of such income poverty as described above. Adequate understanding might be enhanced through education, though the lack of health workers at all levels of the health system makes this unlikely.

The apparent tension between the "public health" approach, which focuses on population-level concerns, and the "individual rights" approach is discussed in the WHO guidelines. It is not implied that the guidelines are deliberately seeking to cause harm—rather that in focusing on the public health message and accepting socioeconomic conditions, the recommendation chosen is not the objectively safest one for infants. Beauchamp and Childress outline the "rule of double effect," wherein a single act has two foreseen effects, one of which is good while the second is harmful. The evaluation of the intervention depends on the nature of the act, its intention, and proportionality between effects—that the good effect must outweigh the bad effect (2001: 129). They emphasize the distinction between the means and effects—that a bad effect not be a means to a good effect. The intent of the recommended approach of maximizing HIV-free survival chances of most infants, i.e. the public health approach, preventing "spillover" etc., can be judged as beneficent. The 2009 guidelines seem paternalistic, asking national policy-makers to specify advised courses of action. They therefore appear to undermine a respect for the autonomy of individual women. This apparent conflict between beneficence and autonomy defines paternalism (Beauchamp and Childress 2001). However, paternalism is further defined by Beauchamp and Childress as:

> ... the intentional overriding of one person's known preference or actions by another person, where the person who overrides justifies the action by the goal of benefiting or avoiding harm to the person whose preferences or actions are overridden (Beauchamp and Childress 2001: 178).

Public health promotion is a multi-factorial process operating at different levels, and therefore interventions are difficult to evaluate (Speller et al. 1997). The guidelines state that women's preference is for the action with best evidence to support it, though they acknowledge that some recommendations are made with weak evidence to support them. The recommendation with the best evidence to support it is that women who are HIV-positive do not breastfeed. That is the recommendation to women in resource-rich contexts. What is recommended for women in resource-poor contexts is a compromise, driven by public health concerns and the acceptance of the status quo of poverty and lack of access to resources. Recommending breastfeeding with ART is the "next best thing," but not the best for individuals. Furthermore, women often do not know what action has the best supporting evidence, nor what that evidence means. Public health workers must interpret and communicate this, again a challenge in such constrained human resource settings. The lack of desired high quality of evidence often pertains to the fact that it is often not ethical or feasible to carry out Randomized Controlled Trials in areas of interest relating to breastfeeding. It is also important to distinguish between a lack of evidence about an intervention and evidence that an intervention is ineffective.

CONCLUSION

The utilitarian 2009 WHO guidelines of recommending national policies of "breastfeeding and ART" offer *probably* the best possible overall public health message. However, there are no impersonal ways of looking at this. This requires an acceptance of the double standard implicit in this recommendation, before even considering the underlying difficulties with implementing exclusive breastfeeding, the barriers to HIV testing, and the difficulties sustaining access to ART. These effectively render the guidelines meaningless, if they were ethically acceptable.

Rejecting that double standard, whereby the same recommendation would apply to all women, means that access to safe water, sanitation, and formula milk, as well as health structures and medication (where required) to ensure maternal health, would have to be "guaranteed"—but by whom? This is the standard required of mothers in developed countries: that they do not breastfeed their babies if they are HIV-positive, even if they are taking ART. While this may be seen to constitute a lack of freedom, it is objectively the safest feeding option to avoid any risk of HIV transmission while also not threatening infant survival from other causes, assuming resource availability for infant formula feeding.

Access to the resources to secure formula, safe water and sanitation are unlikely for those who are HIV-positive in countries such as Malawi because of the social and economic conditions of most people who are HIV-positive. Equally difficult to implement is the exclusive "breastfeeding and ART" option for mothers who know they are HIV positive in resource-poor countries. Globally, five million people do not have access to the ARV treatment they need (WHO 2009a). The majority of those living with HIV are unaware of their status, despite reported increases in testing for women antenatally, linked with cultural and social realities described here. These are uncomfortable realities. Yet even to implement the "double standard" deemed appropriate for mothers in resource-poor countries requires improvements in access to HIV testing, to ART, and the promotion and support of exclusive breastfeeding. If a single (not a double) standard was our goal, then the right of a mother who is HIV-positive to the safest infant feeding option (formula feeding) would be necessary. An impersonal perspective on the double standard affecting infant survival is neither possible nor desirable.

–10–

Breastfeeding and Bonding: Issues and Dilemmas in Surrogacy

Sunita Reddy, Tulsi Patel, Malene Tanderup, Birgitte Bruun Nielsen

Mammals have the longest period of dependency of children on their parents—especially humans. From infancy to adulthood, humans depend on their parents for various kinds of support; physical, financial, emotional, and psychological. This long dependency and closeness engenders social bonding. Of all the human bonds, the maternal bond between the mother and the infant is seen as one of the strongest.

The bonding discourse was extremely popular in the mid-1970s because of its usefulness in the political struggle between the natural childbirth movement and hospital obstetrics. Bonding gave women more control over the birth experience part of natural birth. Bonding is still widely believed to be an established rule for governing the mother's behavior; however, some scholars found this to be conservative fiction, rooted in institutional medicine and popular beliefs about the true nature of womanhood (Eyer 1994). There are various ways in which the bonding is believed to be ensured: by providing support during labor, skin-to-skin contact immediately after delivery, to latching on for the first feeding, continued breastfeeding, and keeping mother and infant together in the first hours and days after delivery (Kennell and McGrath 2005). Breastfeeding practice is reported to foster early post-partum maternal bonding through the process of touch, response, and mutual gazing between the mother and the infant.

Traditionally, a "mother" was defined as one who becomes pregnant through heterosexual contact, gives birth, and raises a child. A woman holding her baby close to her breast, feeding and watching the baby suckle, fondly symbolizes "motherhood." Though motherhood is seen as universal, mothering is culture specific.

New reproductive technologies (NRTs) and gestational surrogacy have changed the meanings of mother and motherhood; motherhood has thus transcended the body boundaries of one single woman to multiple mothers;

biological, social, and carrier–surrogate. The development of science and technology, preservation, conservation, and transportation of gametes, and the world wide web, have made it possible for fluids—be they sperm, embryos, or even breastmilk—to flow across bodily and geographical borders.

New reproductive technologies have dissolved the biological boundaries of reproduction. Transcending the boundaries of natural birth are NRTs, in vitro fertilization (IVF), and surrogacy, which are redefining reproduction. Gamete donation, freezing of gametes, embryo formation and transfer to surrogate's womb, and breastfeeding may be undertaken by different people in different places: outside, in the lab, or inside the body of the intended mother/surrogates (Smajdor 2013).

The advent of NRT, IVF, gamete donation, and surrogacy challenged the "natural" and biological conceptualization of "motherhood" and kinship (Strathern 1992; Franklin and Ragone 1998). For instance, gestational surrogacy, where the surrogate is implanted with fertilized eggs from another woman, created three possible categories of motherhood: the biological mother (the mother who contributes the ovum); the gestational mother (the surrogate); and the social or intended mother (the woman who raises the child) (Pande 2009: 380).

The gender stereotyping, gender-based myths of maternal behavior and maternal instincts of selfless love—the all-consuming maternal instinct—have been disputed by scholars (Scheper-Hughes 1992; Hrdy 2000). The meaning of "mother" and "motherhood" has further changed and is challenged due to NRTs. Competing demands and conflicting strategies are further pronounced in the surrogacy process, between IVF clinics and commissioning parents (CPs), also called intended parents/social parents[1] and surrogates. After the surrogate mother relinquishes the infant, breastfeeding is a major issue, which has not been researched.

Breastfeeding notably symbolizes the most fundamental social bond between the mother and child. Breastfeeding practice is a bio-cultural process connecting women's bodies to infants' bodies; it is socially determined and an essential element in cultural construction of sexuality (Maher 1992; Howard and Millard 1997). Scholars have researched on the themes of sexuality, reproduction, embodiments, and subjective experience linking to breastfeeding in bottle-feeding cultures. The literature on the embodiment and subjective experience of breastfeeding is informed by feminist theory on how the breast is related to self and gendered bodies. However, an interdisciplinary research may provide new perspectives on embodiment and how breastmilk creates social relations (Esterik 2002).

Views on breastfeeding practices have also changed. "Every mother ought to nurse her own child, if she is fit to do it ... No woman is fit to have a child who is not fit to nurse it," counseled the author of a home medical manual in the eighteenth century. A quotation from a century later—"under good medical guidance ... bottle mother may still be a perfect mother ..." (Apple 1987: 3)—shows shifts in childcare practices between nineteenth and mid-twentieth centuries, when babies were bottle-fed. Women's groups and consumers later advocated for baby-friendly hospitals and "breast is best" in order to reclaim power over their own (women's) lives and bodies, and against the medical professionals, mostly men. The discarding of colostrum, position of feeding, exclusive breastfeeding period, and other beliefs and practices in breastfeeding and weaning have been culture-specific and vary within social strata (Eidelman 2012). Anthropological writings have shown different child-rearing and feeding practices across "primitive people" (Wickes 1953a; Reddy 2003), cultures (Mead 1949), and classes (Reddy 2000).

Health-wise, breastfeeding is considered to be the best feed for infants, and has advantages for both babies and mothers. Breastmilk helps in building babies' immunity, which is documented by a host of medical facts. Breastfeeding also helps in preventing and reducing the chances of otitis media, asthma, bronchiolitis, pneumonia, and the likelihood of developing certain serious chronic adult illnesses, such as diabetes (Eidelman 2012). Breastfeeding provides maternal protection against breast cancer and osteoporosis (Yang 1993; Blaauw 1994). Studies have also shown that human milk enhances intellectual, neurological, psychomotor, and social development and is correlated with the development of fewer dental caries among breast-fed toddlers. From a purely health point of view, breastfeeding is still the best form of early human sustenance, especially in a contaminated world (Draper 1996).

Evidence from epidemiological studies shows that breastfeeding develops attachment, security, and enhances affection and desire in mothers for greater proximity with babies, which is corroborated by Gribble (2006) in her study of adoptive mothers' and children's responses through skin-to-skin contact in breastfeeding.

This chapter reflects on the current debates and dilemmas of breastfeeding babies born out of surrogacy. With limited empirical data on this area of research, the chapter analyzes the practices and the perceptions of the clinics in Hyderabad, Delhi, and Anand, where the authors have carried out the study. The dilemma of CPs for the surrogate to breastfeed or not is often a conscious/thought-out decision, taken by the clinics and the CPs, often against breast-feeding by the surrogate. Yet this is not a simple and straightforward decision. It is being imbued with dilemmas emanating from the cultural meanings of motherhood and mother–child bonding.

SURROGACY AND BONDING

The word "surrogate" literally means "substitute" or "replacement." A "surrogate mother" is therefore a "substitute mother": she is a woman who, for financial and/or compassionate reasons, agrees to bear a child for another woman who is incapable or, less often, unwilling to do so herself (Niekerk and Zyl 1995).

Pointing to the surrogate's role, Amrita Pande (2010) termed the surrogate as the "mother–worker," as she is similar to trained subjects in a factory, but is, at the same time, a virtuous mother. Surrogates are counseled and trained to naturalize the transient and disposable nature of their work so that they are disciplined contract workers, but at the same time nurturing, selfless mothers who would take care of the babies inside them. Thus, Pande has interrogated this new form of labor, which is becoming more and more prevalent in India in the form of commercial surrogacy, and how women belonging to poorer families are trained for this market.

Other feminists consider the surrogacy issue debatable and draw out serious ethical issues. Scholars stress threats in global trade in health and several ethical issues pertaining to surrogates and children born through them, and call for debates on these issues (Sama 2009; Qadeer 2010; Saravanan 2013; Tanderup et al. forthcoming).

Recent discussions and debates have been focusing on the rights of the child born through the surrogacy process; the right to citizenship, to know the biological parents (in the case of donor sperms or eggs), to know who carried the child for nine months (surrogates) and the right to breastmilk. From the point of view of the child born through surrogacy, there could be problems later in the child's life should he/she want to know about the identity of a surrogate mother. This becomes a legal problem, as the contract signed assures secrecy and anonymity. The market rules and, further, no one in the entire contracting process speaks for the future of the child (George 1998, quoted in Rosato 2004). The emerging reality is that children born using these technologies are at risk of serious harm, due to risk of high order multiples, from twins to septuplets; because of this they are more likely to be born with low or very low birth weight, as found in our Delhi study (Tanderup et al. forthcoming) and by others (Rosato 2004).

Psychological studies say that bonding develops during the pregnancy and childhood (Bowlby 1973). In-utero bonding is supported by Hindu mythology. There are mythological stories of how experiences of the fetus in the womb have a huge impact on its later life too. The mother who is carrying it for nine months is thus to observe certain desirable prescriptions during pregnancy.

Various rituals are performed for the welfare of the pregnant woman and for the baby. Hindu scriptures mention *"sanskars,"*[2] meaning rituals as well as values. One *sanskar* performed during pregnancy is Garbha Sanskar.[3] Indian mythologies too have depicted lasting influences of the mother's environment on the unborn child, seen later in life after birth, in the stories of Abhimanyu,[4] Prahalad,[5] and Ashtavakra.[6] All cultures have belief systems and prescriptions for the pregnant woman, do's and don'ts for the good of the forthcoming baby. The effect of music, nutrition, and the surrounding environment all are seen as having an impact on the newborn. Baby showers in every culture have huge meaning: blessing the woman so that she will have a healthy baby. Whether these rituals and associated festivities strengthen the mother–child bond is a matter of debate and speculation, but what is clear is the belief among the participants that they bring joy and appreciation to the pregnant woman, and by implication the fetus she carries (Patel 2006).

WET-NURSING PRACTICE

Breastfeeding by a woman other than the biological mother is not a new phenomenon. Also called wet-nursing, it can be traced back to ancient times. Wet-nursing was a deeply ingrained and widely accepted social custom even in ancient civilizations like Egypt, Mesopotamia, and in Roman society. Since "commoners" commonly practiced breastfeeding, royalty, especially in Western Europe, sent their infants for wet-nursing. Historical evidence shows that throughout the period 1500–1800, wives of European aristocracy, gentry, and wealthy merchants and farmers regularly wet-nursed their infants. Usually, a wet nurse came to an infant's home to suckle the baby; in France, infants were sent away to a wet nurse, often miles away, in the country. However, the mortality rate of infants increased (Fildes 1995). Similarly, in the U.K. and U.S.A., breastfeeding was seen as lowly and out of fashion until the 1950s (Apple 1987). Higher- and middle-class women in the U.S.A. hired wet nurses (Golden 1996b).

Selection criteria for wet nurses have varied through the ages and within different cultures. Obviously, breastmilk was believed to have a strong influence on the infant. "Scientific studies" would justify the belief that milk of a "brunette" was better than that of "redhead." There was a belief in the U.S. that women with small breasts were not adequate for breastfeeding, and mannerisms and racial characteristics were transmissible through milk (Baumslag, in Hamosh 1986). Further, beliefs about the importance of wet-nursing were seen in choices based on physically, psychologically, and morally perfect woman (Apple 1987). Breastfeeding of babies born to others is not unknown in rural India, where a baby in need of a feed may be put to the breast of another kinswoman present, if the mother were away for some reason at that point of time (Patel 2006). There is, however, little research on bonding between wet nurses and infants, though it is alluded to in popular literature.

The practice of wet-nursing prevailed without much compulsion among the nobility and aristocracy in Europe and elsewhere, as is the case in surrogacy today. CPs are in a way the new aristocracy, with technologically expressed breastmilk or manufactured bottle feed.

For infants born out of surrogacy, the surrogate may be the wet nurse (as she has carried and delivered the baby, so her body naturally produces breastmilk), provided she is either allowed to or is herself inclined to breastfeed the surrogate baby. It would be interesting to find out why the clinics and the CPs are unwilling for a surrogate to breastfeed the infant she bears. Is it to do with fear of bonding, or sheer inconvenience, or other factors? The following section discusses the competing complexities and strategies in the practice.

SURROGACY AND BREASTFEEDING

Language of "rights" has been constantly used in feminist thinking, be it the right to abortion, surrogacy, breastfeeding, sterilization—i.e. the will of the woman over her body (Rothman 2006). However, in the case of surrogacy, the "right" of the newborn to breastmilk is rarely raised, or even forgotten. In the battle/anxiety over ownership, or claim of ownership of the surrogate baby and assumed bonding developed during breastfeeding, CPs and the clinics deny such infants breastfeeding by the surrogates, though in some cases in the Delhi clinics we found token feeding of colostrum may happen.

Breastfeeding is physiologically and hormonally linked to pregnancy, but neonates born in the surrogacy arrangement are usually deprived of the advantage of breastfeeding. CPs are expressing their wish to breastfeed their babies born through surrogate arrangements by a process of induction of lactation, by which a non-pregnant, commissioning mother is stimulated to lactate.[8] This induction of lactation is proposed by the clinics to commissioning mothers if they show the inclination to breastfeed their babies. Several methods and pharmacologic agents have been used to induce lactation (Biervliet 2012: 412).

Commissioning mothers interested in inducing lactation may not be able to breastfeed exclusively and need to rely on supplements. Under the management of breastfeeding, the commissioning mother is consoled that the breastfeeding *experience* is important, and not the quantity of milk she produces (Biervliet 2012: 413). Dr. Nayna Patel in her surrogacy practice in Anand induces commissioning mothers to produce breastmilk around the time the baby is due, to enable them to breastfeed for health reasons and to bond with the baby.

Some of the studies carried out in India on surrogacy show a clear denial of maternal bonding among surrogate mothers (SMs) in Anand (Saravanan 2010), which is seen as the process of objectification. Saravanan shows that most SMs who had relinquished babies had bonded with them in the process of pregnancy and postnatal care. The SMs were also involved in breast-feeding and tending to the infants after birth, as required by the clinics. Most mothers spent a short while with the babies and the SMs, and their spouses also bonded with the babies until the social/genetic parent arrived. The medical practitioners' argument is that the surrogate is paid for all her services, including infant caretaking, and thus should have no complaints. CPs[9] also feel satisfied, as the doctors remind and counsel the surrogates from the beginning, time and again, that the baby does not belong to them and they would need to relinquish her/him (Saravanan 2010). Clinics deny any kind of bonding development between SMs and the child. Breastfeeding by the surrogate was a CP's choice, not the surrogates. Most CPs did not meet the surrogate after delivery, leaving her feeling miserable; the clinic too provided very little social and psychological support post-relinquishment (Saravanan 2013). A study by Vora (2014) reported surrogates usually breastfeed new-born infants for two to three days after delivery in return for some kind of benefits. Former surrogates were feeding for two weeks or three months after delivery. Pande's study also highlights the narratives of surrogates who breastfed the infants when their CPs wanted them to (Pande 2010). Thus, it is the CPs' will and choice, and not that of the surrogate, that dictates whether the neonate will be breastfed by the surrogate mother, and for how long.

BREASTFEEDING BY SURROGATES IN HYDERABAD AND DELHI IVF CLINICS

In the studies conducted by the authors,[10] the surrogates are conditioned to hand over/relinquish the baby to a couple without any feeling or attachment. The experiences of surrogate mothers and the views of doctors in the two cities Delhi and Hyderabad differs.

A qualitative study was conducted in the four clinics of Hyderabad and 28 women engaged in surrogate services. The surrogates were well conditioned, tutored, and counseled by the clinics. In Hyderabad clinics, the practice was not to show the baby to the surrogate after delivery. As most of the births are by caesarean section, the child is immediately removed from the surrogate and handed over to the CPs.

Only in a few cases, where foreigner CPs have to take the infant overseas with them and the surrogate has to sign papers at an embassy, does she tend to see the baby. The view of the doctors in Hyderabad is that there is no point showing the baby to the mother, as her job was to carry it and hand it over. They were told that they are like an "*almirah*," where one keeps and from where one removes clothes; similarly, the embryo is implanted and the baby is removed after nine months. Time and again, surrogates are reminded of the fact that they should not feel attached to the baby, as it is for the CPs that they are bearing, and for which they are being remunerated. The following narratives show the views, perceptions, and practices of relinquishing the baby and detaching the surrogates from the process of surrogacy. Referring to a surrogate, a counselor, who is also a dietician in one clinic said:

> She has taken a big responsibility and she knows about it. She knows she is doing good for someone who cannot conceive. She takes care with trust and not with "Why should I do it?" attitude. She has a feeling of responsibility. She is mentally prepared from the beginning; she is ready to give up the child after birth, she just has to complete the process and go. She has no bond with the baby, no feelings till the last moment.

Venkatamma, a surrogate who delivered twin babies, said:

> I was given sedation and they covered my eyes; I could hear the cry, I removed the cover partly and saw both the kids. I never saw them after that. I thought of taking a photo, but could not ... Other women used to take pictures from their mobiles, when they go for signing; since I did not sign, I never got the chance to take photos. Till now I am asking, if I can see the pictures of the kids, sir told "*inkemundamma, pillenti choostavu, inke aipondi, vallu ame chestunaro*," meaning what is there now, what will you do after seeing them, who knows, what they are doing.

After ten days, they removed Venkatamma's stitches, and sent her home. "I don't have any more feelings, I got my money. It was only when other mothers say '*ido na papa, ido na papa*,' meaning this is my child, this is my child, by showing pictures, that I too feel like having a picture," she expressed sadly.

According to an agent:

In some hospitals, the doctors do not allow surrogates to see the baby. Nusratbee has seen the baby, when she went to airport. They wanted her to take photo along with the baby. Some hospitals started showing babies. The surrogate mother should be prepared mentally that it is not her baby and she should not develop any feelings towards the baby. It is very difficult but that's what they should do.

A surrogate mother said:

Even if we wish to see the baby, as per the rules they do not allow to see the baby after birth. If we think we own baby for one percent the parents have ninety-nine percent ownership. It is not my baby anyway. At hospital when we join they tell us clearly that we cannot see the baby after delivery. When the CPs comes from foreign countries they take the mothers to the airport to sign. Maybe at that point they see the baby.

Another surrogate expressed her desire to see the baby, but was apprehensive about bonding. She said:

They tell us in the beginning that they will not show the baby. I want to see the baby at least once after delivery. I know that it is not my own baby, even though I wish to see once. But if I see I may develop attachment. I do have my own children; I need to be satisfied with that.

Another mother expressed her fears of attachment, but still desired to see the child and give a goodbye kiss. She said:

I feel it is better not to see them, if we see, it is difficult to leave them. A woman told that the baby whom I delivered looks like me. That time I wish to see the baby, I thought for two days. I asked the doctors to show the baby. The doctor said: "What do you do, if we show the baby?" [She answered] I kiss the baby, I cannot see any more in my life.

Regarding breastfeeding, one surrogate felt:

"I think it is better for the baby to be with the surrogate for one to three months and breastfed; in that way baby can be healthy."

Contrary to the above view, another mother said:

"I feel it is not good to stay with baby for three months; if we stay and breastfeed the baby, it is too hard to leave them. We may develop affection towards them and cannot leave them."

Carrying to full term, where the surrogate's flesh, blood, nutrition, and bodily fluids are shared between mother and the fetus, and where the fetus is alive and kicking and so much physical attachment is experienced, is not seen as bonding. It is seen in an objective manner, associated with an object, like the "*almirah*," a simile or metaphor for the womb. Most SMs thought that the critical moment of bonding came about on viewing the baby at birth: whether the baby resembled the SM or not, her bond in utero peaks to its maximum on seeing the baby soon after delivery. But this viewing is precisely what is disallowed in Hyderabad hospitals, much to the regret of most SMs. Eye contact is prioritized over the contact of the innards of the human body, and the womb and the fetus in it. Breastfeeding is thus linked to the belief that viewing is bonding, as this chapter shows.

In Delhi, a mixed-method study was carried out in 18 fertility clinics, in which 20 doctors, and seven agents from four agencies, and 14 surrogate mothers were interviewed. There were varying opinions about breastfeeding by the surrogates, but they were interested in feeding colostrum to the baby on the CPs' demand. On being asked whether a newborn is breastfed by the surrogate, a doctor from D1[11] clinic in Delhi said:

See, we actually avoid it. We definitely give them the colostrum, the first milk (60 percent CPs ask for it), which comes out from the surrogate mother, because some of the CPs are very much particular they want the first colostrum to be provided to their babies. So we are giving them, but breastfeeding is a kind of emotional attachment, so there is no point of taking the advantage from the surrogate to do such a thing. Because at least she has carried for nine months, so if we allow her to give the breastfeed it is not the right thing. But yes, this is again all about what the commissioning parents want. So instead of giving the direct breastfeed we take the milk from the pump and give the baby.

In the same clinic, D1, another doctor said:

The newborns are not breastfed; instead the newborns are given supplements. The SM's lactation is down regulated with injection of pregenova an estrogen analog.

In a bigger hospital, where IVF clinic D2 is located, the doctors said:

The SM is not allowed to have contact at all—therefore we cannot do kangarooing after delivery. Some CPs have contract with the SM to deliver breast milk so she will send the breast milk to them. If there is no contract, cabagolin is given to the SM for three days to stop lactation.

In another clinic, D3, the doctor said:

> The newborn is breastfed by the SM, especially if she is a relative of the CP. Sometimes the CP comes one week or ten days after the delivery so the SM has to feed the baby. After this, the baby is top fed with substitute.

This shows that it is the surrogate's responsibility to take care of the infant, in case of a delay in delivering the baby to the CPs. In another clinic, D4, the doctor said:

> After delivery the child is on top feeds. The newborn is directly handed over to the CP. If the SM kept the child for a short time it would be much harder for her to hand over the child. The SM in India is not the same kind as in the western countries. Here they only do it for the money, they need the money so badly, that they don't want to take any problems or get emotionally involved.

The perception of the doctor is that due to poverty in India the SMs opt for surrogacy purely for economic reasons and thus there are no issues of emotional attachments, unlike in the West, where surrogacy may be altruistic, and thus open to emotional bonding.

Another doctor from clinic D5, where the surrogates do not see the child after delivery, expressed similar views, reiterating that poverty makes surrogates more practical and devoid of emotions, or rather they will show different kinds of emotion. Only if she demands to see the baby will they allow her to. The reason, the doctor said, for this denial was CPs' fear that the surrogate would get attached to the child, and that this would create problems. He added, however,

> These girls, because they are poor, have other kinds of emotion, not to say they don't have any, but of another kind. So the money is the big thing. She will not put her emotions into the child.

The following two cases show that undue advantage can be taken from both sides, by the SM in the first case and the CPs in the second case. Dr. K. shared a case where the CPs were a nice, simple couple. They let the surrogate see the baby and suddenly the surrogate wanted to see the child every day. Then the surrogate's husband also wanted to see the child every day. The doctor had to tell the SM's husband that this was not the way it works; that the SM did it for the money and her part was over now.

One clinic, D6, reported a different experience, where the CP asked the surrogate to take care of the baby for six months, which the clinic did not allow—they felt this was very unreasonable. The doctor said:

> Letting [the] surrogate feeding the baby for six months, how can we allow that? If the emotional attachment becomes [great], then … what will happen to her family? Six months she will stay in their house with a little one to breastfeed or every day you will send a bottle with a driver to go and collect the milk and get it for the baby. That is unreasonable!

In another clinic, D7, in Delhi, as in Hyderabad, they do not allow the surrogate to see the child, as they fear this causes bonding and heartburn and may lead to warmth and maternal instinct. The doctor reported that:

> Once they have delivered, that instinct will always be there. It would be easier to forget if you have physically not seen the child. You know, once you have physically seen and in your mind's eye, you have a picture, you will always tend to associate with that …

Doctors from Delhi and Hyderabad clinics explained how they keep the surrogate from developing any bonding through frequent counseling and pep talks:

> … at all points everybody is counseling the surrogate … you are actually doing a very noble cause … you obviously have no claim on the child … it is not your child … it's just that you are a carrier, but you are doing a very noble deed.

A doctor from clinic D2 said:

> … I really don't know how to put this, but all along, her brain has been conditioned to feel that she is the star of the show. And she is doing a very noble deed, which she indeed is, to give away the child. So, by the time she actually delivers, she looks at herself as somewhat of a heroine who has done the good deed and now she is, you know in a euphoria of her own because, you know they are the class to whom the two lakhs or three lakhs or four lakhs is a lot of money. So, you know that there is going to be emotional sequel or psychological sequel, you have to start making the person look at things in a different manner. And it is how you condition them, the CPs condition them or how the agency conditions them, which actually results in very little heartburns at the end of the day.

In clinic D2, however, the doctor expressed the view that it is the agent's responsibility to take care of the surrogate:

> ... either the surrogate's husband tackles it or the agency tackles it or they control themselves, or the CP also possibly has some role. Because, I know that CPs have taken the breast milk from the surrogates over time, let's say over one and half month or so. So I suppose, they must be having some interaction. I really don't know how ...

It is important to mention that surrogates too are often not especially interested in any bonding with the babies. They are clear enough in their discussions with agents even before they decide to try to be surrogates that the babies they carry are not their own and that they are helping someone who can't have a baby. Such an understanding is further reinforced during the pregnancy, with doctors and counselors reiterating the relinquishing logic.

Yet the doctors bear a lurking suspicion that breastfeeding may lead to emotional bonding between the surrogate and the child, and that this may make it difficult for the SM to part with the baby. Thus, conditioning her from the beginning is important. In the case of Delhi, unlike that of Hyderabad, there is evidence to show that CPs have been asking for colostrum feeding and in some cases breastfeeding for a few months. In Hyderabad, there is a uniform policy of not breastfeeding the baby, and they avoid showing the baby to the surrogate mother in the first instance itself. As mentioned earlier, the view in Gujarat stands in striking contrast to that in Hyderabad, and somewhat in Delhi clinics too. The doctor in Anand is very confident about the question of bonding through breastfeeding. She arranges for several surrogates to be taken to hotels after she discharges them, as the CPs have requested that the baby be breastfed by the surrogate. The doctor ensures that enough money is paid to the surrogate for this service, and she was very categorical in her statement that she found no case of emotional bonding, where a surrogate wished not to relinquish a baby who she had breastfed after delivery, in her decades-long surrogacy practice. She has several cases of women who are surrogates three times over and who have encouraged other kinswomen from their families to work as surrogates.

Surrogates usually do not breastfeed the baby more out of fear of bonding, thus causing unwanted trouble for centers or hospitals where births happen. In Hyderabad, these are mostly places other than IVF/fertility centers, unlike in Delhi, where babies are delivered in the IVF center itself. The surrogates too are desperate to get back home to their "own" children, and family might also be a consideration. Yet surrogates in Anand (Gujarat) often breastfeed babies they deliver upon extra payments, without any of the above considerations complicating the issue further.[7] In view of the criticality for health of the neonate, this may make for a case that surrogates who carry for nine months could feed the baby for a few more days or months. Several reasons mentioned above obviate breastfeeding of a surrogate baby. The fears, anxieties, issues, concerns, and competing strategies have emanated from the above interviews.

DISCUSSION

The research thus shows it is invariably the choice and the decision of the CPs to ask for breastfeeding. However, this is also guided by the clinics, differently in different cities. In Hyderabad, there is no possibility of even showing the baby to the surrogate, let alone breastfeeding, in order to avoid any kind of contact and thereby any kind of bonding. However, in Delhi and Anand, the choice lies with the CPs and the willingness of the surrogate. Colostrum feeding is given priority for the benefit of the child, and breastmilk is given for a few days or weeks, mostly through extraction of milk. The doctors and the surrogates held different views about bonding during breastfeeding. Also, clinical preferences vary as does the perception of bonding through breastfeeding, not breastmilk.

The debate over bonding as being "natural"' once again comes to the fore, where, in the case of the surrogates, they are conditioned to be mother–worker and to be alienated from the baby and not to develop any kind of emotional attachments (Pande 2010). The experiences of the surrogates in Hyderabad too shows that they are curious to see the baby, but do not feel attached, and are counseled enough. They also prioritize their own children, for whom they took up this contract. Even though mythological stories express the strong influence of the mother on the fetus, in surrogacy, even seeing the baby seems to develop bonding between the two and is thus avoided. Ironically carrying for nine months is not seen as bonding.

The involvement of monetary transactions transforms the meaning of a highly emotional experience in commercial surrogacy. This perpetuates the perception that a surrogate mother who bears for nine months for a payment does not bond with the fetus, as per the clinician and the CPs. But when it comes to breastfeeding the child, the fear and anxiety of the CPs and the IVF specialists are that *this* may lead to bonding, making the relinquishing of the child more difficult, and thus denying the child the right to be breastfed. Breastfeeding, which is culturally seen to develop a bond between the mother and child, is best avoided in commercial surrogacy by either not breast-feeding at all, or at best collecting and feeding.

Debates on the rights of the child born through surrogacy, and in general for IVF babies, and their right to breastmilk are picking up. Breastmilk banks are in the process of being set up, as is being contemplated for example in Anand. The expelling and pumping of breastmilk and keeping it stored to feed the infant can go on for at least one month, thereby benefitting both the surrogate, allowing her to regain her reflexes and not take lactation suppressants, and the child who gets colostrum and milk during this critical period. Breastmilk, too, can be stored, like any other products under certain temperatures and for a certain period.[12]

It is important to see that the shift from traditional surrogacy to gestational surrogacy has played an important role in separating and minimizing the bonding of the surrogate to the child, especially when this arrangement is commercial in nature, and the infant is being carried to term for a fee. There is reiteration of the fact that the surrogate has no right to claim the baby or show any kind of bonding with the baby. This is unlike traditional surrogacy—where the surrogate is also the genetic mother, having more reasons to bond and difficulty relinquishing, as seen in the long-drawn-out supreme court case of Baby M in the U.S.[13]—in India; with commercial gestational surrogacy, clinics make a strong point of saying that there is no reason for mother and child to bond, as surrogates are mere "carriers."

In commercial gestational surrogacy, the main concern is to have a baby for the CPs; breastfeeding the infant is a secondary or a non-issue. It is interesting to see that bonding during pregnancy by the surrogate is overlooked, whereas breastfeeding is avoided due to a fear of bonding between the SM and the child and her inability to relinquish, thus complicating the surrogacy contract once the baby is born. Even the importance of colostrum feeding is brushed aside; so few children are breastfed anyway in commercial surrogacy. As one doctor said, "It is unreasonable to ask the surrogate to breastfeed, for she has done her job of carrying and delivering." However, we have been experimenting with breastmilk, formula milk, wet-nursing and now milk banks and there are no "right or wrong" answers—it is how CPs and the IVF specialists feel, interpret, and act. The moot question is, what about the child's right to breastmilk?

–11–

Breastmilk Donation as Care Work

Katherine Carroll

The prevalence of human milk banks (HMBs) and the amount of donor breastmilk medically prescribed in neonatal intensive care units (NICUs) is steadily growing in Western Anglophone nations.[1] Non-profit HMBs accept voluntary, unpaid donations of breastmilk from healthy women. After screening the donors, pasteurizing, and testing their breastmilk, and then bottling and labeling it, HMBs provide breastmilk to NICUs that care for sick or premature infants. These infants benefit from donor breastmilk (DBM) when their own mothers are unable to provide sufficient volumes of breastmilk. One of the main reasons for using DBM for this cohort of infants is to prevent the severe, costly, and sometimes fatal gastrointestinal disease called necrotizing entero-colitis, the prevalence of which is drastically reduced when preterm infants are fed a diet of breastmilk rather than formula[2] (Schanler et al. 2005).

Across the U.S., the U.K., and Australia the HMB donation guidelines ("the guidelines") with which milk donors must comply are very similar. For example, donors are required to avoid the regular use of alcohol, be non-smokers, and be free of most prescription medications. In many cases donors must also limit their daily caffeine intake and abstain from most herbal teas and medications. The guidelines used in the U.S., U.K., and Australia also require particular hygiene practices. For example, donors must ensure that their breasts are clean prior to expressing[3] breastmilk, and that the pump equipment is appropriately cleaned and sterilized before use. Furthermore, at the time of expressing milk, the donor and her household must be free from any contagious illness, such as influenza. Once milk is expressed the guidelines also stipulate certain labeling and frozen storage procedures to ensure that breastmilk is transported safely, without bacterial growth or contamination, and with full traceability from donor to the HMB.

In this chapter I argue that breastmilk donors engage in work *and* a significant amount of care in order to meet the requirements of the donation guidelines. Without this "care work," the liters of donated milk provided to

HMBs would simply not exist,[4] nor would the "safety" of this milk be optimized (Carroll 2014). Expressing and donating breastmilk have each been cast as work (Stearns 2010; Mulford 2012; Gerstein Pineau 2013; Carroll 2014), yet unlike oocytes and sperm (see Almeling 2011), little research has been conducted on the actual practices engaged by milk donors (National Institute for Health and Care Excellence 2010). Osbaldiston and Leigh (2007) found that donors who pump their breasts in order to stimulate lactation donate significantly more milk than those who do not. Similarly, Arnold and Borman (1996) state that the majority of donors are those who express milk because they need to go to work and wish to leave breastmilk for their infants. These studies highlight that the most viable donors are those who are available for regular periods of pumping on a once- to twice-daily basis, with the specific intent of donating that milk. Such opportunities are associated with the stay-at-home mother or a mother with flexible or accommodating work arrangements.

Linking individual practices with class and motherhood ideologies, American sociologist Gerstein Pineau (2013) highlights the time and effort involved in producing breastmilk and the value the bottled breastmilk accrues as a symbol of the effortful regimes undertaken and of the commitment to one's infant (Gerstein Pineau 2013). Gerstein Pineau (2013) argues that milk donation is a product of the child-centered, labor-intensive, and financially expensive "intensive motherhood" ideology where mothers become moral actors responsible for staving off all possible risks and optimizing their children's development (Faircloth 2013). The moral value afforded to breastmilk as "good mothering in a bottle," Gerstein Pineau (2013: 62) argues, is a form of identity work and is a major motivation for milk donation to HMBs. This is an important sociological insight and contribution to inquiry into milk donation, as it counters the dominant characterization of milk donors as simply altruistic and in possession of a bountiful supply of breastmilk that is in excess of their infants' needs (Arnold and Borman 1996; Azema et al. 2003; Osbaldiston and Leigh 2007; Estevez de Alencar and Fleury Seidl 2009).

Breastfeeding, lactation, and motherhood are also often cast as "natural" (Zizzo 2013) or a "state of being" that harbors "automatic reserves of knowledge and expertise" (Maher 2005). Terms such as "surplus" naturalize the existence of breastmilk as an "involuntary physiological functioning of the reproductive body" (Zizzo 2013: 79). These characterizations of motherhood and lactation ignore the fact that milk production and the transfer of it to another body is accomplished through not only physiological means (pregnancy, birthing, and supply–demand mechanism of lactogenesis), but through time spent breastfeeding or through the use of a breast pump

(Faircloth 2013). Mothers and donors, for instance, classify pumping as physical and emotional "hard work" (Stearns 2010; Gerstein Pineau 2013), and similarly women also define motherhood itself in terms of the tasks and activities they perform on a daily basis (Bartlett 2005; Maher 2005). While altruism and "surplus" milk[5] are undoubtedly involved in milk donation, the overuse of such terminology propagates the notion of an inherent motherly altruism and obfuscates donor motivations and practices that are mediated by social structures such as class and race, and by the identity work enacted by women in conversation with "intensive," "good," and "natural" motherhood ideologies. Therefore simply referring to DBM as surplus, and to donation as altruistic, renders as invisible the various practices that created "surplus" breastmilk for donation. Moreover, such terms do not attend to the authenticity of the work mothers invest as they critically imbibe or rally against the normative infant feeding standards set by intensive motherhood.

INTRODUCING THE MILK DONORS: AN ACCOUNT OF THE METHODOLOGY

As part of a larger research study into DBM and HMBs for preterm infants in NICUs, I interviewed 25 milk donors[6] in the U.S. and conducted ethnographies of three HMBs and three NICUs located in the U.S. and Australia, an account of which can be read elsewhere[7] (Carroll 2014). However, for the purposes of providing additional detail of how I conducted the interviews for the topic discussed in this chapter, it is important to note that I did not observe the very private practice of donors expressing their breastmilk for donation. Rather, I asked donors about what expressing milk for donation to a HMB involved. This position is somewhat problematic for political and methodological reasons. First, it reveals the invisibility that the task of expressing milk occupies in contemporary Anglophone society, despite it being a foundational practice that many women engage in to achieve the "gold standard" of breastmilk feeding (Stearns 2010). Second, asking about rather than observing practice is problematic because turning care practices into words risks obliterating all the non-verbal components of care (Mol, Moser et al. 2010: 10). To redress this, during the hour-long in-depth semi-structured interviews, I asked women what was actually involved in being a milk donor, as above all else I was interested in what milk donors *actually did*. Therefore throughout the interview I used my identity as a childless female in her thirties with a genuine interest in, and respect for, breastfeeding to gain deeper appreciation of, and access to, the intricacies of everyday milk donation. Typically, I prefaced my more direct questions about producing and storing extracorporeal breastmilk by confessing my naivety as a non-mother:

Tell me ... I am not a mother, I have never lactated and I have never donated milk ... so what is it like to use a breast pump? What do you actually do?

I noted that many of the donors responded to this question. They would brighten, lean forward, and engage with me. Some donors relished the opportunity to tell a childless female of similar age about the secret world of motherhood. Some donors gave lengthy and at times humorous stories about *exactly* what it was like to pump one's breasts for their milk. Others remained more private but diligently described personalized routines at home, work, and while on vacation. Through these interviews donors became their own ethnographers (Mol 2003: 15), which granted me access to the private and often-solitary practice of expressing breastmilk for donation. Of importance to the exploration of care practices in this chapter, donors' stories not only included *how it felt* to express their milk but *what was done*. As this chapter will show, donors revealed how they were mindful of their milk production in relation to their own infant's needs, segregating milk for the HMB, and that this was a continually negotiated process with their fluid, milky, lactating body, and their identity as a mother and donor.

The donors participating in this research can be classified into three broad cohorts: those who give to the milk banks "excess" milk that their infant did not need; those who fully breastfed their baby and choose to express milk explicitly for donation; and those mothers who provide milk but no longer have a baby in their care. The majority of donors belonged to the first category; they donated milk that they considered to be surplus to their infant's needs, or a byproduct of the time and care invested in producing sufficient volumes of breastmilk for their own infant. Most commonly, these donors had to return to work while their infant was still breastfeeding, and in order to continue to provide their child with breastmilk, the donor would express her milk using an electric breastmilk pump. The expressed milk was then brought home from work, frozen, and kept as a store so that it could be fed to the baby while the mother was at work.

I've been back at work part-time for six weeks now ... Mondays I pump enough that I hope will be sufficient for while I'm gone the rest of the week, so the other times I'm pumping and I'm assuming he won't drink it, so as soon as I get home, I put it in the little bags for the donors. [Adriane]
I pump what I make, and if I have extra, I give it. [Brit]

I'm just going to keep a three-month stash. That's my goal. So every time I hit a month and I haven't used it, I'll need to donate the next month. [Sheila]

All donors who were expressing their breastmilk while at work carefully calculated the amount they believed would meet the needs of their infant in the short and medium term, and the rest they deemed able to be donated to the HMB. Although the original care work invested by these donors was directed towards their own infant (Gerstein Pineau 2013), at the moment of their milk donation to the HMB, the donors' care work was also conferred upon many of the unknown future recipient infants of the milk. In this sense, it is easy to see how the individualized child-centered care enacted by women as part of intensive motherhood can stretch anonymously across vast geographic and spatial locales, and can even transcend the established kinship and community networks of the donor (Boyer 2010).

In contrast, the second most prevalent donor category explicitly stated that they expressed breastmilk with the prime purpose of donation. These donors did not need to express any breastmilk for their own infant as the infant was fed fully at the breast and not taking milk from a bottle. Lindy, a mother of two, explained her deliberate decision to become a milk donor after the recent birth of her daughter:

It was just making the commitment and thinking, "I am going to do this." I would generally pump first thing in the morning. I would have nursed her, and I would be pumping in front of my son. He liked it: "Are you going to pump milk for the babies?" Yep, I'm going to pump my milk! I think it was just a mental commitment that I was going to make it happen as a priority. [Lindy]

The third category of donors provided milk that was generated in very different circumstances. Aileen became a milk donor after engaging in a gestational surrogacy arrangement with friends. As part of her surrogacy, Aileen decided that she would also provide breastmilk for the baby. For the first eight weeks of the baby's life, Aileen expressed her breastmilk and gave it to the genetic mother of the child, who then fed the baby with Aileen's milk. When the baby and its genetic parents returned to Europe, Aileen continued to express her breastmilk for a further eight weeks, and provided it to the local HMB. In the other two cases, breastmilk donation was as a result of infant death. The lactating body will continue to produce milk after an infant dies and needs careful lactation management to express the milk to prevent discomfort and health complications for the mother, such as mastitis. Two donors I interviewed were mothers of premature infants who had died in the

NICU. Both bereaved donors needed to express their milk, which they then chose to donate to the HMB. In both cases, donation was primarily motivated by self-care. They reported that expressing their breastmilk enabled them time to nurture their maternal bodies in private, and expressing their milk gave them a routine at a time of complete and utter grief.

PRACTICES AND CARE WORK: A FEMINIST FRAMEWORK

Although care is part of daily life, there is insufficient scholarly attention to the importance of care (Mol 2010). The notion of "care work" highlights the often-invisible or unrecognized labor enacted by women in the domestic sphere, a prime example of which is breastfeeding and lactation (Waring 1988). Unpaid domestic care work is removed from the measures and recognition of the market economy, and therefore it is often invisible, ignored, or radically undervalued as a legitimate form of labor (Dickenson 2001; England 2005). Care work can be defined as the work involved in unpaid family and community caregiving, and domestic chores (Mulford 2012: 124). It can also include more immaterial tasks, such as motivating, humoring, explaining, acknowledging, praising, and connecting emotionally with individuals (Jespersen, Bonnelycke et al. 2013). Motherhood typifies care work. It can include cleaning, cooking, shopping, raising children (Waring 1988; Mol, Moser et al. 2010), breastfeeding (Waring 1988; Smith 2004; Smith and Ingham 2005; Smith and Forrester 2013), and expressing and storing breastmilk (Mulford 2012; Smith and Forrester 2013). These tasks are bound by three common factors: women's unpaid domestic caregiving, the instrumental tasks of caring, and affective relations between the carer and the cared-for (England 2005).

"Care work" is significant as it defines care as not simply natural and uncomplicated, but consisting of hard physical, mental, and emotional investments between two or more bodies (Mol 2008; Mulford 2012: 127). However, the use of the term "care" also contains "normative components of altruism and compassion, nurture and suffering" (Beasley and Bacchi 2005). Some feminists view care work as oppressive and strip it of any sentimentality; however, this position also denies the enjoyment and pride that that some women find in their daily work (Abel and Nelson 1990; England 2005). Thus feminist scholars face difficulties as they seek "simultaneously to challenge oppressive structures of mothering, recognize women's work as mothers and to rethink the activities of mothering" (Maher 2005).

Coined in the public sphere, the terms "work" and "labor" aim to draw care out of the relatively invisible private sphere and highlight its benefits to capitalist economies (Abel and Nelson 1990). Although politically useful, such rational terminology is also problematic as what constitutes caring is presumed to be known and therefore *actual* care practices risk being overlooked, eroded, or even lost (Mol, Moser et al. 2010: 9). Moreover, the terms work and labor also focus attention on the actors of caring rather than the activities themselves (Fisher and Tronto 1990). To counter this, a complex characterization of caring as a heterogeneous practice that is constituted by time, material resources, knowledge, and skill is required (Fisher and Tronto 1990: 41). To exemplify how this may be taken up in the field of healthcare, the study by Jespersen et al. (2013) is particularly useful. In a randomized control trial (RCT) investigating a diet and exercise regime to treat overweight and obesity, Jespersen and colleagues found that the researchers charged with managing participants invested an array of care practices, including humoring, explaining, motivating, and praising. Importantly, these played a critical role in ensuring participants' adherence to the RCT protocol and were integral to the success of the treatment protocol itself in producing weight loss among participants (Jespersen, Bonnelycke et al. 2013). A second example of heterogeneous practices as integral to success in healthcare are the everyday self-care practices invested by patients with diabetes, both in the home and in the clinic (Mol 2008: 8–9). Mol's study celebrates the significant productivity of patients in managing their own care, an attribute that is often only awarded to carers or health professionals (Hor, Godbold et al. 2013). The methodology of these studies exemplifies how one must start with what people do rather than "will" or "intend" to do when investigating care work (Mol 2008: 10).

Rather than referring to abstract or normative identities of care and motherhood in interviews with donors, I used a notion of care that examines how it is done in everyday practice (see Maher 2005; Mol 2008, 2010; Mol, Moser et al. 2010). In this chapter I reach beyond the material production and pumping of breastmilk as a literal representation of care for infants (Swanson, Nicol et al. 2012; Gerstein Pineau 2013) and instead explore the subtle and sophisticated care practices donors enact in order to provide breastmilk deemed suitable for donation. Practices can be explained, understood, and analyzed from different standpoints, which "places us in a particular kind of relationship with the ... practice" under investigation (Green 2009). In this chapter donors' practices are framed through a feminist perspective of "care work" and are defined as donors' "doings, sayings, and relatings," including any use of material artifacts (Green 2009) such as breast pumps, storage bags, and freezers. This approach does not individualize practices or frame them as being enacted in isolation. Practices are shaped by wider social, political, and cultural influences (Green 2009), and, in the case of milk donors, these include broader motherhood and infant feeding discourses, cultural beliefs about breastmilk (Gerstein Pineau 2013), interactions with HMB staff, and compliance with donation guidelines. It is this framework of care, from the perspective of donors themselves, that I now use to explore and analyze the care work involved in milk donation to HMBs.

THE CARE WORK OF MILK DONATION

In order to present the sequential care work donors engage in throughout the process of donation, it is perhaps most obvious to start with the donation guidelines themselves. To ensure their compliance with the guidelines, donors reported regularly reviewing them or contacting staff at the HMB for any additional clarification:

> Some people, I think, are able to do it pretty easily, and not get worried about it. But I was more wrapped up in all the rules, and making sure I did it right. I don't want to accidentally do anything wrong, or contaminate anything … so I'm a real rule follower, and there were some rules that I just didn't want to mess up. [Lindy]
> I'm pretty uptight, so, I keep a pretty close tab on everything. The first month I was reading the guidelines all the time, every day or two before I pumped, just to make sure that I hadn't done anything, that I hadn't had a cup of tea or something and not thought about it. Just to make sure that it was like a habit of "okay, make sure you wash, make sure you wipe down the breast" and all these things, until it really became a habit. [Ally]
> They [the HMB staff] were very helpful by email. I could always just say, "Hey, I need to take this medicine. Can you remind me …?" [Kasey]

In their accounts of involving the guidelines in their daily life, donors frequently described being "mindful," "conscious," "aware," or "thinking twice about them":

> It's a little bit of effort to be mindful, "Oh yeah, I have a headache. Do I want to take something for it, or not? But I need to take something for it. So when can I donate again?" You have to be a little bit more mindful, but it's not bad. I understand why the regulations are there. [Jackie]
> I'm not one to take Advil or aspirin, but for a lot of people, that is part of their

life: you get a headache, you take something. But when you're a milk donor, you really have to think about it. You have to keep yourself pure and clean, because you are giving to babies that are sick. So yeah, I think it's a commitment, and you have to be conscious of it. You can't just pop open an Advil because you have a headache. You have to go then look at the sheet and find out how many hours after your milk is ok, and if you have alcohol you have to wait a full 12 hours. So it makes you think twice about what you do, you know? [Margaret]

The hardest part, for me, was being aware of who I was around that was sick, or noticing if my baby had a fever, or if my husband was sick. It wasn't that hard to follow the guidelines. It was just like, "ok, today I can't." It wasn't that hard at all. Like, I would try to avoid medication unless it was like, "ok, I really have to take something in order to get rid of this headache." Or if my allergies were really bad, I'd be like, "ok, one pill takes however many hours … it'll be ok!" I do remember consciously thinking about that after I started donating. [Brit]

The donors' accounts of actively recalling or re-reading the guidelines or, alternatively, consulting with HMB staff suggests that it is not only following guidelines that is part of care work, but that their mindfulness or attention to them in the first instance is an integral part of the care work that donors enact. Such mindfulness is a further example of the immaterial caring tasks that ensure the successful implementation of programs in the health sector. Another such example is the practice of abstaining from certain behavioral or dietary preferences by donors, for example, the consumption of coffee or certain herbal teas, and foregoing some medications during times of discomfort, such as having a headache. Abstinence requires a degree of effort on the part of donors, particularly because some sacrifices would not normally be made by donors for their own infant:

The only thing is to not drink the herbal teas. So I do like chamomile tea. So I haven't had any herbal tea, which I normally would drink. And then there's been a couple of times where I've had a sip, you know, less than an ounce of wine, and so I always make sure I wait the 24 hours. So if I've had a little bit of wine with dinner, I don't donate for the next day. So I will nurse him first before dinner, and then have a like, the ounce of wine, and then it's a couple of hours before I nurse him, and he seems fine. [Ally]

Most people say, "I couldn't do it!" because it is a change in lifestyle, right? I like to drink chamomile tea at night. Can't drink that. I really had a problem with limiting caffeine to 24 ounces with the two kids. If you drink two big cups of tea, you are almost there! And then in the afternoon I would need, like, a little boost, and it was just really hard. I was always right at the edge of 24 fluid ounces of caffeine. [Lindy]

> I noticed that because I get headaches pretty frequently, and usually Ibuprofen works better for them, but if I remember right, it seemed like with Ibuprofen it took longer for it to get out of your system than it would with the Tylenol, so I would try and drink a lot of water and do other things to get rid of my headache before I would take medication. And it wasn't for *my* baby. I mean, she was fine! It was purely for donating. [Brit]

While these donors referred to the work involved in abstaining from tea, coffee, alcohol, and some medications, other donors found abstinence to be easy as it did not require a change from their usual lifestyle, or from what they were already doing for their own baby:

> I guess I don't usually have that stuff anyway, so it didn't seem like a big deal. I'm not a drinker, I don't drink wine. I don't drink tea, and I don't have a lot of herbs, and I always try to stay off medications anyway. I don't think it was a big deal, because you shouldn't be doing it anyway because you're giving your milk to your own kid, so you shouldn't be downing the booze anyway! [Arty]
> There were not really any changes for me. I'm not a coffee drinker, I forgot what the other guidelines were, but it wasn't anything I had to change. I don't ever take any medications, so it was fine. [Aileen]

As a consequence of donors' care work being constituted by careful practices, the vast majority of donors were stricter with the milk they produced, expressed, and stored for donation than with the milk they produced, expressed, and stored for their own baby. When I presented this as paradoxical to the donors, they unanimously corrected me, verbalizing a series of sequential logics. First, donors explained that the recipient of their breastmilk donated to the HMB would be a small, fragile, preterm, and immune-compromised infant:

> They use it for the young babies, so it really, really, needs to be as sterile as possible, and nothing in the blood, nothing that you are taking. You need to keep it as clean as possible. And I understand that. [Lindy]
> I've definitely been pretty strict myself about not giving them any milk if I thought there's a chance, because I keep thinking about these preemie babies, and gosh, I don't want to chance passing these little babies something when they're already so small and delicate! [Selina]
> Having had a baby in NICU, I'm pretty strict about it, because I think, "If that were my child in there, I would want to know what's in their diet." [Angie]
> The babies that are getting it … are ones that are more fragile, more sensitive … and there need to be limits and safeguards to really take care of those little

babies. I think they're [the HMB] just watching out to make sure that they get the best product in these little babies that they can. [Arty]

Second, by contrasting their own healthy, community-dwelling and robust baby with the imagined intended recipient of their milk donations, donors explained that it was not that purer milk was going to the HMB, but that "ordinary" breastmilk was perfectly suited to their own infant:

> I wouldn't even think twice about giving [donor's daughter] something with Ibroprofen because the amount is so miniscule, and I hate to admit it, but I am also that person who would dilute milk. Like, if I felt I'd had too much to drink in that milk for my own daughter … I would just mix it with milk that had no alcohol in it. I know it sounds so awful, but I totally would because I have these big healthy babies. I just don't see how it would impact them. But the other, I'm not going to mess around with. I think some of the documents that they gave us from the milk bank were really very clear. Like, these babies cannot tolerate anything and you can put the kids at risk if you do that. So I take it pretty seriously. It was easy to separate the two—you just label it, and move on. [Moggie]
>
> My baby—he had a rough start but he's awesome now, and he's fine, so these things wouldn't bother him. [Ally]
>
> My baby's fine, she's healthy. Whereas, being in the NICU for a year, I saw how fragile those babies were and how one little thing can really mess them up for a month or more. You know, it's not like a couple of days where they're a little off. It's long term, what could happen. And so I think that really helped me to see what really needed to be done in order to help protect them. [Brit]

With so many references to keeping one's self and one's milk pure or clean, it is clear that donors' care work is enacted in relation to the broader notion of the "pure maternal body" (Hausman 2011). Born into a world increasingly defined by risk and contamination, infants are characterized by purity and innocence (Hausman 2011), a position that is heightened by infant prematurity or hospitalization. This positions the breastfeeding mother, and now the breastmilk donor as a potential conduit for the contamination of infant purity (Hausman 2011). This notion is already commonplace among pregnant women who are advised to avoid certain foods and exposure to toxins for the sake of the growing fetus (Hausman 2011; Washburn 2014). Moreover, such ideals of maternal purity continue to be promoted post-partum by targeting breastfeeding mothers who are increasingly self-monitoring health behaviors and their local environment (Washburn 2014). This trend is also clearly articulated by donors to the extent that it calls forth practices that some donors would not otherwise enact in the production of extracorporeal breastmilk for their own infant.

The vigilance invested by the majority of donors in following donation guidelines is also evident in their action of withholding or discarding breastmilk from donation when their milk does not comply:

> I couldn't assure that I didn't take any Advil that day or the baby didn't have a runny nose that day, I couldn't remember that far back, so we decided that we would just feed the baby what has been frozen and I would go ahead and donate what I was pumping out at work, and in the evening before I went to bed. [Jackie]
> I decided he wasn't going to be able to use it, contacted the milk bank, they said no because of the fenugreek. It's a herbal supplement they don't want. They don't want anything. So my mom was here and we just threw it all away! [Emily]

The value that milk accrues, partly as a result of the efforts enacted, is one reason that women seek to donate their milk rather than discard it (Arnold and Borman 1996; Gerstein Pineau 2013). Thus, care does not always equate to affection, sympathy, and kindness directed toward another body, but also toward the donor's self.

Notions of purity, risk, and contamination are also played out in donors' hygiene practices. Milk donors are asked to be aware of hand hygiene and ensure they clean their breasts and breast pump before expressing. Some donors explained in great detail their personalized routines to ensure the milk is expressed in the most hygienic way possible:

> It's been kind of tricky because no one in the house can be sick! So just making sure that he's well, and then just getting the equipment ready. You have to make sure that it's either when he's taking a nap, or when he's really happy and situated, because you've got to get the pump out and get it all set up, and the worst thing is when you get it on and he starts fussing! Just getting things done, making sure the equipment's all cleaned … so you wash it, and you also do it with the sanitizing bags they give you in the microwave, so you make sure that's all dried, da-da-da, and then setting up, and after that, making sure you're storing it pretty quickly and doing the proper—they give you paper to make sure you're doing it as sanitary as possible, and store it … It's not no effort. Yeah. It's a little bit more effort than if I was doing it for him, but not that much, because you know, you're not quite as concerned about the sanitary aspect, because breastfeeding, you just breastfeed, whereas before you do that you have to wash the nipples and all that, and make sure your breasts are clean right before you do it. Yeah it's just a little bit more effort, but the main thing is just cleaning the pump and doing all that. [Jacqueline]
> At first I was not overwhelmed, but there was a lot to remember, on how to keep things clean and proper techniques. After a while it just became routine, and it wasn't that big of a deal. And I was kind of doing the same thing for Frankie

anyway, trying to be keeping everything clean, and making sure that once it was pumped it went right to the freezer, right to the fridge, so that it wasn't going to sit out. [Anne]

Once breastmilk had been expressed, donors explained that they also designed systems for adhering to the donation guidelines for storing and labeling their milk. Labeling and storage are also reliant upon donors' mindfulness of what she has ingested and whether or not household members have been sick.

Like, if I could donate it, I would just automatically put my number there, and if I couldn't donate it, I wouldn't. So that way I wouldn't get confused. [Brit]
Sometimes it's hard to keep track of, like, if you take an Ibuprofen, I just wouldn't label it with my donor number, and I would put it in my stash, because I kept a stash for when I had babysitters, and I had no issue giving my daughter milk that had Ibuprofen or even a glass of wine actually. I just wouldn't label it with a number and then it wouldn't get put into that bin. [Moggie]

Donors devised careful regimes of separation to ensure that milk suitable for donation to the HMB was kept apart from that which was intended for their own infant. During one interview, Jess, who is a nurse and mother of one, invited me to see her freezer and her system of segregation between milk for her son, and milk for the HMB. While showing me her freezer she explained:

These bags are a light purple color, and the milk bank ones are very blue, and they want me to stand them upright, so they sit differently. They're a different kind of plastic. And they have my name on and donor number written across the top in case I have any doubts! I have two different bags. I have the milk donor bag and I have the one I use to freeze milk, and so depending on what I have done in the last 24 hours depends on which bag I freeze it in. So, like, if I've taken Panadol because I have a headache, then that goes in that bag. [Jess]

The materials utilized by donors play a central role in their care work. Donors referred to their pump kits, microwaves, sterilization kits, fridges, and freezers. For milk labeling, donors also referred to the role of the differently colored plastic storage bags and marker pens for dating and segregating their milk. Donors also recounted in great detail their systems for demarcating areas in their freezers that are solely for storing milk for donation. By putting into words donors' regular use of these various material artifacts, the practices that constitute care work that would otherwise remain a hidden routine of domestic labor are now positioned as integral to milk donation.

CONCLUSION

In this chapter, the sheer number of practices that donors describe, and the detail with which they do so, reveals that the care work of donating milk to a HMB is a nuanced and heterogeneous activity. Many donation practices involve "doing," such as taking time to express milk, and partaking in cleaning and hygiene regimes. Other practices are less visible to an observer, and involve donors recalling donor guidelines, being mindful of their diet, withholding inappropriate milk from donation, and abstaining from certain medications, caffeine, and alcohol. Collectively, these careful practices constitute donors' care work.

Care has been criticized for reaffirming a dichotomy between those who are cared for and those doing the caring, thereby falsely creating an asymmetry that houses fragility on the one side and altruistic generosity on the other (Beasley and Bacchi 2005). Putting the care practices of milk donation into words is politically important as they can now obtain a presence in the distant sites "from where they are governed" (Mol 2010: 229). For instance, HMBs, health authorities, clinicians, and parents can now draw on what donors *actually do* to enrich their understandings, tinker with, or govern the specificities of care (Mol 2010) that donors practice.

Importantly, although donation guidelines are necessarily oriented towards the vulnerable recipient of donor milk, the specificities of care articulated in this chapter can blur the carer–cared-for dichotomy if they are used to inform and focus discussion on how lactating women themselves could be cared for as they continue to provide this important but largely invisible service to infants hospitalized in NICUs. This chapter presents a "logic of care" that takes the mortal and vulnerable body as its starting point (Mol 2008) and respects the donor's body as productive and competent (Mol 2010). By attuning ourselves to the donors' practices, the donor is now cast as an active agent whose practices may become increasingly visible in the production and donation of safe breastmilk. Importantly, donors' everyday care work should be integral to the deliberations associated with future policy-making on milk banking and the development of donation guidelines.

Acknowledgments

An Australian Research Council Discovery Grant DP110103025 (Chief Investigator, Dr. Katherine Carroll) and an Endeavour Fellowship funded this research. I would like to thank the University of Technology, Sydney Communication Studies Writing Group and Dr. Catherine Robinson for their valuable feedback on this chapter.

–12–

Women and Children First? Gender, Power, and Resources, and their Implications for Infant Feeding[1]

Vanessa Maher

THE RISE IN INTEREST IN BREASTFEEDING

There has been an exponential rise over the last few decades in the amount of attention devoted to breastfeeding, including the number of books and articles written. Some of these works have been dedicated to denouncing the damaging effects on children of the spread of bottle-feeding and the use of infant formula. In countries in which the greater part of the population has no access to a supply of safe drinking water or refrigeration, the bottle of formula becomes a vehicle of contamination and disease. In the wake of many infant deaths attributable to formula feeding and the subsequent public outcry, international legislation was passed to prohibit the advertising and promotion of infant formula (WHO 1981). Important organizations such as the WHO and UNICEF established guidelines for the promotion of breastfeeding wherever possible, since it was considered to confer important health advantages on babies and to prevent their falling victim to various diseases (WHO UNICEF 1989). However, advocates of breastfeeding were thrown into disarray in 1985 as the worldwide HIV/AIDS epidemic picked up speed and it was discovered that, in about a fifth of cases, the HIV virus (or one of the different HIV viruses) was transmitted from mother to child through breastmilk, and that the longer a child was breast-fed by an HIV-infected mother, the more likely the baby was to contract HIV/AIDS (see White 1999: 32; Piot UNAIDS 2001).

Whereas the immunological benefits of breastfeeding versus formula feeding had been established for a range of diseases threatening infants, in particular those giving rise to diarrhea, breastmilk suddenly appeared to be the vehicle of one of the most feared viruses to affect humankind. The choice for mothers seemed to be between opting for a long agony for a child infected with HIV through breastmilk or feeding the infant formula and risking its rapid death by diarrhea. Edith White suggests that many mothers expressed a preference for the second course of action (White 1999: 155, quoting Nicholl et al. 1995). However, for mothers in resource-poor settings, this meant giving up breastfeeding as a time-tested method of contraception, risking having more children.[2]

Never has it been so clear that there is no optimal solution to infant feeding in the modern world and that women's circumstances have a deter-mining influence on how they feed their babies and on the outcomes of their behavior. Thus our subject is not breastfeeding or bottle-feeding, or the recent spread of milk banks in different countries, or how medical advances or the HIV/AIDS epidemic have affected or been affected by these phenomena, or what women's choices are. We turn our attention rather to how women's infant feeding choices are limited, enhanced, or oriented by the circum-stances in which they live.

ECONOMIC, DEMOGRAPHIC, AND POLITICAL DISTINCTIONS BETWEEN COUNTRIES

Edith White, who has spent a lifetime promoting women's health and breast-feeding, points out in an authoritative work on the subject of breastfeeding and HIV/AIDS that it is useful to make several distinctions at the outset of our discussion (White 1999: 45). First, we must make distinctions among populations who live in resource-poor, resource-rich, and "emergent" countries. These countries differ not only as far as resources are concerned, but also demographically, and the problems posed by infant feeding are peculiar to each context. We may usefully compare the demography of the United States as a resource-rich country with that of Zambia as an example of a resource-poor country, and that of Brazil as an "emergent country" (*CIA World Fact Book* 2011).

In 2011 the total fertility rate in the United States was 2.06 children per woman, in Zambia it was 5.98, and in Brazil 2.18. There were 13.83 births per 1,000 population in the United States, 44.08 in Zambia, and 17.79 in Brazil.[3] The infant mortality rate in the United States was 6.06/1,000 births, in Zambia 66.6, and in Brazil 21.17. The life expectancy in the United States was 78.37, in Zambia 52.36 years, and in Brazil 72.53 years. On the other hand, the percentage of adults living with AIDS aged 15–49 was 0.6 in the U.S.A., 13.5 in Zambia, and 0.6 in Brazil, while those known to be infected in

Table 1: Comparative demographic data (Source: *CIA World Fact Book 2011*)

	U.S.A. (resource-rich)	Zambia (resource-poor)	Brazil "emergent"
Total fertility rate/ woman	2.06	5.98	2.18
Births/1,000	13.83	44.08	17.79
Infant mortality/1,000 births	6.06	66.6	21.17
Life expectancy/ years	78.37	52.36	72.53
Percentage adults living with AIDS aged 15–49	0.6	13.5	0.6
Total adults living with AIDS aged 15–49	1,200,000	980,000	730,000
Total population	312,000,000	13,800,000	203,400,000

the United States are 1,200,000 (out of 312 million), but in Zambia 980,000 (out of 13.8 million), in South Africa 5,600,000 (out of 49 million), but in Brazil 730,000 (out of 203.4 million) (see Table 1).

It is clear not only that the experience of women and children in these countries varies enormously, but also that the demographic structure and economic resources of Brazil, which we have described as an "emergent" country, are more similar to those of the United States than to those of Zambia. Some of the problems posed by the transmission of HIV/AIDS in breastmilk or by the feeding of premature and underweight infants may be dealt with in similar ways in the United States and in Brazil. But there are also resource-poor, resource-rich, and "emergent" social categories within a single country and, indeed, the resources to which we refer may be qualitatively, rather than quantitatively, differentiated: different kinds of employment, education, healthcare, gender relations, or kinship and belief systems may make it culturally appropriate to feed children in particular ways. In this volume we have several illustrations of all these differences.

METHODOLOGICAL PROBLEMS

Edith White points out that the terms used in the discussion of infant feeding are also differentiated and may lead to confusion. There are many differences between doctors' and researchers' language, midwives' language, and anthropologists' language and "discourse." The meanings of the concepts used—exclusive feeding, dominant breastfeeding, mixed feeding, formula feeding, and above all demand feeding—differ from profession to profession and may be alien to the mothers whose behavior they attempt to describe or influence. If the "experts" cannot agree on the meanings of the terms, it is difficult to believe that the women questioned as to their breastfeeding behavior grasp the sense of the queries to which they are replying. For this reason, we cannot be sure what the "statistics" on infant feeding really mean, because they are rarely based on direct and continuous observation.

The terms also mean different things in different cultural contexts. Fiona Dykes suggests, for example, that demand feeding in Britain is really time-dominated and so poles apart from the demand feeding practiced by Australian Aborigines or Kalahari desert wanderers (quoted in Crowther et al. 2009). We should "understand the power of our culturally embedded desire for orderliness and timeliness" and that "our hospitals are run like factories according to a deeply engrained institutional culture." But Gujerati women living in Britain say that "there is no time here" and that is why they stop breastfeeding. They experience notions of time as a form of external control on their choices (Crowther et al. 2009: 64).

ADVOCACY AND AGENCY IN THE LITERATURE ON BREASTFEEDING

It is useful to distinguish between the discourse of the advocates of breast-feeding and that of other researchers on infant feeding behavior and its outcomes who stress the need for women to acquire the "capability" to make the decision best suited to their circumstances (agency). As our authors point out, resource-poor countries often have high rates not only of maternal ill health and mortality but also of infant mortality due to causes other than HIV, such as malnutrition, diarrhea, and infectious and respiratory diseases, which flourish in more general conditions of poverty and the lack of sanitation and water. In this essay we will see that advocacy of breastfeeding emerges in particular in relation to women in resource-rich countries in which breast-feeding is not widely practiced. Breastfeeding advocates also tend to sustain the creation of milk banks.

The "research on agency" discourse tends to take into its compass women in resource-poor countries and communities and the economic and social constraints on women's decision-making, factors that the advocacy discourse does not often consider. Edith White writes that:

... advocacy for breast-feeding is not the same as advocacy for Third World women, especially when there is the problem of transmission of HIV. To advocate for universal breast-feeding is not the same as to advocate for women's right to make their own informed infant feeding decisions. (White 1999: 65; see also Carter 1995: 235)

Indeed, "agency" dialogue is not the same as "advocacy" dialogue and offers different frameworks for interpreting the controversy over infant formula.

In spite of their concern for women and children in resource-poor countries, the guidelines of international organizations such as WHO and UNICEF have been closer to breastfeeding advocacy than to agency discourse. The intent of the recommended approach (which is to maximize HIV-free survival chances for all infants) can be judged as benevolent, but the 2009 guidelines appear to show little respect for the autonomy of individual women. This apparent contradiction between benevolence and lack of respect for women's autonomy defines paternalism (Desclaux and Alfieri, Chapter 8).

THE PENDULUM OF POLICY

There has been confusion in policies and practice since 1985, when the transmission of AIDS through breastmilk was first discovered, while organizations hesitated to pass on to the field the medical discoveries and pondered suggestions for practice. Matthews (Chapter 9) points out the information *lag* lasting from 1991–8, between the time the guidelines were published, the time they filtered through to health personnel, and then to the women concerned. International agencies did not withdraw the imperative instruction to breastfeed, although new data on the transmission of AIDS through breast-feeding had become available many years before. Transmission rates were known in 1991, but only in 1998 did this knowledge produce a new policy statement on infant feeding. In 2001 the options were reduced to two—either exclusive breastfeeding with early weaning and possibly antiretroviral (ART) therapy, or formula feeding.

Matthews also highlights a *practice drag*, which was due to the persistence of contradictory messages and the inertia of government policies and propaganda as well as the embarrassment and resistance of health personnel and of the women themselves, who had previously been won over (you might say "converted") to a policy subsequently considered to be ill-advised (Matthews, Chapter 9). All the rhetoric evoking human rights, ethics, maternal affection, and responsibility for the life and death of children was brought to bear each time on health personnel, governments, and the women themselves, in order to convince them to promote or adopt one mode of infant feeding first and then its opposite in the presence of HIV/AIDS, both modes often in contradiction with local norms of kinship and maternal behavior. Researchers have noted the "polarization" of concepts in health personnel's discourse as breastfeeding is pitted against bottle-feeding. This dualism tends to delegitimize certain options, but those possible are many, and more "fuzzy" (Desclaux and Alfieri, Chapter 8). White lists the options open to HIV-infected mothers as:

> ... one feeding generic formula, feeding regular commercial formula, feeding homemade formulas or animal milks or semisolid foods, brief breast-feeding followed by rapid and complete cessation of breast-feeding, wet-nursing, the use of anti-retroviral drugs to treat mothers or babies, feeding mother's own expressed and heat-treated breastmilk, feeding heat-treated breastmilk from donors. (White 1999: 163)

The recommendation for HIV-infected women is exclusive breastfeeding and early weaning. Mixed feeding (breast and bottle or other supplementary feeding) is considered the worst option. However, in White's opinion, there is no society in the world where "exclusive breast-feeding" is normally practiced: women generally adopt different methods of feeding at different times, and often "mixed feeding." The WHO and other agencies often claimed to fear a "spill-over effect" to non-infected women, if HIV-infected women were advised not to breastfeed. For example, it was feared that a shift to formula, to stem the spread of HIV, might have repercussions in other fields, or cause a decline in the general rate of breastfeeding among women not affected by HIV and a rise in the infant morbidity rates related to the use of formula. One African health expert argues that the "WHO did not do its research on how African women feed babies when their mothers are unable to breast-feed and assumes that they cannot make decisions on their children's health." As for the "spill-over effect," "women had actually been spilling over into the non-breast-feeding group since the 1980s and it had nothing to do with formula distribution; there wasn't any" (Machekanyange 1997, in White 1999: 148).

ARE MOTHERS IN A POSITION TO MAKE INFORMED DECISIONS?

Women, according to WHO 2006 guidelines, should be helped to make their own informed decisions. In Europe, the kind of information to which most "informed mothers" have access is largely breastfeeding advocacy literature. When I perused recently the shelves of large bookshops in European and British university cities, I was struck by the fact that most works on breast-feeding consisted of "why to do it" and "how to do it" manuals, mainly addressed to mothers. These texts could be classified under the heading of "popular health" and, in contrast to the literature available in the 1990s, which still emphasized feeding intervals and quantities, such manuals are more likely to have realistic and practical advice as to how to breastfeed. However, they insist that "breast is best" and do not weigh up the advantages of one method of infant feeding against another for mothers in different social and economic contexts. Material on breastfeeding is rarely to be found in the scientific or medical sections of bookshops. This could suggest that medical students are not expected to be aware of the scientific and policy dilemmas posed by breastfeeding in the contemporary world, but rather to have assimilated "the advocacy discourse" and to encourage women to apply it. For most members of the medical profession, breastmilk is a biological substance transferred from mothers to children, and they do not consider its social or cultural meanings.

WHAT PREVENTS MOTHERS FROM BREASTFEEDING? SOCIAL CONTROL AND IDEAS OF THE "GOOD MOTHER"

It is partly because of this lack of awareness of the social and cultural meanings of breastfeeding that health experts in European countries, who had previously considered that the dissemination of information and a policy of promotion of breastfeeding would be decisive, have been disappointed by the statistics on breastfeeding. In a Wellcome Trust seminar held in London in 2007 entitled "The Resurgence of Breastfeeding," some participants who had been promoting breastfeeding in Britain for years felt that great strides had been made, but others deplored the lack of progress.

The breastfeeding statistics in the United States are also puzzling. Since the adoption in 2000 of the U.S. Health and Human Services Blueprint of Action on Breastfeeding, there has been a national campaign to encourage women to breastfeed for as long as possible and preferably "exclusively" for six months. Repeating almost the same phrases in these different years, in 2007 and 2010 Reuters reported the news issued by the Center for Disease Control and Prevention that there had been a "record rise" to 75 percent in initial breastfeeding. However, half of these mothers resorted to formula in the first week, and only 11 percent continued to feed "exclusively" up to six months. Common-sense views of breastfeeding in the States, perhaps affected by the long history of wet-nursing in Europe, do not appear to favor maternal breastfeeding. The problem of how common sense is formed has occupied social scientists for centuries but is ignored by many health experts (see Debucquet and Adt, Chapter 5). Should that common sense be changed—and by whom? As Karen Moland has pointed out in her work on the Chagga of Kilimanjaro, Tanzania, and as I myself wrote many years ago, the mode of infant feeding that women adopt in any given setting is related to cultural beliefs and many important social relationships (Maher 1992; Moland 2004). To change them is to threaten those relationships and question those beliefs, including local definitions of "the good mother." In resource-poor settings in which women commonly breastfeed for one or two years, but not exclusively, to adopt exclusive breastfeeding and rapid weaning or bottle-feeding will not only stigmatize them as "bad mothers" but also jeopardize many important relationships.

Richer countries, among them the United States and many European countries, have adopted the WHO guidelines in some form as part of their national health policies (see UKAMB and NHS documents). In these countries women are encouraged to breastfeed and those who choose not to do so are considered to be "bad mothers," and, increasingly, blamed for not giving their children the best start in life. (The exceptions are women with AIDS, who are discouraged from breastfeeding.) Breastfeeding is presented as a corrective or even a form of prevention of social and economic ills, although evidently these have economic and political, not biological or physiological, causes and need to be addressed by an input or redistribution of economic and political resources.

Many women in resource-rich countries have access to adequate health facilities and are greatly influenced by expert medical advice, which is generally in line with national health policies. In the United States, women in under-privileged groups, such as African Americans or Native Americans, who, for complex historical reasons, breastfeed less than others, are often judged to fall short of widespread expectations of "the good mother" and so held responsible for the social problems of the young in their communities (Blum 1999).

GENDER, POWER, AND RESOURCES

The effect of gender is rarely mentioned in connection with breastfeeding. As I have pointed out in earlier publications, the roles not only of male medical advisors but also of husbands and fathers are important in permitting, enjoining, or limiting breastfeeding, in determining the way in which it is done, by whom, and the time of weaning (Maher 1992). Even today, Senegalese migrant women in Verona say that it is the father or grandfather of the child who decides when it should be weaned; also. that a woman who exclusively breastfed her baby would be considered neglectful. She and other relatives should give water and paps from an early age (Faggionato 2010). Many groups expect the father to abstain from sexual activity during breastfeeding. This is not the same as the more common post-partum abstinence period for the mother only.

Men in some societies may be regarded as the "owners" of the milk and may incur milk kinship ties through their wife or mother breastfeeding other men's children. And, of course, so-called "structural milk kinship" (and often fostering and godparenthood) was arranged by men and accrued to men through their wife's nursing a child of another man. Societies vary in the degree to which fathers take responsibility for the child's welfare. To illustrate this point, we may mention that in many countries the distribution of food and other resources within the family is inequitable. Adult men are favored and the life expectancy of women and children is affected negatively. Men may limit or enhance women's access to resources but, obviously, they have an important influence on their sexual experience and its reproductive outcomes. A high infant mortality rate is likely to be associated with high fertility and increased social and physical burdens for women. We will see below that the tendency to ignore gender relations and men's roles may seriously affect national and international health policies and their outcomes but also hamper our under-standing of women's infant feeding and other behavior in the presence of HIV/AIDS. WHO guidelines are that health personnel should advise women with HIV/AIDS to adopt exclusive breastfeeding unless "replacement feeding is acceptable, feasible, affordable, sustainable and safe," but these conditions are rarely to be found.

Women cannot "choose" when their possibilities are foreclosed. Then they are an easy scapegoat for their children's plight. One of the main causes of children being born underweight and pre-term is the undernourishment, overwork, and ill health of their mothers. However, the solution to this problem lies in addressing gender inequalities, such as women's lack of land rights and access to food and other resources (Sweetman 2006). They own only 1 percent of the landed property in the world. Women do not hold title to land even where, as in Africa, they are the main food producers, but gain access to land through their husbands or male relatives. It is these relatives who make decisions and receive compensation if the land is used for non-agricultural purposes. The plight of HIV/AIDS widows who lose access to land on their husbands' deaths has often been pointed out (Nduati 2001). The current wave of "land grabbing" in Africa and Latin America by multinational corporations and the governments of resource-rich countries for the cultivation of biofuels has had a devastating impact on women's access to land and on the prices of food crops (Sweetman 2006).

WET-NURSING

Just as men tend to control breastfeeding, so historically they have often controlled wet-nursing. Italy is a case in point. Klapisch-Zuber analyzed the Florentine *ricordanze*, account books kept by men in professional and merchant families, from 1360–1530. Children were separated at birth from their mothers and sent to wet nurses, chosen and paid by the father, and for the period he deemed fit. The father controlled all communication with the wet nurse and her husband (Klapisch-Zuber 1985). Wet nurses from the Veneto were often hired in the nineteenth and even twentieth centuries by rich families in Milan or other cities, but the terms of their engagement were transacted by their fathers-in-law, who tended to pocket their earnings. The mothers appear as marginal figures *vis-à-vis* patriarchal structures, the wet nurses earning the lasting resentment of their own children, left for years without a mother (Perco 2010).

Joan Sherwood (2010) has pointed out that an ideology of maternal nursing dominated eighteenth-century Europe, despite the prevalence of wet-nursing. Doctors blamed puerperal illnesses on women's failure to breastfeed, though for decades puerperal fever was spread by the doctors themselves. Wet nurses were hired not only by well-to-do families, but in the years after the Renaissance also by people of other urban categories, in particular in Italy, and at least from the fifteenth century onwards by hospitals and orphanages in order to feed premature and orphaned babies. "Wet-nursing was a highly organized industry organized by the state as early as the thirteenth century" (Matthews Grieco 1991: 17). With the spread of syphilis in France in the eighteenth century, healthy wet nurses were asked to feed syphilitic orphans, thereby often contracting the disease themselves. Furthermore, they were instructed to take mercury. This was supposed to pass through their milk and cure the syphilitic baby, but often irremediably damaged the health of the wet nurse herself (Sherwood 2010). The idea that breastfeeding is embedded in motherhood resulted in Europe from particular health policies which used the rhetoric of motherhood even while they employed non-maternal nursing as a form of "technology" (Sherwood 2010; Pomata 1980: 497–542). When wet-nursing was managed by the medical profession in nineteenth- and twentieth-century European hospitals, authority was invested in male doctors. The wet nurses were hirelings who had to obey the doctors and were criticized if they nursed the children of relatives or friends on their own initiative.

Pomata (1980) examined the personal records of unmarried mothers in lying-in hospitals in Rome, as well as medical and obstetrical material from foundling hospitals, in order to reconstruct the experience of mothers and children and the attitudes of doctors and administrative staff towards them. Important changes took place at the end of the ninteenth and the beginning of the twentieth centuries. In fact, while the civil code initially allowed parents to remain anonymous, maternity gradually became a "social obligation"[4] and mothers were pressured to assume responsibility for illegitimate offspring. No such pressures were exerted on fathers who remained anonymous. In the 1920s the medical debate came to see artificial feeding, often resulting in gastroenteritis, as the main cause of mortality among illegitimate offspring (these estimated to be a quarter of all born in 1933). The illness of the babies was used to exhort mothers to accept their illegitimate children in order to breastfeed and bring them up according to medical dictates, and sometimes to feed other children in the orphanages associated with the hospitals. Paradoxically, wet-nursing—even though doctors were against it because it was believed to spread syphilis—justified the keeping of records on lower-class women and gave doctors the right to inquire into their sexual behavior. The Wasserman test for syphilis (introduced in 1906) enabled doctors to know if a woman was infected. Rarely were women informed of their condition, since this would have made it more difficult for hospitals to find wet nurses, and they could have claimed higher rates of pay. The doctor intervened "to control contagion" but blamed the spread of syphilis on women's promiscuity. Though men were obviously infecting women, as in the case of prostitutes, by law only women were regularly examined for venereal diseases.

Pomata (1980) wrote of a particular *structure of attention* in the medical profession and in the general population. Although TB, like other infectious diseases, was widespread during the early decades of the last century and devastating for children, its implications for breastfeeding were seldom discussed. The close contact between mother and child required for exclusive breastfeeding increased the probability of a TB-infected mother passing her illness to her child through her breath, but the rhetoric on the maternal duty to breastfeed and the attention paid to syphilis prevented any measures being taken, since these would have required the separation of mother and child and the recourse to other forms of feeding. Breastfeeding was considered to be endangered by promiscuous sexual behavior. Pomata (1980) points out that the sanction was only on women using their sexual capacities promiscuously, but in a mercantile culture this could not be prevented.

As other writers have pointed out, there are many parallels between the history of the medical management of syphilis in Europe and the management of HIV/AIDS in Africa and elsewhere. The discovery that HIV/AIDS can be transmitted through breastmilk has led to the testing, control, and stigmatization of women for their sexual behavior and their inadequacy as mothers. No such discourse seems to be directed towards men. The structure of attention tends to make women appear to be responsible for the death of their children. Such stigmatization derives both from the attitudes of the medical and health agencies and from the women's local and social environment. Few attempts seem to be made to defend women from the effects of severe gender inequality, although such a policy might help them to resist AIDS, avoid commercial and unprotected sex, and above all bear fewer and healthier children.

MILK KINSHIP, MILK BANKS, AND THE CONFUSION OF KIN

Wet-nursing is sometimes linked in the discussion of breastfeeding to the institution of milk kinship, which is found in different societies with different implications. Perhaps the main distinction worth making is that in societies that recognize milk kinship, nursing another woman's child is viewed positively; in Morocco, the milk may even have magic and curative properties. In stratified European societies, in contrast, wet-nursing has often signified social inequality and the fear of the contamination of one social category by another. Although commercial wet-nursing is mentioned in medieval Islamic texts, in Muslim societies most non-maternal breastfeeding is viewed positively as a gift that creates kinship (Gil'adi 1999). Kinship has many social and political functions and milk kinship is one way of forging alliances based on trust and loyalty. I think it is important to consider this in the light of Peter Parkes's (2006) work on the history of the Hindu Kush in North Pakistan and on what he calls alternative kinship structures, but also in relation to gender. Fosterage, milk kinship, and godparenthood (Altorki 1980; Goody 1983; Khatib-Chahidi 1992; Parkes 2006) are considered structurally equivalent by Parkes. Hammel writes of such "alternative structures among Christian and pre-Christian Serbs and in general in the Balkans." The idea of milk kinship in the Hindu Kush is that of accumulated links that create networks of allegiance over the generations, overriding rival and stratified patrilineal and segmentary formations. These networks are counterbalanced or reinforced by hypergamous marriages linking together different levels of the society. In comparable contexts, kinship—constructed through either fosterage or godparenthood—thus constituted a politically vital regime of replicable allegiances between kin groups and houses analogous to that of prescriptive marital alliances among the Kachin of Highland Burma (Parkes 2006: 28–9). In the Hindu Kush, there could never be enough property or produce to go round and milk kinship allowed rival sibling princes to create networks of allegiance which would allow them to seize power. "Milk kinship arguably held this fissiparous kingdom together in pre-colonial times; as one hugely quarrelsome foster-family, a literally 'galactic' (i.e., milk-connected) polity" (Parkes 2006: 26–7). It would be interesting to see how this applies in the warlord-torn Hindu Kush today. In the Mediterranean many forms of dyadic milk relationship are apparently unlinked to structure and lack political implications, except that in wet-nursing (but not always with milk kinship) the milk-giver is usually of inferior status to the milk-taker (Pomata 1980; Parkes 2006). It is difficult to gauge the long-term implications of feeding others' children at the expense of one's own. However, it is important to note that, even in twentieth- and twenty-first-century contexts, milk kinship emerges not only as a Muslim or Middle Eastern institution.

In some parts of Albania, particularly in the north, the political use of milk kinship has had some currency until recently and certainly some Albanian women breastfeed one another's children, even today. In Gambia, milk circulates within but not between tribes, serving to create boundaries between them. Women do not give or take milk from women of other "tribes." Kinship terms in these contexts may be used for people with whom there is no genealogical/biological relationship but with whom there are forms of collaboration and common interests. Breastfeeding, in any case, is considered to create relationships. Parkes's discussion omits every reference to women cross-nursing on their own account and whether in the long run this could have structural implications. However, for many women, kinship is a relationship of "closeness" created by various means, and among them is breastfeeding. Not breastfeeding may serve to reinforce political and religious boundaries across certain lines.

Wet-nursing in Europe, in contrast, appears to have been rife with suspicion and exploitation. Wet nurses were poor women who breast-fed children that were not theirs, usually at the expense of their own. Although their milk often kept children alive, it was considered potentially "dangerous" by mothers and doctors alike. It did not create kinship; rather it reinforced the symbolic separation between families with different economic and social destinies. In Europe and the United States, negative attitudes to women breastfeeding in the male-dominated public space may have had an important impact on their infant feeding choices.

WET-NURSING AND MILK BANKS

Little love was lost between mothers and wet nurses either in Europe in the eighteenth and nineteenth centuries or in the United States in the twentieth century. Doctors too regarded them with suspicion and contempt. Since they were poor women, great importance was attached to ensuring that their habits and characters were not detrimental to the children. Wolf (1999) maintains that the association of breastfeeding with poor women discouraged well-to-do mothers in Chicago from breastfeeding their own children, and these attitudes were carried over to the first milk banks in the United States. Although midwives persuaded mothers to donate their milk to the milk station, attempting to lift the mercenary stigma and represent the relation between donor and receiver as a "moral transaction," receiving women were not generally grateful to the donors:

> By 1929 at least twenty American cities provided bottled breastmilk to sick and premature infants through human milk stations ... milk stations began where wet- nursing ended, amidst class rancour, nativism, racism and distrust of human milk. (Wolf 1999)

The solution to the contemporary dilemma over breastfeeding during the HIV/ AIDS pandemic is sometimes seen to lie in the direction of the establishment of milk banks and the recruiting of healthy donors of breastmilk for those children who would risk death or debilitating diseases from being fed formula or non-human milk. However, it is here that our ploy of distinguishing between countries with different demographic structure and resource endowments becomes crucial. Some resource-rich countries are better endowed with milk banks than others and obviously they are of different capacities. Almost all of them are not commercial. The women who give their milk are regarded as donors, and their milk is ideally a gift to an unknown baby, though often it is used for their own.

However, these are countries with a history of non-maternal nursing and relatively early weaning. In the first several decades of the twentieth century many women fed formula to their infants according to a rigid timetable.

Nowadays, health services encourage breastfeeding, but may advise or even oblige HIV-infected mothers to feed formula to their children. Milk banks are used not so much for the children of HIV-infected mothers as for the needs of premature and sick infants. In these countries, advanced medical technology allows even extremely premature infants to survive. Many babies are delivered by caesarean section (around 30 percent in Europe and in the United States), making breastfeeding more difficult to establish. In the United States many babies from disadvantaged groups, such as African Americans and Native Americans, are born underweight (less than 2.5 kilos), and these too may have feeding problems and may benefit from donor milk. But in resource-poor countries, where most women would normally breastfeed for long periods, the most urgent problem is seen to be that of preventing the transmission of HIV/AIDS through breastmilk. So the problems of resource-rich countries in which milk banks help to solve the problem of premature births and the unintended consequences of advanced medical technology appear at first sight to be different from the main concern of resource-poor countries in Africa, namely the transmission of HIV/AIDS.

Milk banks have often been considered too expensive for resource-poor African countries where the health budget is $11 per year per person, compared to $2,000 per person in the United States. Milk banks require facilities for testing women for diseases, such as hepatitis or HIV, which can be transmitted through breastmilk, for collecting, storing, testing, freezing milk, melting it over water, testing it again for bacterial cultures, freezing, distributing it, and finally feeding the milk to the baby. A pre-term infant may not need human milk from a milk bank for as long as the child of an HIV-affected mother because, if she is lucky, her mother may be able to feed her after a few weeks. In this way, a given quantity of milk could provide for the needs of more pre-term infants than infants at risk from HIV. Remarkable work has been done by physicians and health personnel in Brazil, an "emergent country" with pockets of extreme deprivation. Milk banks in Brazil have existed in an unorganized way since the 1930s, but since the 1980s they have been developed with determination and did not shut down, like those of other countries, in the 1980s and 1990s during the HIV/AIDS epidemic. Between 1980 and 2008 they have helped to reduce infant mortality from around 90/1,000 to 22/1,000. In 1998 the Brazilian Milk Bank Network of 193 local and regional milk banks was set up, distributing milk to nearly 200,000 sick and premature children every year, providing counseling and promoting breastfeeding among local mothers and helping mothers of pre-term infants to establish their own supply. There is no need to test for HIV since it is eliminated by the pasteurization process, but missing ingredients may have to be added. The Brazilian Milk Bank network has announced:

> We are discussing how to adapt our work to Africa. But there are crucial differences, due to climate conditions, conditions of health and hygiene, important questions for the cold chain. Once collected, milk has to be kept at a low temperature, and this is more complicated in Africa.

To establish milk banks on a scale large enough to meet the requirements of the vast numbers of HIV/AIDS-infected mothers in Africa or other resource-poor countries seems a formidable task. But this may be a question of perspective and, as with wet nurses and syphilis in nineteenth-century Europe, such a perspective may stem from the tendency of organizations and local communities to avoid "community responsibility" and to blame women for their children's fate, focusing on a disease seen as sexual in origin, and so stigmatizing women and issuing unrealistic directives rather than listening to what they have to say. What they say is that they need more food. The primary cause of the death of children under one year old is not their mother's HIV but their mother's hunger and overwork, to which we may attribute many pre-term births.

The children of HIV-infected women, however, have a higher risk of low birth weight, pre-term delivery, and perinatal mortality. Ruth Nduati (2001) and others point out that people with HIV have a high metabolic level and need extra food that few of them receive or have energy enough to procure. Lactation is another demand on HIV-infected women's energies. In a randomized Kenyan study carried out between 1992 and 1998, HIV-infected women who breastfed for an average of 17 months lost weight and had a threefold risk of dying (10 percent) compared to those who did not breastfeed. A total of 69 percent of these deaths were attributable to breastfeeding. In studies in Tanzania these outcomes have been impeded by the distribution of micronutrients (Nduati 2001, citing Fawzi et al.).[5]

Ruth Nduati writes:

> In Africa, reduced transmission of HIV has not translated into improved survival of children of HIV-infected women. In addition to preventing viral transmission, much more needs to be done to improve the well-being of young infants in Africa. We must target *women* [my emphasis] to improve birth outcomes and the nutritional status of children. We can improve lactation performance and improve survival of mothers so there are fewer orphans. (Nduati 2001: 58)

The lack of resources for women translates into a high rate of pre-term and underweight babies, and then high rates of perinatal mortality. Most neonatal deaths (99 percent) occur in the developing world. There are 13 million pre-term births worldwide every year, of which 27 percent end in death (about 3.5 million), compared to 2 million deaths from HIV/AIDS. The deaths of 3.5 million babies, to which we may add 3.2 million stillbirths, are caused by pre-term births. A total of 7.5 percent of births in high-income countries are pre-term, 8.8 percent in middle income, 12.5 percent in least-developed regions, and 25 percent in Africa. In the United States 1 in 8 children (12 percent) is born before 37 weeks' gestation, but 18.4 percent of babies born to African Americans are pre-term, and 13.5 percent among Native Americans and Alaskans (Lawn et al. 2010). The trend is upwards. The American rates went up from 10.6 percent in 1990 to 12 percent in 2005, and in Brazil from 4 percent in 1983 to 12 percent in 2004. A trend analysis in Canada suggests that a significant part of this increase is due to caesarean section for poor fetal growth. Lawn et al. declare:

> The numbers discussed in this report are largely on par with the issues considered the greatest priorities in global health today and indeed larger than some that receive major attention, such as two million annual HIV/AIDS deaths. Yet pre-term birth and particularly stillbirth are not included among global priorities. (2010: 20)

If we add to these figures the large number of orphans whose mothers die in childbirth or from other causes, the problem of finding a way to feed infants when their mothers cannot do so looms large. Although the scale of this problem seems to defy solution by means of milk banks only, there have been some courageous initiatives in Africa that have tended to show that the provision of human milk to needy infants is a question of organization and creativity rather than of a vast and expensive technical apparatus.

Dr. Peter McCormick, working in Cameroon, discovered that several factors compounded the risks for children, chief among them high maternal mortality and malnutrition (Arnold 2010). In West Africa, 40 percent of children under the age of five die. Mothers are often sick at birth or don't lactate readily. For pre-term babies, the "kangaroo mother" is unheard of. Because of kin and gender hierarchy, women cannot make decisions for themselves and their babies. In hospitals, pediatricians are responsible for finding milk for needy, sick, or pre-term infants, otherwise they violate the UN Convention on the Rights of the Child. They must find a way to bridge the time between birth and the establishment of breastfeeding and provide milk for orphans.

One way in which McCormick did this was to look for surrogate mothers (they might be aunts or even grandmothers) and encourage relactation. In spite of the HIV/AIDS pandemic, in Cameroon, as in the rest of the world, exclusive breastfeeding is uncommon and the hospital staff is often unaware of its importance. McCormick set up milk banks following the example of Anna Coutsoudis in South Africa, who inaugurated a system of pasteurizing donated breastmilk for HIV orphans (Arnold 2010).

Coutsidis and McCormick demonstrated that the costs need not be high. Breastfeeding mothers have to be persuaded to donate their milk, and parents to accept it, which, as we will see below, is not easy. Hospitals need labs for bacterial screening and their staff a place to pasteurize donated milk. The apparatus has to be simple and the program sustainable and self-perpetuating.

McCormick described how the hospital staff persuaded healthy mothers (identified by a questionnaire) at infant welfare clinics to give their milk and 50 percent agreed to do so. The samples of milk were incubated overnight on blood agar. Simple apparatus from UKAMB (single-bottle pasteurizer) was purchased in the U.K. at a price affordable by the small trust founded by McCormick and shipped to recipient hospitals, together with low-cost plastic bottles and sterile lab containers. Glass bottles from a local hotel were collected, washed, and sterilized using electric kettles. All this equipment was put in a sturdy container. The total cost of each kit was $1,000, including shipping. Protocols were formulated for the expression of donor milk, the hand hygiene of donors and nurses, and for pasteurization. The HIV virus is destroyed by pasteurization for 30 minutes at 62 degrees Celsius and thermo-sensitive stickers on bottles provide proof that the right temperature has been maintained. Five Cameroonian hospitals adopted these procedures and set up milk banks.

How much milk was provided? McCormick calculated that five clinics of 40 mothers and babies each could provide 500 liters a year if half of the mothers became donors. "This is a worthwhile low cost, low technology, small scale life-saving project, tailored to the need of a resource-poor world" (Peter McCormick, Volunteer Children's Physician, Founder, Beryl Thyer Memorial Africa Trust) (Arnold 2010: 374).

In 2009 the population of the United States was estimated at 310 million, with only 34,000 liters banked—68 times the product of the five Cameroon milk bank kits for around 18 times the population (though with a different demographic profile), and so proportionally only about four times as much. So, *in theory*, in Cameroon they would only have to provide 15 more kits to reach the same level as the United States. *In practice*, we are dealing with populations with different levels of nourishment and general health, living in different conditions, as the Brazilian milk banking experts pointed out.[6]

WHAT DO WOMEN THINK?

In many African countries women persist in breastfeeding babies in the way they always have because they cannot afford or have no access to formula, or because to change the way they feed would cause them to be identified as HIV-infected, a result which in some cases may bring about divorce or social ostracism (Moland 2004: 91–2). Women do not like being tested because they think that to be found to be HIV-positive can only worsen their position vis-à-vis their husband, kin, and community, and it is difficult to see how being tested will save their children. Even in the absence of men, young women are usually not "autonomous," but are subordinate to and dependent on mothers and mothers-in-law, who condition their options. In a Kenyan study, although 98 percent of mothers breastfed, only 34 percent said they would be willing to breastfeed exclusively for three months, only 9 percent would choose to heat-treat expressed breastmilk, only 12 percent would consider using a milk bank, considering it culturally unacceptable, and only 35 percent would allow a wet nurse to feed her child. Most women did not know how to modify cows' milk for infant consumption. A sample of women in South Africa thought all babies had been infected with HIV by breastfeeding, but 77 percent went on breastfeeding all the same, and in Tanzania so did 95 percent of a sample of mothers affected by HIV/AIDS (Thairu 2001: 63–72).

The WHO 2009 guidelines state that women's preference is for the action with the best evidence to support it, though they acknowledge that some recommendations are made with weak evidence to support them. The evidence is weak because the statistics are unreliable. How many are affected by AIDS in African countries? The lack of reliable information leaves the way open for suspicion, rumors, and adverse propaganda. In south-western Tanzania, traditional healers consider that AIDS is a foreign disease that can be treated only by foreign medicines. In Malawi this is also the case: the term EDZI is "meaningless" in local terms (Matthews, Chapter 9). For Central, East, and West Africa, AIDS is an American disease sent to control family size, or even a "government disease." Senegalese women consider that the government's withdrawal of formula or the change of policy in favor of exclusive breastfeeding and ART is a ploy on the part of agencies that can provide a solution, but consider that African women and children matter less than European or American ones.

THE ROLE OF MIGRATION IN SPREADING AIDS, DESTABILIZING BREASTFEEDING, AND DISCOURAGING CROSS-NURSING

In some breastfeeding societies, such the Tanzanian Wagogo in the first half of the twentieth century, a check on the quality of breastmilk was provided by the fact that the partners of men and women were known. Each married woman had an institutional lover who, like her husband, was obliged to observe a post-partum taboo on sexual intercourse when she was breast-feeding (Mabilia 2006). A woman's baby might give and receive milk from a limited number of others, whose observance of the taboos, like that of their menfolk, was known to her and them. The restrictions on the number of partners and the notoriety surrounding the sexual behavior of both men and women made it easier to space births and limit eventual illnesses. This system collapsed with the growth of salaried work and migration to the towns of men, and in the 1980s and 1990s AIDS began to spread. We may say that migration brings about the demise of community controls on sexuality, especially on those that involve men in ensuring the safety of breastfeeding. Migration, on the other hand, is a source of cash and consumer goods. Many women who began to feed formula to their children could hardly have done so without the remittances of migrants, whether national or international. Migrants live in countries with different habits and opportunities. The falling rates of exclusive breastfeeding in countries such as Morocco (20 percent at four months in 1987, 10 percent in 2009, see UNICEF 2010) may be due not only to the entry of women into the labor market but also to their increasing familiarity with non-breastfeeding habits in other countries. On the positive side, migrants may be able to promote and finance projects like those described by Peter McCormick (Arnold 2010).

In Italy an association of students and professionals from Guinea-Bissau, many of whom are nurses, doctors, chemists, and laboratory technicians, was founded two years ago. I attended a meeting in Verona where they declared their intention of helping to improve health facilities in their home country. Since the rate of infant mortality in Guinea-Bissau is the highest in West Africa, it would seem that the provision of small milk bank kits and the training of local personnel in using them could be an excellent start.

However, the best approach would empower women by dealing directly with those economic, social, and political factors that prevent them from being able to make decisions in their own interest or avoid risky and unprotected sex or childbearing. In Verona I have come to know the members of the NGO Child in India Institute, which has operated for nearly 40 years in West Bengal and other areas of India for the benefit of women and children, and has fund-raising branches in different countries, including Italy. Its founder, the medical physician Dr. Samir Chaudhuri, has received several international rewards, and has gradually built up a team to run a network of clinics for mothers and children and educational projects for street children and the children of poor families. His intent has been to reduce the enormous number of children born pre-term and underweight by providing care and food for pregnant mothers, and for mother and child until the child is two years old. One project to this end is called "Adopt a Mother." The scheme is now part of a government program and involves millions of women and children living in poverty. It does not limit its approach to a clinical one, but addresses gender inequalities across the board.

As a development of the work of CINI (Children In Need Institute), the initiative Child and Woman-Friendly Communities has recently signed an agreement with the Panchayat and Rural Development Department of the government of West Bengal to train 25,000 women from mutual help groups, who will transfer their knowledge in the field of health and the nutrition of mothers and babies to around 200,000 women. The groups will also be given loans to undertake economic activities to improve their individual incomes and together promote development in the villages. The women will undertake enquiries and assessment of needs in their own communities, they will be involved in the preparation of school meals, in the maintenance of birthing clinics in the local health centers, and will act as local health workers and midwives. A project of social marketing has been set up to launch Nutrimix, a low-cost food to combat child malnutrition. The link between income-generating activities and those aimed at promoting child survival and protection is intended to overcome conditions of abject and deeply rooted poverty. By reinforcing the partnership with government decision-makers, the women get involved in decision-making processes as citizens with rights (Riggio, in Maher [ed.] 2011). In this way, by tackling general problems related to gender, power, and resources, women may acquire real decision-making capacity. By intervening earlier in a negative reproductive cycle, funds, lives, and human dignity may be saved.

Notes

FOREWORD

1 This is a concept I am further elaborating in a book I am writing with Richard O'Connor, called the *Dance of Nurture*.
2 Please note there are two authors named Wolf who have published on breast-feeding issues: Jacqueline H. and more recently and controversially Joan B.
3 This is an interview and therefore should be recognized as an off-the-cuff remark. The research between breastfeeding and allergies has been contro-versial (see Matheson et al. 2012). Pediatric gastroenterologist and food allergy researcher with Murdoch Children's Research Institute in Australia Professor Katie Allen has been widely quoted in saying experts now believe "that breastfeeding neither causes nor prevents food allergy."
4 There are a number of examples of food made using human milk. For instance, in 2010, Daniel Angerer served a "Mommy's Milk Cheese" at his restaurant, Klee Brasserie in New York, which had been made from his partner's breastmilk. In 2011 another widely publicized example occurred with the opening of "The Lady Cheese Shop," a temporary art installation by Miriam Simun, a graduate student at New York University, who offered samples of cheese made from human milk. That same year, in London at Icecremists, a breastmilk-infused and flavored ice cream, originally called "Baby Gaga," was sold. In March 2012 these stories inspired a workshop held at Keele University in the U.K., entitled "The Baby Gaga Saga: Regulation of Human Products and the Politics of Breastfeeding." The opening paper was presented by Dr. Tanya M. Cassidy, one of the editors of this volume.

INTRODUCTION

1 Considered to be the father of ethnography, Malinowski's (1922) most famous ethnographic work was published only a few years prior to Mead's work on Samoa.
2 The use of the word "breastmilk," as one word, is common in the lactation advocacy and research community, particularly in Australia. In North America there is a movement towards wanting to use the term "human milk," as Penny Van Esterik points out in the foreword of this volume.

CHAPTER ONE

1   It is important to note that the amount of milk obtained by pumping does not accurately reflect the amount that a breastfeeding infant can remove from the breast.

CHAPTER TWO

1   The overwhelming majority of breastmilk donors are female and also identify as women and mothers. However, evidence from ongoing milk sharing research demonstrates that breastmilk donors may also include persons who describe their gender as male, transgendered, and/or queer.
2   Other terms for milk sharing that are commonly used include "peer-to-peer," "casual milk sharing," "cross-nursing," "modern wet-nursing."
3   The University of Massachusetts Breastmilk Lab is run by Dr. Kathleen Arcaro, http://www.breastmilkresearch.org
4   This quote appeared on one of the Eats on Feets Facebook pages in 2013, and is ascribed to Shell Walker, the Phoenix, Arizona midwife who began the organization in 1991 as a local exchange network. Eats on Feets is said to be a play on Meals on Wheels, an often-government-supported and community-administered food service provision.

CHAPTER FOUR

1   A condensed version of this article appears as Faircloth, C. (2013), "'Intensive Motherhood' in Comparative Perspective: Feminism, Long-term Breastfeeding and Attachment Parenting in London and Paris," in C. Faircloth, D. Hoffman, and L. Layne, L. (eds) *Parenting in Global Perspective: Negotiating Ideologies of Kinship, Self and Politics*. London and New York: Routledge.
2   These are women who practice an "attachment parenting" philosophy in addition to being members of LLLI. Classification is based on statistics and responses derived from the questionnaire—that is, those women breastfeeding their children beyond a year—as well as the author's observations at groups meetings and interviews.
3   These statistics should be read cautiously. "Initiation" means that the baby is put to the breast once. After one week in the U.K., over a third of women are not breastfeeding, and by six weeks, that figure is well over half (DH, Infant Feeding survey 2005). These were the rates correct at the time of research from the DH and MS surveys (Ministère de la Santé 2005). The most recent *report* at the time of research available in France (2002), however, puts the rate of initiation

at 52 percent with an average duration of 10 weeks: www.sante.gouv.fr/htm/ pointsur/nutrition/allaitement.pdf) (last accessed April 2, 2009).

4 An organization based in France with 30 member countries including France, Germany, Italy, Japan, New Zealand, Australia, the U.K. and the United States committed to democracy and the market economy.

5 The following statistics are taken from the data set http://stats.oecd.org/ wbos/default.aspx?DatasetCode=LFS_D (accessed December 2, 2008).

6 This was the case at the time of research; recent (2008) measures have extended standard maternity leave to one year. See: http://www. direct.gov.uk/en/Parents/Moneyandworkentitlements/WorkAndFamilies/ Pregnancyandmaternityrights/DG_10029285 (accessed December 2, 2008), now at https://www.gov.uk/maternity-leave.

7 These are the national, standardized rates of maternity leave. Some women— particularly in the U.K. sample—had more generous maternity packages. Women also have the option of taking extended periods of unpaid leave.

8 www.babyfriendly.org.uk/page.asp?page=213 (accessed February 26, 2009). Now at www.unicef.org.uk/BabyFriendly/About-Baby-Friendly/ Breastfeeding-in-the-UK

9 http://www.lllfrance.org/allaitement-information/hopital-ami-bebe.htm# (accessed April 23, 2009).

10 Save Solidarilait, which is more strictly a campaigning organization.

11 Indeed, the word "Parenting" as a description of a genre of literature is in debate, which is an interesting social comment in itself. Some informants would use *Parentalité* (the state of being a parent, which renders 400,000 hits on Google.fr) in place of *Parentage* (accessed April 23, 2009).

12 There are, of course, criticisms of pumping from another perspective, in that it is seen as a way of doubling the labor women have to carry out—to both express and bottle feed—becoming another pressure point for women who can't (or don't want) to breastfeed (Blum 1999).

13 "Quand Superwoman Rentre à la Maison." http://www.elle.fr/elle/societe/ les-enquetes/quand-superwoman-rentre-a-la-maison/la-fin-du-feminisme/ (gid)/740943 (accessed April 23, 2009).

14 http://www.guardian.co.uk/world/2010/feb/12/france-feminism-elisabeth-badinter (accessed November 3, 2010). See also http://www.guardian.co.uk/ commentisfree/2011/apr/01/france-breast-breastfed-baby-death for an interesting comment piece on breastfeeding in France (accessed January 15, 2013).

CHAPTER FIVE

1 Please note this chapter was translated by Chadai Cassidy Boulos, with Tanya Cassidy.

2   This chapter deals with NUPEM sociological and anthropological task that has been carried by LESMA-AUDENCIA Laboratory, whose head is Mohamed Merdji.
3   An intermediary ideal-type has also been found (see Table 2), but in this chapter we will be focusing on the two extreme ideal-types because of the higher internal consistency of mothers' discourses.

CHAPTER SEVEN

1   UNICEF published an extensive report with current percentages in 2013.

Qur'anic verses on breastfeeding and wet-nursing.

(1): The mothers shall give suck
For two whole years,
If the father desires
To complete the term.
But shall bear the cost
Of their food and clothing
On equitable terms.
No soul shall have
A burden laid on it
Greater than it can bear.
No mother shall be
Treated unfairly
On account of the child.
Nor father
On account of the child,
An heir shall be chargeable
In the same way.
If they both decide
On weaning,
By mutual consent,
And after due consultation,
There is no blame on them.
If they decide
On a foster mother
For your offspring,
There is no blame on you,
Provided ye pay (the mother)
What ye offered,
On equitable terms.
But fear God and know

That God sees well what ye do.
(Ali 1983: 93; chapter 2, verse 233)

(2): Prohibited to you
(For Marriage) are
Your mothers, daughters,
Sisters; father's sisters,
Mother's sisters; brother's daughters,
Sister's daughters; foster-mothers
(Who gave you suck), foster-sisters;
Your wives' mothers;
Your step-daughters under your
Guardianship, born of your wives
To whom ye have gone in,
No prohibition if ye have not gone in;
(Those who have been)
Wives of your sons proceeding
From you loins;
And two sisters in wedlock
At one and the same time,
Except for what is past;
For God is Oft-forgiving,
Most Merciful.
(Ali 1983, 186; chapter 4, verse 23)

(3): The day ye shall see it,
Every mother giving suck
Shall forget her suckling-babe,
And every pregnant female
Shall drop her load (unformed):
Though shalt see mankind
As in drunken riot,
Yet, not drunk: but dreadful
Will be the Wrath of God.
(Ali 1983: 850; chapter 22, verse 2)

(4): So We sent this inspiration
To the mother of Moses:
"Suckle (they child), but when
Thou hast fears about him,
Cast him into the river,
But fear not nor grieve:
For We shall restore him
To thee, and We shall make

Him one of Our apostles."
(Ali 1983: 1003; chapter 28, verse 7)

(5): And We have enjoined on man
(To be good) to his parents:
In travail upon travail
Did his mother bear him.
And in years twain
Was his weaning: (hear
The Command), "Show gratitude
To Me and to thy parents:
To Me is (they final) Goal."
(Ali 1983: 1083; chapter 31, verse 14).

(6): We have enjoined on man
Kindness to his parents:
In pain did his mother
Bear him, and in pain
Did she give him birth.
The carrying of the (child)
To his weaning is
(A period of) thirty months.
At length, when she reaches
The age of full strength
And attains forty years,
He says, "O my Lord!
Grant me that I may be
Grateful for Thy favour
Which Thou hast bestowed
Upon me, and upon both
My parents, and that I
May work righteousness
Such as Thou mayest approve;
And be Gracious to me
In my issue. Truly
Have I turned to Thee
And truly do I bow
(To Thee) in Islam."
(Ali 1983: 1370; chapter 46, verse 15)

(7): Let the women live
(in *'iddat*) in the same
Style as ye live,
According to your means:

Annoy them not, so as
To restrict them.
And if they carry (life
In their wombs), then
Spend (your substance) on them
Until they deliver
Their burden; and if
They suckle your (offspring)
Give them their recompense:
And take mutual counsel
Together, according to
What is just and reasonable.
And if ye find yourselves
In difficulties, let another
Woman suckle (the child)
On the father's behalf.
(Ali 1983, 1564–5; chapter 65, verse 6)

CHAPTER EIGHT

1   Research program ANRS 1271, held by Aix-Marseille University (CReCSS: Centre de Recherche Cultures, Santé, Sociétés, JE 2424) and Institut de Recherche pour le Développement (UMI TransVIHMI), and funded by Agence Nationale (française) de Recherche sur le Sida et les hépatites virales.
2   The infant was exposed during 14 months to non-exclusive breastfeeding, when his mother was highly immunodepressed, a situation with a very high risk of HIV transmission.
3   "Old women" is a respectful term used in French-speaking African countries to name old women with reference to the knowledge they hold, especially regarding care, that they apply in their household, or as a more or less specialized activity.
4   A terracotta pot used as a container for liquids.
5   This may include barks, roots, or various parts of vegetal species usually sold and kept dry and used as herbal teas.

CHAPTER TEN

1   The parents who commission the baby through surrogacy have been named differently in different studies. This paper uses CPs (commissioning parent, who commissions the child), but they are also called intended parents (IPs) and social parents, as they are going to rear the child.

2 It is difficult to define *sanskar*, but simply it means to purify, to refine, to supplement, to brighten, to adorn inner conscience.

3 Garbha Sanskar can be traced back to ancient Hindu texts like the Vedas, which date to 1500–500 BCE. It also finds reference in the Mahabarata, which was written roughly 400 BCE. Garbha Sanskar also finds place in traditional ayurvedic medicine as a guide for pregnant women in prenatal education, the practice of which will result in a well-balanced and health baby http://www.babycenter.in/a1049729/mythology-behind-garbha-sanskar (accessed February 23, 2014).

4 There are various interesting mythological stories about the Garbha Sanskar. A very well-known story is of Abhimanyu, son of Arjuna, from the Mahabarata. When Arjuna's wife was pregnant with their son, Abhimanyu, Arjuna told her about how to penetrate the "Chakravyuh," a particular war formation. When Abhimanyu became a young man and a warrior in the "Kurukshetra" war, he remembered his father's story and was able to employ the strategy that he had heard his father tell his mother while he was in her womb. Abhimanyu could not listen to the strategy of coming out of the Chakravyuh, as his mother fell asleep in the middle of the story. And thus, when Abhimanyu grows up, he fiercely battles and enters the Chakravyuh, but dies, as he was not aware of the exit from this whirlpool of soldiers.

5 Another story is of Prahlad from the Puranas. Prahlad was born into a family of demons who were wreaking havoc on the Gods in heaven. His mother listened to devotional prayers and stories about Lord Vishnu while he was in her womb. As a result, he became a devotee of Lord Vishnu. He stood by good and renounced all evil. This led to the downfall of his demon father's evil empire.

6 Another interesting story is of Ashtavakra, which means "eight disfigures." Ashtavakra's mother Sujata wanted her son to be the most intelligent sage there ever was, so she would sit in on the classes taught by her father and husband while she was pregnant. In a class taught by her husband, the unborn baby spoke up and corrected his father, Kahoda. Kahoda, feeling insulted, cursed his son to be born deformed, so Astavakra was born physically challenged. But as he had taken part in the classes of his learned father and grandfather while in the womb of his mother, he was a genius. The story goes on to say that because of his intelligence he was able to fix his physical handicap. So in the end he became a handsome man as well as the most intelligent sage of his time.

7 The second author interviewed Dr. Nayana Patel, from Anand Gujarat, who is a pioneer in the establishing commercial surrogacy in India.

8 In pregnancy estrogen and progesterone prepare the breast in association with prolactin, the principal lactogenic hormone produced by the anterior pituitary gland. Other hormones involved in lactation are oxytocin, which is released by nipple-stimulation involving in the let-down reflex.

9 Saravanan uses intended parents for CPs.

10 The study in Hyderabad was conducted by the first two authors who are principal investigators and the study in Delhi was conducted by all four, with the third author as principal investigator.

11 To maintain confidentiality, the Delhi clinics have been named as D1, D2, D3, D4 and so on.

12 Justbreastfeeding.com gives different categories of breastfeeding guidelines and information about how to store breastmilk. It is to be kept at room temperature (66–72 degrees Fahrenheit) for 0–4 hours; cooled milk frozen in ice packs (59 degrees Fahrenheit) for 0–24 hours; refrigerators (32–9 degrees Fahrenheit) for 5–7 days; milk in a self-contained freezer (below 32 degrees Fahrenheit) for 3–4 months; or, if it is deep frozen (at 0 degrees Fahrenheit) for 6 months.

13 In the New Jersey Supreme Court in 1988, the case of Baby M, the genetic mother, Mary Beth Whitehead, carried and bore (traditional surrogacy) a child for the genetic father and his wife. She had been inseminated artificially with the father's sperm. During and after pregnancy, Mary Beth Whitehead changed her mind, and tried to keep custody of the child herself.

CHAPTER ELEVEN

1 Currently there are 16 non-profit milk banks in the U.S.A. and Canada that are aligned with, and operate according to, the voluntary safety guidelines set down by the Human Milk Banking Association of North America (Human Milk Banking Association of North America 2011, Updegrove 2013a). In the United Kingdom there are 12 HMBs supported by the United Kingdom Association for Milk Banking (UKAMB), which operate in accordance with National Institute for Health and Care Excellence (NICE) safety guidelines (National Institute for Health and Care Excellence 2010). In Australia there are five HMBs, but unlike the in U.K. and the U.S.A., there is no national advocacy association that co-ordinates the ideal operating guidelines for HMBs in Australia. Instead, Australian HMBs operate within a confluence of regulatory systems recommended by the NICE and HMBANA guidelines, Hazard Analysis and Critical Control Points (HACCP) system safety procedures, and relevant state and federal governmental legislations (Hartmann et al. 2007; Carroll and Herrmann 2012).

2 Feeding with breastmilk enables infants to avoid bovine-based proteins present in infant formula and it also offers benefits such as enhanced immunity and gastrointestinal development (Sullivan et al. 2010).

3 In Australia the term "express" is used and in the U.S. the term "pump" is used. Given the international focus of this research the terms express/ing and pump/ing are used interchangeably throughout.

4 Of the 25 donors I interviewed, the amount of milk donated from each individual woman ranged from 2 liters to 30 liters, with a mean of 11.5 liters per donor.

5 Academic literature as well as websites pertaining to milk banks and milk banking associations refer to DBM as "surplus," "spare," or "extra." HMBANA's website, for example, combines the notions of excess milk with altruism: "Lactating women who find that they have more milk than their own baby needs are endowed with something extraordinary: the ability to help another baby thrive" https://www.hmbana.org/ (accessed December 20, 2013).

6 All 25 of the donors interviewed were American-born; 24 were white, and 1 was of Indian descent. Ten donors worked in the healthcare sector, four were stay-at-home mothers, three worked clerical jobs, and the others were scattered across education, IT, business, and sales. In addition to providing milk to the HMB, half of the donors had either offered milk (and it was refused) or successfully provided milk to others, including neighbors, friends, or through internet-facilitated breastmilk sharing programs.

7 Human Research Ethics Committee and Institutional Review Board approval was granted by the University of Technology, Sydney and by the relevant hospital research sites.

CHAPTER TWELVE

1 This chapter owes much to the papers of Alice Desclaux, Gervaise Debucquet, Rossella Cevese, Anne Matthews, Abdullahi El Tom, and Tanya Cassidy, delivered at the EASA workshop The Breast Milk Problem: Cultural Considerations when Mother's Own Milk is Unavailable, for which I acted as discussant. The workshop was organized at Maynooth, Dublin in 2010 by Tanya Cassidy and Abdullahi El Tom.

2 Though women with AIDS are less fertile.

3 Gaps in registration of infants at birth, especially in some African countries, are currently being corrected with the help of UNICEF projects for the integration of civil registration with health services.

4 UNICEF figures presenting the apparent rise of exclusive breastfeeding in some countries can be misleading. They plot the number of babies under six months of age being exclusively breastfed. Such data are meaningless since the baby could be breastfed exclusively for one day or three weeks or for six whole months, and all of these will appear in the statistics as "exclusively breastfed." So to the uninitiated reader it might appear that the number of children being exclusively breastfed for six months has increased: http://www.childinfo.org/breast-feeding_progress.html (accessed January 25, 2012).

5 However, Nduati claims that, given adequate counseling, HIV-affected women in Kenya feed formula to their children relatively safely (UNAIDS 2001).

6 This research provoked much debate (see Coutsidis et al. 2002) and a WHO statement assessing the evidence for and against (see UNAIDS 2001).

Bibliography

Abel, E. and Nelson, M. (1990), "Circles of Care: An Introductory Essay," in E. Abel and M. Nelson (eds) *Circles of Care: Work and Identity in Women's Lives*. Albany: State University of New York: 4–34.

ABM (2010), "ABM clinical protocol #8: human milk storage information for home use for full-term infants." *Breastfeeding Medicine* 5(3): 127–30.

Akre, J. E., Gribble, K. D., and Minchin, M. (2011), "Milk sharing: from private practice to public pursuit," *International Breastfeeding Journal* 6(8): 1–3.

Akuse, R. M. and Obinya, E. A. (2002), "Why healthcare workers give prelacteal feeds." *European Journal of Clinical Nutrition* 56: 729–34.

Ali, Y. (1983), *The Holy Qur'an: Text, Translation and Commentary*. Brentwood MD: Amana Corp.

Almeling, R. (2011), *Sex Cells*. Berkley CA: University of California Press.

Altorki, S. (1980), "Milk kinship in Arab Society: an unexplored problem in the ethnography of marriage." *Ethnology* 19: 233–44.

Anderson, N. (2012), "American university professor breast-feeds sick baby in class, sparking debate." Washington Post, September 11.

Andrews, T. and Knaak, S. (2013), "Medicalized mothering: experiences with breast-feeding in Canada and Norway." *The Sociological Review* 61: 88–110.

Antier, E. (2003), *Vive l'éducation!* Paris: Laffont.

Appadurai, A. (1986), *The Social Life of Things: Commodities in Cultural Perspective*. Cambridge: Cambridge University Press.

Apple, R. (1987), *Mothers and Medicine: A Social History of Infant Feeding, 1890–1950*. Madison WI: University of Wisconsin Press.

Aria, M. (2008), "Le aporie della donazione del sangue: un dono che non fa amici," in F. Dei, M. Aria, and G. L. Mancini (eds) *Il dono del sangue: per un'antropologia dell'altruismo*. Ospedaletto PI: Pacini: 193–217.

Arnold, L. and Lockhardt Borman, L. (1996), "What are the characteristics of the ideal human milk donor?" *Journal of Human Lactation* 12(2): 143–5.

Arnold, L. D. W. (2010). *Human Milk in the NICU: Policy into Practice*. Sudbury MA: Jones and Bartlett Publishers.

Auerbach, K. G. (1991), "Breastmilk versus breastfeeding: product versus process." *Journal of Human Lactation: Official Journal of International Lactation Consultant Association* 7(3): 115–16.

Avishai, O. (2004), "At the pump." *Journal of the Association for Research on Mothering* 6(2): 139–49.

—(2011), "Managing the Lactating Body: The Breastfeeding Project in the Age of Anxiety," in P. Liamputtong (ed.) *Infant Feeding Practices*. Bronx NY: Springer Science+Business Media, LLC: 23–38.

Azema, E. and Callahan, S. (2003). "Breast milk donors in France: A portrait of the typical donor and the utility of milk banking in the French breastfeeding context." *Journal of Human Lactation*, 19(2): 199–202.

Badinter, E. (1981) [1980], *The Myth of Motherhood: A Historical View of the Maternal Instinct* (trans. Roger De Garis). London: Souvenir Press.

—(2010), *Le Conflit: Le Femme et la Mère*, Paris: Flammarion.

Balsamo, F., De Mari, G., Maher, V., and Serini, R. (1992), "La produzione e il piacere: medici e madri a Torino," in V. Maher V. (ed.) *Il latte mateno. I condizionamenti culturali di un comportamento*. Torino: Rosenberg & Sellier.

Bardin, L. (1983), *L'analyse de contenu*. Paris: PUF.

Barston, S. (2012), *Bottled Up: How the Way We Feed Babies Has Come to Define Motherhood and Why it Shouldn't*. Berkeley: University of California Press.

Bartlett, A. (2005), *Breastwork*. Sydney: University of New South Wales Press.

Baumslag, N. (1986), "Breastfeeding: cultural practices and variations," in M. Hamosh and A. S. Goldman (eds) *Human Lactation 2:* Maternal and Environmental Factors. New York: Plenum Press: 621–42

Baumslag, N and Michels, D. L. (1995), *Milk, Money, and Madness: The Culture and Politics of Breastfeeding*. Westport: Bergin & Garvey.

Beasley, C. and Bacchi, C. (2005), "The political limits of 'care' in re-imagining interconnection/community and an ethical future." *Australian Feminist Studies* 20(46): 49–64.

Beauchamp, T. L. and Childress, J. F. (2001), *Principles of Biomedical Ethics* (5th edn). Oxford: Oxford University Press.

Bell, S. E. (1987), "Changing ideas: the medicalization of menopause." *Social Science and Medicine* 24(6): 535–42.

Beneduce, R. (1998), *Frontiere dell'identità e della memoria: Etnopsichiatria e migrazioni in un mondo creolo*. Milano: Franco Angeli.

Berer, M. (1999), "Reducing perinatal HIV transmission in developing countries through antenatal and delivery care, and breastfeeding: supporting infant survival by supporting women's survival." *Bulletin of the World Health Organization* 77(11): 871–7.

Bernie, K. (2014), "The factors influencing young mothers' infant feeding decisions: the views of healthcare professionals and voluntary workers on the role of the baby's maternal grandmother." *Breastfeeding Medicine* 9(2): 56–62.

Berry, N. J. and Gribble, K. D. (2008), "Breast is no longer best: promoting normal infant feeding." *Maternal and Child Nutrition* 4: 74–9.

Biervliet, F. P and Atkin, S. L. (2012), "Lactation by a commissioning mother in surrogacy," in K. Sharif and A. Coomaramy (eds) *Assisted Reproduction*

Techniques: Challenges and Management Options. West Sussex: Wiley Blackwell: 412–16.

Bila B. M. (2011), *Genre et médicament dans le contexte du sida au Burkina Faso,* Ph.D. in anthropology, University Paul Cézanne of Aix-Marseille.

Blaauw, R., Albertse, E. C., Beneke, T., Lombard, C. J., Laubscher, R., and Hough, F. S. (1994), "Risk factors for development of osteoporosis in a South African population." *South African Medical Journal* 84: 328–32.

Bland, R. M., Little, K. E., Coovadia, H. M., Coutsoudis, A., Rollins, N. C., and Newell, M. L. (2008), "Intervention to promote exclusive breastfeeding for the first six months of life in a high prevalence area." *AIDS* 22: 883–91.

Bland, R. M., Rollins, N. C., Coutsoudis, A., and Coovadia, H. M. (2002), "Breastfeeding practices in an area of high HIV prevalence in rural South Africa." *Acta Paediatrica* 91: 704—11.

Blum, L. M. (1993), "Mothers, babies, and breast-feeding in late capitalist America: the shifting contexts of feminist theory." *Feminist Studies* 19(2): 291–311.

—(1999), *At the Breast: Ideologies of Breast-feeding and Motherhood in the Contemporary United States.* Boston: Beacon Press.

Blum, L. M. and Vandewater, E. A. (1993), "'Mother to mother': a maternalist organization in late capitalist America." *Social Problems* 40(3): 285–300.

Blystad, A. and Moland K. A. (2009), "Technologies of hope?: motherhood, HIV and infant feeding in eastern Africa." *Anthropology and Medicine* 16(2): 105–18.

Bobel, C. (2002), *The Paradox of Natural Mothering.* Philadelphia: Temple University Press.

Bode, L., Kuhn, L., Kim, H. Y., Hsiao, L., Nissan, C., Sinkala, M., Kankasa, C., Mwiya, M., Thea, D. M., and Aldrovandi, G. M. (2012), "Human milk oligosaccharide concentration and risk of post-natal transmission of HIV through breastfeeding." *American Journal of Clinical Nutrition* 96(4): 831–9.

Boltanski, L. (1969), *Prime éducation et morale de classe.* Paris: Editions de l'EHESS.

—(1971), Les usages sociaux du corps. *Les Annales* (1): 205–33.

Bosi, M. L. M. and Machado, M. T. (2005), "Breastfeeding: a historic rescue [Amamentacao: um resgate historico]." *Cadernos Escola de Saude Publica* 1(1): 471–7.

Bourke, J. (1990), "Dairywomen and affectionate wives: women in the Irish dairy industry, 1890–1914." *The Agricultural History Review* 38(2): 149–64.

Bowlby, J. (1958), "The nature of the child's tie to his mother." *International Journal of Psycho-Analysis* 39: 350–73.

Boyer, K. (2010), "Of care and commodities: breast milk and the new mobile biostructures." *Progress in Human Geography* 34(1): 5–20.

Bramwell, R. (2001), "Blood and milk: constructions of female bodily fluids in western society." *Women and Health* 34(4): 85–96.

Brinsden, P. R. (2003), "Gestational surrogacy." *Human Reproduction Update* 9(5): 483–91.

Britton, C. (1998), "'Feeling letdown': an exploration of an embodied sensation associated with breastfeeding" in S. Nettleton and J. Watson (eds) *The Body in Everyday Life*. New York: Routledge, 64–81.

Browner, C. H. (2000), "Situating women's reproductive activities." *American Anthropologist* 102(4): 773–88.

Burawoy, M. (2005), "For public sociology." *American Sociological Review* 70(1): 4–28.

Butte, N. Lopez-Alarcon, M., and Garza, C. (2002), *Nutrient Adequacy of Exclusive Breastfeeding for the Term Infant During the First Six Months of Life*. Geneva: World Health Organization.

Caritas Italiana—Fondazione Migrantes (2010), *Dossier 1991–2010: per una cultura dell'altro*. Roma: IDOS.

Carroll, K. (2014), "Body dirt or liquid gold?: how the 'safety' of donated breast milk is constructed for use in neonatal intensive care." *Social Studies of Science*, 44(3): 466–85.

Carroll, K. and Herrmann, K. (2012), "Introducing donor human milk to the NICU: lessons for Australia." *Breastfeeding Review* 20(3): 19–26.

Carsten, J. (2000), *Culture of Relatedness: New Approaches to the Study of Kinship*. Cambridge: Cambridge University Press.

Carter, P. (1995), *Feminism, Breasts and Breast-feeding*. Basingstoke: Palgrave.

Cassidy, T. M. (2010), "100 Years of Human Milk Banking." *Proceedings International Human Milk Banking Conference*, Milan, Italy.

—(2012a), "Making 'milky matches': globilization, maternal trust and 'lactivist' online networking," *Journal of the Motherhood Initiative* 3(2): 226–40.

—(2012b), "Mothers, milk, and money: maternal corporeal generosity, social psychological trust, and value in human milk exchange." *Journal of the Motherhood Initiative* 3(1):96–111.

—(2013), "HIV/AIDS and Human Milk Banking: Controversy, Complexity and Culture Around a Global Social Problem," in Tanya M. Cassidy (ed.) *Breastfeeding: Global Practices, Challenges, Maternal and Infant Health Outcomes*. New York: Nova Science Publishers, Inc.

Cassidy, T. M. and El Tom, A. O. (2010), "Comparing Sharing and Banking Milk: Issues of Gift Exchange and Community in the Sudan and Ireland," in Alison Bartlette and Rhonda Shaw (eds) *Giving Breast Milk: Body Ethics and Contemporary Breastfeeding Practice*. Toronto: Demeter Press: 110–21.

Cavallo, S. (1983), "Strategie politiche e familiari intorno al baliatico: il monopolio dei bambini abbandonati nel Canavese tra Sei e Settecento." *Quaderni storici* Anno XVIII: 391–421.

CDC (2012), *Breastfeeding Among U.S. Children Born 2000–2009 CDC National Immunization Survey*, retrieved from http://www.cdc.gov/breastfeeding/data/nis_data/ (accessed June 20, 2012).

Cheyney, M. (2011), 'Reinscribing the birthing body: homebirth as ritual performance', *Medical Anthropology Quarterly, 25*(4): 519–542.

Chinkonde, J. R., Hem, M. H., and Sundby, J. (2010), "HIV and infant feeding in Malawi: public health simplicity in complex social and cultural contexts." *BMC Public Health* 12: 700.

Chodorow, N. J. (2003), "'Too late': ambivalence about motherhood, choice, and time." *Journal of the American Psychoanalytic Association* 51(4): 1181–98.

Clarke, M. (2005), "Islam and 'New Kinship': An Anthropological Study of New Reproductive Technologies in Lebanon." D.Phil., University of Oxford.

—(2006), "Islam, kinship and new reproductive technology." *Anthropology Today* 22(5): 17–20.

—(2007), "The modernity of kinship." *Social Anthropology/Anthropologie Aociale* 15(3): 287–304.

Clemons, S. N. and Amir, L. H. (2010), "[online survey data] Breastfeeding women's experience of expressing: a descriptive study." *Journal of Human Lactation* 26(3): 258–65.

Clifford, J. and Marcus, G. (1986), *Writing Culture: The Poetics and Politics of Ethnography.* Berkeley CA: University of California Press.

Clinical Report of the Rotunda Hospital (1958), Dublin: Rotunda Hospital.

Condon, D. (2006), "Ireland's only human milk bank," Irish Health.com (accessed September 13, 2014).

Cone, T. E. (1976), *200 Years of Feeding Infants in America.* Columbus OH: Ross Laboratories.

Conrad, P. (1992), 'Medicalization and social control', *Annual Review of Sociology,* 18: 209–232.

—(2007), *The Medicalization of Society: On the Transformation of Human Conditions into Treatable Disorders,* Baltimore, MD: Johns Hopkins University Press.

—(2013), "Medicalization: Changing Contours, Characteristics, and Contexts," in W. C. Cockerham (ed.) *Medical Sociology on the Move: New Directions in Theory.* Dordrecht: Springer.

Conte, É. (2000a), "Énigmes persanes, traditions arabes: les interdictions matrimoniales dérivées de l'allaitement selon l'ayatollah Khomeyni," in J.-L. Jamard, E. Terray, and M. Xanthakou (eds) *En substances: textes pour Françoise Héritier.* Paris: Fayard: 157–81.

—(2000b), "Mariages arabes: la part du féminin." *L'Homme* 154–5: 279–307.

Countdown to 2015 (2014), "Country level data for Malawi." http://www.countdown2015mnch.org/country-profiles/malawi (last accessed February 3, 2014).

Coutsoudis A., Coovadia, H., Pillay, K., and Kuhn L. (2001), "Are HIV-infected women who breastfeed at increased risk of mortality?" *AIDS* 15: 653–5.

Coutsoudis, A., Coovadia, H., and Wilfert, C. (2008), "HIV, infant feeding and more perils for poor people: new WHO Guidelines encourage review of formula feeding policies." *Bulletin of the World Health Organization* 86(3): 210–14.

Crowther, S. M., Reynolds, L. A., and Tansey, E. M. (eds) (2009), *The Resurgence of Breast-feeding 1975–2000.* Wellcome Trust Centre Seminar 2007.

D'Onofrio, S. (2004), "L'épaule et le cœur: allaitement et symbolique du corps en Sicile," in F. Héritier and M. Xanthakou (eds) *Corps et Affects*. Paris: Odile Jacob: 151–68.

Daly, M. W. (2007), *Darfur's Sorrow: A History of Destruction and Genocide*. Cambridge: Cambridge University Press.

Davis-Floyd, R. E. (1992), *Birth as an American Rite of Passage*. Berkeley and Los Angeles CA: University of California Press.

—(1994), "The technocratic body: American childbirth as cultural expression." *Social Science and Medicine* 38(8): 1125–40.

Davis-Floyd, R. E. and Sargent, C. F. (eds) (1997), *Childbirth and Authoritative Knowledge: Cross-Cultural Perspectives*, Berkeley and Los Angeles CA: University of California Press.

Davis, J. R. (2004), "Bad breast feeders/good mothers: constructing the maternal body in public." *Berkeley Journal of Sociology* 48: 50–73.

Daycare Trust (2005), *Childcare Costs Surveys*. Available at http://www.daycaretrust. org.uk/pages/childcare-costs-surveys.html (accessed September 6, 2012).

De Leonardis, O. (2009), *Le istituzioni: come e perché parlarne*. Roma: Carocci.

De Micco, V. (2002), *Le culture della salute: Immigrazione e sanità: un approccio transculturale*. Napoli: Liguori.

De Singly, F. (2009), *Comment aider l'enfant à devenir lui-même?* Paris: Colin.

Dei, F., Aria, M., and Mancini, G. L. (2008), *Il dono del sangue: per un'antropologia dell'altruism*. Ospedaletto PI: Pacini.

Demetrio, F., Monteiro da Silva, Maria da Conceicao, Chaves-dos-Santos, S. M., and Oliveira Assis, A. M. (2013), "Meanings attributed to breastfeeding in the first two years of life: a study with women from two municipalities in the Reconcavo Baiano region of Bahia, Brazil." *Revista De Nutricao–Brazilian Journal of Nutrition* 26(1): 5–16.

Department of Health. (2005), *Infant Feeding Survey 2005*, London: Department of Health.

Derrida, J. (1981), "Plato's pharmacy," *Dissemination* (tr. Barbara Johnson). London: The Athlone Press.

Desclaux A. and Alfieri C. (2008), "Allaitement, VIH et prévention au Burkina Faso: les déterminants sociaux ont-ils changé?" *Science et Technique, Série Sciences de la santé, Hors série 1, Sida, santé publique et sciences sociales. Vingt ans d'épidémie et de recherche au Burkina Faso*: 117–26.

—(2009), "Counseling and choosing between infant-feeding options: overall limits and local interpretations by health care providers and women living with HIV in resource-poor countries (Burkina Faso, Cambodia, Cameroon)." *Social Science and Medicine* 69(6): 821—9.

—(2010), "Facing Competing Cultures of Breastfeeding: The Experience of HIV-Positive Women in Burkina Faso," in P. Liamputtong (ed.) *Infant Feeding Practices: A Cross-cultural Perspective*. Springer: New York: 195–210.

—(2013), "L'annonce du statut VIH de l'enfant: expériences des mères et interprétations des soignants au Burkina Faso," in A. Hardon, A. Desclaux, and J. Lugala (eds) *Disclosure in the Times of ART: Why, When, How and to Whom? Special Issue SAHARA (Social Aspects of AIDS Research in Africa)* 10(1): S81–S92.

Desclaux A., Crochet S., Querre M., and Alfieri C. (2006), "Le 'choix informé' des femmes séropositives qui doivent alimenter leur enfant : interprétations locales, limites et nouvelles questions," in A. Desgrées du Loû and B. Ferry (eds) *Sexualité et procréation confrontées au Sida dans les pays du Sud*. Paris: CEPED: 245–62.

Desclaux A. and Taverne B. (eds) (2000), *Allaitement et VIH en Afrique de l'ouest: De l'anthropologie à la santé publique*. Paris: Karthala.

Desjarlais, R. and Throop, J. C. (2011), "Phenomenological approaches in anthropology." *Annual Review of Anthropology* 40: 87–102.

Dettwyler, K. A. (1995a), "A Time to Wean: The Hominid Blueprint for the Natural Age of Weaning in Modern Human Populations," in P. Stuart-Macadam and K. A. Dettwyler (eds) *Breastfeeding: Biocultural Perspectives*. New York: Aldine de Gruyter, 39–73, 167–217.

—(1995b), "Beauty and the Breast: the Cultural Context of Feeding in the United States," in P. Stuart-Macadam and K. A. Dettwyler (eds) *Breastfeeding: Biocultural Perspectives*. New York: Aldine de Gruyter.

—(2004), "When to wean: biological versus cultural perspectives." *Clinical Obstetrics and Gynecology* 47(3): 712–23.

Dickenson, D. (2001), "Property and women's alienation from their own reproductive labour." *Bioethics* 15(3): 205–17.

Doherty, T., Chopra, M., Jackson, D., Goga, A., Colvin, M., and Persson, L. A. (2007),"Effectiveness of the WHO/UNICEF guidelines on infant feeding for HIV positive women: results from a prospective cohort study in South Africa." *AIDS* 21: 1791–7.

Dolto, F. and Muel, A. (1977), *L'éveil de l'esprit*. Paris: Aubier.

Douglas, M. (1967), *De la souillure: études sur la notion de pollution et de tabou*. Paris: La Découverte.

—(1975), *Purezza e pericolo*. Bologna: Il Mulino

Douglas, S. and Michaels, M. (2004), *The Mommy Myth: The Idealization of Motherhood and how it has Undermined All Women*. New York: Free Press.

Draper, S. B. (1996), Breast-feeding as a sustainable resource system. *American Anthropologist* 98(2): 258–65.

Dreyfus, H. L. (2000), "Merleau-Ponty's critique of Husserl's (and Searle's) concept of intentionality," in L. Hass and D. Olkowski (eds) *Rereading Merleau-Ponty: Essays Beyond the Continental–Analytic Divide*. Amherst NY: Humanity Books, 33–52.

Druckerman, P. (2012), *Bringing up Bébé: One American Mother Discovers the Wisdom of French Parenting*. London and New York: Penguin Books.

Dunn, T. D. T., Newell, M. L., Ades, A. E. and Peckham, C. S. (1992), "Risk of human immunodeficiency virus type 1 transmission through breastfeeding." *Lancet*. 340: 585–8.

Durkheim, É. (1963), *L'éducation morale*. Paris: PUF.

Dykes, F. (2002), "Western medicine and marketing: construction of an inadequate milk syndrome in lactating women." *Health Care for Women International* 23(5): 492–502.

—(2005), "'Supply' and 'demand': breastfeeding as labour." *Social Science and Medicine* 60(10): 2283–93.

Dykes, F. and Williams, C. (1999), "Falling by the wayside: a phenomenological exploration of perceived breast-milk inadequacy in lactating women." *Midwifery* 15(4): 232–46.

Earner-Byrne, L. (2007), *Mother and Child: Maternity and Child Welfare in Dublin, 1922-60*. Manchester: Manchester University Press.

Edwards, R. (2002), "Conceptualizing Relationships between Home and School in Children's Lives," in R. Edwards (ed.) *Children, Home and School: Regulation, Autonomy or Connection?* London: RoutledgeFalmer.

Ehrenreich, B. and English, D. (1978), *For Her Own Good: 150 Years of the Experts' Advice To Women*. New York: Anchor Books.

Eidelman, A. I. (2012), "Breast-feeding and the use of human milk: an analysis of the American Academy of Pediatrics 2012." *Breastfeeding Medicine* 7(5): 323–4.

El Guindi, F. (2012), "Suckling as kinship." *Anthropology News* 53(4): 10–13.

El Tom, A. O. (1996), "Traditional practices and perinatal health in a Sudanese village." *CURARE: Journal of Medical Anthropology, Special Issue on Ethnomedical Perspectives on Childhood* 9: 1–30.

—(1997), "Vowing to Survive: Socio-economic Changes in Burush, Western Sudan," in F. Ibrahim, D. Ndagala, and H. Ruppert (eds) *Coping with Resource Scarcity: Case Studies from Tanzania and Sudan*. Geowissenschaftliche Arbeiten: University of Bayreuth: 239–73.

—(1998), '"Female circumcision and ethnic identification in Sudan with reference to the Berti of Darfur." *GeoJournal* 46: 163–70.

—(2005), "Darfur people: too black for the Arab–Islamic project of Sudan: parts I and II." *Irish Journal of Anthropology* 9: 1–18.

Electronic Dictionary of the Irish Language (eDIL), http://www.dil.ie/

Eljamay, E. (1981), *Siouti Collection of Prophetic Speeches*. Beirut: Dar Elfikr.

Ellis, C. and Bochner, A. (1999), "Bringing emotion and personal narrative into medical social science." *Health* 3: 229–37.

—(2000), "Autoethnography, Personal Narrative, Reflexivity: Researcher as Subject," in N. K. Denzin and Y. S. Lincoln (eds) *Handbook of Qualitative Research* (2nd edn). Thousand Oaks CA: Sage: 733–68.

Ellis, Carolyn (1999), "Heartful autoethnography." *Qualitative Health Research* 9(5): 669–83.

Engebretsen, I. M. S., Wamani, H., Karamagi, C., Semiyaga, N., Tumwine, J., and Tylleskar, T. (2007), "Low adherence top exclusive breastfeeding in Eastern Uganda: a community based cross-sectional study comparing dietary recall since birth with 24-hour recall." *BMC Paediatrics* 7: 10.

England, P. (2005), "Emerging theories of care work." *Annual Review of Sociology* 31: 381–99.

Ensel, R. (1999), *Saints and Servants in Southern Morocco*. Leiden: Brill.

Esping-Anderson, G. (1999), *Social Foundations of Post-industrial Economics*. Oxford: Oxford University Press.

Estevez de Alencar, L. C. and Fleury Seidl, E. M. (2009), "Breast milk donation: women's donor experience." *Revista de saude publica* 43(1): 70–7.

EU Project on Promotion of Breastfeeding in Europe (2004), *Protection, Promotion and Support of Breast-feeding in Europe: A Blueprint for Action*. Luxembourg: European Commission, Directorate Public Health and Risk Assessment, available at http://ec.europa.eu/health/ph_projects/2002/promotion/fp_promotion_2002_frep_18_en.pdf (accessed September 15, 2014).

Eyer, D. (1992). *Mother-infant bonding: A scientific fiction*. New Haven, CT: Yale University Press.

Faggionato, M. (2010), *La relazione madre-bambino e l'allattamento. L'esperieinza in un asilo nido visto in una prospettiva interculturale*. M. A. Thesis, University of Verona.

Faircloth, C. (2009), "'Culture means nothing to me': thoughts on nature/culture in narratives of 'full-term' breastfeeding." *Cambridge Anthropology* 28(2): 63–85.

—(2010), "What science says is best: parenting practices, scientific authority and maternal identity." *Sociological Research Online* Special Section on "Changing Parenting Culture" 15(4), http://www.socresonline.org.uk/15/4/4.html (accessed September 6, 2012).

—(2011), "It feels right in my heart: affect as accountability in narratives of attachment." *The Sociological Review* 59(2): 283–302, May, http://onlineli-brary.wiley.com/doi/10.1111/j.1467–954X.2011.02004.x/abstract (accessed September 6, 2012).

Faircloth, C. (2013), *Militant Lactavism?* Attachment Parenting and Intensive Motherhood in the UK and France. New York: Berghahn.

Faircloth, C. Hoffman, D., and Layne, L. (eds) (2013), *Parenting in Global Perspective: Negotiating Ideologies of Kinship, Self and Politics*. London and New York: Routledge.

Falkner, N. (1944), "Report of the Rotunda Hospital." *Irish Journal of Medical Science* 6(224): 234–371.

Fenske, M. and Bendix, J. (2007), "Micro, macro, agency: historical ethnography as cultural anthropology." *Journal of Folklore Research* 44(1): 67–99.

Fentiman, L. C. (2009), "Marketing mothers' milk: the commodification of breast-feeding and the new markets for breastmilk and infant formula." *Nevada Law Journal* 10(29): 29–81.

Ferguson, S. J. and Parry, C. (1998), "Rewriting menopause: challenging the medical paradigm to reflect menopausal women's experiences." *Frontiers: A Journal of Women Studies* 19(1): 20–41.

Fildes, V. A. (1986). *Breasts, Bottles and Babies: A History of Infant Feeding.* Edinburgh: Edinburgh University Press.

—(1988), *Wet Nursing: A History from Antiquity to the Present*, Oxford: Basil Blackwell.

—(1995), "The culture and biology of breastfeeding: an historical review of Western Europe," in P. C. Macadam and K. A. Dettwyler (eds) *Breastfeeding: Biocultural Perspectives.* New York: Walter De Gruyter Inc.: 101–26.

Finkler, K. (2001), "The kin in the gene: the medicalization of family and kinship in American society." *Current Anthropology* 42(2): 235–63.

Fischer, T. P. and Olson, B. H. (2013), "A qualitative study to understand cultural factors affecting a mother's decision to breast or formula feed." *Journal of Human Lactation* 30(2): 209–16.

Fischler, C. and Masson, E. (2008), *Manger: Français, Européens et Américains face à leur alimentation.* Paris: Odile Jacob.

Fisher, B. and Tronto, J. (1990), "Toward a Feminist Theory of Caring," in E. Abel and M. Nelson (eds) *Circles of Care: Work and Identitiy in Women's Lives.* Albany: State University of New York: 35–62.

Flint, J. and De Waal, A. D. (2005), *Darfur: A Short History of a Long War.* London: Zed Books.

Fonseca, J. B. (2007), 'Book reviews: Lwanda politics culture and medicine in Malawi (2005)." *Africa Today* 54(1): 122–3.

Foster, K., McAllister, M., and O'Brien, L. (2006), "Extending the boundaries: autoethnography as an emergent method in mental health nursing research." *International Journal of Mental Health Nursing* 15(1): 44–53.

Fouda, G., Jaegera, F. H., Amosa, J. D., Hoa, C., Kunza, E. L., Anastia, K., Stampera, L. W., Liebla, B. E., Barbasb, K. H., Ohashic, T., Moseleyd, M. A., Liaoa, H., Erickson, H. P., Alama, S. M., and Permara, S. R. (2013), Proceedings of the National Academy of Sciences of the United States of America 110(45): 18220–25.

Fouts, H. N., Hewlett, B. S., and Lamb, M. E. (2012), "A biocultural approach to breastfeeding interactions in Central Africa." *American Anthropologist* 114(1): 123–36.

Franklin, S. and Ragoné, H. (eds) (1998), *Reproducing Reproduction: Kinship, Power, and Technological Innovation.* Philadelphia PA: University of Pennsylvania Press.

Furedi, F. (2002), *Paranoid Parenting: Why Ignoring the Experts May be Best for Your Child.* Chicago: Chicago Review Press.

Geertz, C. (1989), *Margaret Mead 1901-1978: A Biographical Memoir.* Washington, DC: National Academy of Sciences.

Geraghty, S. R., Heier, J. E., and Rasmussen, K. M. (2011), "Got milk? Sharing human milk via the internet." *Public Health Reports* 126: 161–4.

Geraghty, S. R., McNamara, K. A., Dillon, C. E., Hogan, J. S., Kwiek, J. J., and Keim, S. A. (2013), "Buying human milk via the Internet: just a click away." *Breastfeeding Medicine* 8(6): 474–78.

Gerstein Pineau, M. (2013), "Giving Milk, Buying Milk: The Influence of Mothering Ideologies and Social Class in Donor Milk Banking," in T. Cassidy (ed.) *Breastfeeding:* Global Practices, Challenges, Maternal and Infant Health Outcomes. New York: Nova Publishers, 61–79.

Ghaly, M. (2010), "Milk banks through the lens of Muslim scholars: one text in two contexts." *Bioethics*. Article first published online: November 23, 2010; DOI: 10.1111/j.1467–8519.2010.01844.x, available at http://onlinelibrary.wiley.com/doi/10.1111/j.1467–8519.2010.01844.x/abstract (accessed February 1, 2011).

Gil'adi, A. (1999), *Infants, Parents and Wet Nurses@ Medieval Islamic Views on Breast-feeding and their Social Implications*. Leiden: Brill NV.

Giles, F. (2002), "Fountains of love and loveliness in praise of the dripping wet breast." Journal of the Association for Research on Mothering 4(1): 8–18.

—(2004), "'Relational, and strange': a preliminary foray into a project to queer breastfeeding." *Australian Feminist Studies* 19(45): 301–14.

Ginsburg, F. and Rapp, R. (1991), "The politics of reproduction." *Annual Review of Anthropology* 20: 311–43.

Giugliani, E. R. J. (2002), "Rede nacional de bancos de leite humano do Brasil: tecnologia para exporter." *Jornal de Pediatria (Rio de Janeiro)* 78(3): 183–4.

Goffman, E. (1959), *The Presentation of Self in Everyday Life*. New York: Doubleday.

Gojard, S. (2000), L'alimentation dans la prime enfance: diffusion et réception des normes de puériculture. *Revue Française de sociologie* 41(3): 475–512.

Golden, J. (1996a), "From commodity to gift: gender, class, and the meaning of breast milk in the twentieth century." *Historians* 59: 75–87.

—(1996b), *A Social History of Wet Nursing in America: From Breast to Bottle*. Cambridge: Cambridge University Press.

Goody, J. (1983). *The Development of the Family and Marriage in Europe*. Cambridge: Cambridge University Press.

GRADE (n.d.), *Grading of Recommendations Assessment, Development and Evaluation Group*, www.gradeworkinggroup.org (last accessed February 3, 2014).

Green, B. (2009), "'Introduction: Understanding and Researching Professional Practice," in B. Green (ed.), *Understanding and Researching Professional Practice*. Rotterdam: Sense Publishers: 1–19.

Greiner, T. (1999), "The HIV challenge to breastfeeding." *Breastfeeding Review* 7 (3): 5–9.

Greiner, T., Van Esterik, P., and Latham, M. C. (1981), "The insufficient milk syndrome: an alternative explanation." *Medical Anthropology* 5(2): 232–47.

Gribble, K. D. (2006), "Mental health, attachment and breastfeeding: implications for adopted children and their mothers." *International Breastfeeding Journal* 1(1): 5.

—(2007), "Hot Milk Debate part 6: Dr Karleen Gribble, "http://www.youtube.com/watch?v=QByhsCw_L2g (accessed September 11, 2014).

—(2013), "Peer-to-Peer Milk Donors' and Recipients' Experiences and Perceptions of Donor Milk Banks." *Journal of Obstetric, Gynecologic, and Neonatal Nursing* 42(4): 451–61.

—(2014a), "Perception and management of risk in Internet-based peer-to-peer milk-sharing." *Early Child Development and Care* 184(1): 84–98.

—(2014b), "'I'm Happy to Be Able to Help:' Why Women Donate Milk to a Peer via Internet-Based Milk Sharing Networks." *Breastfeeding Medicine* 9(5): 251–6.

—(2014c), "'A better alternative': why women use peer-to-peer shared milk." *Breastfeeding Review* 22(1): 11–21.

Gribble, K. D. and Hausman, B. L. (2012), "Milk sharing and formula feeding: infant feeding risks in comparative perspective." *Australasian Medical Journal* 5(5): 275–83.

Guerra de Almeida, J. A. (2013), personal communication.

Gunnlaugsson, G. and Einarsdottir, J. (1993), "Colostrum and ideas about bad milk: a case study from Guinea-Bissau." Social Science Medicine 36: 283–8.

Gustafsson, L., Aits, S., Onnerfjord, P., Trulsson, M., Storm, P., and Svanborg, C. (2009), "Changes in proteasome structure and function caused by HAMLET in tumor cells." *PLoS One* 4(4): e5229. E-pub April 14, 2009.

Gutierrez, D. E. and De Almeida, J. A. G. (1998), "Human milk banks in Brazil." *Journal of Human Lactation* (14)4: 333–5.

Halfmann, D. (2012), "Recognizing medicalization and demedicalization: discourses, practices, and identities." *Health* 16(2): 186–207.

Harris, B. J. (2002), *English Aristocratic Women, 1450–1550: Marriage and Family, Property and Careers*. Oxford: Oxford University Press.

Harris, H., Weber, M., Chezem, J., and Quinlan, M. (2005), "Human milk banking: neonatologists' opinions and practices." *Pediatric Research* 58(4): 821.

Hartmann, B., Pang, W., Keil, A. D., Hartmann, P. E., and Simmer, K. (2007), "Best practice guidelines for the operation of a donor human milk bank in an Australian NICU." *Early Human Development* 83: 667–73.

Hassan, N. (2010), "Milk markets: technology, the lactating body, and new forms of consumption." *WSQ: Women's Studies Quarterly* 38(3–4): 209–28.

Hassiotou F., (2013), "Science interviews: breast milk stem cells." *The Naked Scientist: The University of Cambridge*, http://www.thenakedscientists.com (accessed April 17, 2014).

Hassiotou, F., Beltran, A., Chetwynd, E., Stuebe, A. M., Twigger, A. J., Metzger, P., Trengove, N., Lai, C. T., Filgueira, L., Blancafort, P., and Hartmann, P. E. (2012), "Breastmilk is a novel source of stem cells with multilineage differentiation potential." *Stem Cells,* October 30(10): 2164–74.

Hathout, H. (2005), "Islamic perspectives in obstetrics and gynaecology." Available at http://www.islamset.com/bioethics/obstet (accessed February 14, 2011).

Hausman, B. L. (2006), "Contamination and contagion: environmental toxin, HIV/ AIDS, and the problem of the maternal body." *Hyaptia* 21(1): 137–56.

—(2011), *Viral mothers: breastfeeding in the age of HIV/AIDS*. Ann Arbor MI: University of Michigan Press.

Hays, S. (1996), *The Cultural Contradictions of Motherhood*. New Haven and London: Yale University Press.

Héritier, F. (1994), "Identité de substance et parenté de lait dans le monde arabe," in P. Bonte (ed.) *Épouser au plus proche: inceste, prohibitions et stratégies matrimoniales autour de la Méditerranée*. Paris: Éditions de l'École Des Hautes Études en Sciences Sociales: 149–64.

—(1996), *Masculin, féminin la pensée de la différence*. Paris: Odile Jacob.

Hinde, K. and German, B. (2012), "Food in an evolutionary context: insight from mother's milk," *Journal of the Science of Food and Agriculture* 92: 2219–23.

HIV, "Infant feeding and more perils for poor people: new WHO guidelines encourage review of formula milk policies." *Bulletin of the World Health Organisation,* 86: 210–214Top of Form

Ho, C. J., Storm, P., Rydstrom, A., Bowen, B., Alsin, F., Sullivan, L., Ambite, I., Mok, K. H., Northen, T., and Svanborg, C. J. (2013), "Lipids as tumoricidal components of human alpha-lactalbumin made lethal to tumor cells (HAMLET): unique and shared effects on signaling and death," *The Journal of Biological Chemistry* 288(24): 17460–71.

Hoddinott, P. Tappin, D., and Wright, C. (2008), "Clinical review: breastfeeding." *British Medical Journal* 336: 881–7.

Holy, L. (1974), *Neighbours and Kinsmen: The Berti of Darfur*. London: C. Hurst.

Hor, S., Godbold, N., Collier, A., and Iedema, R. A. (2013), "Finding the patient in patient safety." *Health* 17(6): 567–83.

Hotz, C. and Gibson, R. S. (2001), "Complementary feeding practices and dietary intakes from complementary foods amongst weanlings in rural Malawi." *European Journal of Clinical Nutrition* 55: 841–9

Howard, M. and Millard, A. (1997), *Hunger and Shame: Child Malnutrition and Poverty on Mount Kilimanjaro*. New York: Routledge.

Hrdy, S. B. (2000), *Mother Nature: Maternal Instincts and how they Shape the Human Species*. London and New York: Ballantine Books.

Human Milk Banking Association of North America (HMBANA) (2011), *Guidelines for the Establishment and Operation of Donor Human Milk Bank*. USA: HMBANA.

Inhorn, M. C. (2003a), "Global infertility and the globalization of new reproductive technologies: illustrations from Egypt." *Social Science & Medicine* 56(9): 1837–51.

—(2003b), *Local Babies, Global Science: Gender, Religion, and In Vitro Fertilization in Egypt*. New York: Routledge.

—(2006), "Defining women's health: a dozen messages from more than 150 ethnographies." *Medical Anthropology Quarterly* 20(3): 345–78.

INSD (Institut National de la Statistique et la Démographie) and ICF International. (2012), *Enquête Démographique et de Santé et à Indicateurs Multiples (EDSBF-MICS IV)*. Ouagadougou, Calverton: INSD and ICF.

Irish Business and Employers' Confederation. (2007), *Business Perspectives on Future Dairy Policy: A Discussion Document Compiled by the Irish Dairy Industries Association*. Dublin: Irish Business and Employers Confederation, Dublin. Available from: www.fdii.ie/ (accessed May 9, 2010).

ISTAT, (2011), *Popolazione straniera residente*, http://demo.istat.it/strasa2010/index.html (accessed February 2, 2011).

Jansson, M. (2009), "Feeding children and protecting women: the emergence of breastfeeding as an international concern." *Women's Studies International Forum* 32: 240–48.

Jelliffe, D. B. and Jelliffe, E. F. (1988), "HIV and breastmilk: non-proven alarmism," Journal of Tropical Pediatrics 34: 142–142.

Jespersen, A., Bonnelycke, J., and Eriksen, H. H. (2014), "Careful science?: bodywork and care practices in randomised clinical trials." *Sociology of Health and Illness*, 36(5): 655–69.

Jodelet, D. (1987), "Le sein laitier, plaisir contre pudeur?" *Communication* 46: 356–78.

Jodelet, D. and Ohana, J. (2000), "Représentations sociales de l'allaitement maternel, une pratique de santé entre nature et culture," in G. Petrillo (ed.) *Santé et société: la santé et la maladie comme phénomènes sociaux*. Lausanne-Paris: Delachaux et Niestlé: 139–65.

Johnson, S., Leeming, D., Lyttle, S., and Williamson, I. (2012), "Empowerment or regulation: women's perspectives on expressing milk," in P. Hall Smith, B. L. Hausman, and M. Labbok (eds) *Beyond Health, Beyond Choice: Breastfeeding Constraints and Realities*. New Brunswick: Rutgers University Press, 180–9.

Jones, E. and King, C. (2005), *Feeding and Nutrition in the Preterm Infant*. London: Churchill Livingstone.

Jones, F. (2003), "History of North American donor milk banking: one hundred years of progress." *Journal of Human Lactation* 19(3): 313–18.

Kasenga, F., Hurtig, A. K., and Emmelin, M. (2007), "Home deliveries: implications for adherence to nevirapine in a PMTCT programme in Malawi." *AIDS Care* 19(3): 646–52.

Kaur, S. D. (2003), *The Complete Natural Medicine Guide to Breast Cancer*. Toronto: Robert Rose Inc.

Keim, S. A., McNamara, K. A. and Kwiek, J. J. "Microbial Contamination of Human Milk Purchased Via the Internet". *Pediatrics* 2013; 132:5 e1227-e1235; published ahead of print October 21, 2013, doi:10.1542/peds.2013-1687.

Kelleher, C. M. (2006), "The physical challenges of early breastfeeding." *Social science and medicine* 63(10): 2727–38.

Kelly, F. (1988), *A Guide to Early Irish Law*. Dublin: Institute for Advanced Studies.

Kennell, J. and McGrath, S. (2005), "Starting the process of mother–infant bonding." *Acta Paediatrica* 94(6): 775–7.

Khatib-Chahidi, J. (1992), "La parentela di latte nell'Iran musulmano sciita," in V. Maher (ed.) *Il latte materno: I condizionamenti culturali di un comportamento.* Torino: Rosenberg & Sellier: 119–42.

Kirkman, M. and Kirkman, L. (2001), "Inducing lactation: a personal account after gestational surrogate motherhood between sisters." *Breastfeeding Review* 9(3): 5.

Klapisch-Zuber, C. (1985), *Women, Family and Ritual in Renaissance Italy.* Chicago: University of Chicago Press.

Koch, J. T. (2006), *Celtic Culture: A Historical Encyclopedia Volumes 1–5.* California: ABC-CLIO Inc.

Kukla, R. (2005), *Mass Hysteria, Medicine, Culture and Women's Bodies.* New York: Roman and Littlefield.

—(2006), "Ethics and ideology in breastfeeding advocacy campaigns." *Hypatia* 21(1): 157–80.

Labbok, M. H. (2013), "Breastfeeding: population-based perspectives." *Pediatric Clinics of North America* 60(1): 11–30.

Labiner-Wolfe, J., Fein, S. B., Shealy, K. R., and Wang, C. (2008), "Prevalence of breastmilk expression and associated factors." *Pediatrics* 122 Suppl. 2:S63–8.

Lawn, J. E., Gravett, M. G., Nunes, T. M., Rubens, C. E., Stanton, C., and the GAPPS Review Group (2010), "Global report on preterm birth and stillbirth (1 of 7): definitions, description of the burden and opportunities to improve data BMC." *Pregnancy and Childbirth* 10 (Supp. 1): S1, http://www.biomedcentral.com/1471–2393/10/S1/S1 BMC (accessed February 23, 2010).

Layne, L. (2013), "Intensive Parenting Alone: Negotiating the Cultural Contradictions of Motherhood as a Single Mother by Choice," in C. Faircloth D. Hoffman, and L. Layne (eds) (2013), *Parenting in Global Perspective: Negotiating Ideologies of Kinship, Self and Politics.* London and New York: Routledge: 213–29.

Layne, L. and Aegnst, J. (2010), "'The Need to Bleed?' A Feminist Technology Assessment of Menstrual-suppressing Birth Control Pills," in L. Layne, S. Vostral, and K. Boyer (eds) *Feminist Technology.* Champaign, IL: University of Illinois Press.

Lazenbatt, A. (2013), "Child health: quantitative study—other: for vulnerable families, continued postnatal care, provided by family midwives, is associated with improved maternal care and parent–child relationship." *Evidence-Based Nursing,* 16(4): 104–5.

Le Breton, D. (1990), *Anthropologie du corps et modernité.* Paris: PUF.

Lecourt, D. (2003), *Dictionnaire de la pensée médicale.* Paris: PUF.

Lee, E. (2007a), "Health, morality, and infant feeding: british mothers' experiences of formula milk use in the early weeks." *Sociology of Health and Illness* 29(7): 1075–90.

—(2007b), "Infant feeding in risk society." *Health, Risk and Society* 9(3): 295–309.

—(2011), "Breast-feeding advocacy, risk society and health moralism: a decade's scholarship." *Sociology Compass* 5(12): 1058–69.

Lee, E. and Bristow, J. (2009), "Rules for Feeding Babies," in S. Day Sclater, F. Ebtehaj, E. Jackson and M. Richards (eds) *Regulating Autonomy: Sex, Reproduction and Family*. Oxford: Hart: 73–91.

Leigh, B., Mwale, T. G., Lazaro, D., and Lunguzi, J. (2008), "Emergency obstetric care: how do we stand in Malawi?" *International Journal of Gynaecology and Obstetrics* 101: 107–11.

Lepore, J. (2009), "Baby food." *New Yorker* 84, January 19: 34–9.

Lévi-Strauss, C. (1949), *Les structures élémentaires de la parenté*. Paris: PUF.

Liamputtong P. (ed.) (2010), *Infant Feeding Beliefs and Practices across Cultures*. New York: Springer.

Libamba, E., Makombe, S., Harries, A. D., Schouten, E. J., Kwong-Leung Yu, J., Pasulani, O., Mhango, E., Aberle-Grasse, J., Hochesang, M., Limbambala, E., and Lungu, D. (2007), "Malawi's contribution to '3 by 5': achievements and challenges." *Bulletin of the World Health Organization* 85(2): 156–60.

Libamba, E., Makombe, S., Mhango, E., de Ascurra Teck, O., Limbambala, E., Schouten, E. J., and Harries, A. D. (2006), "Supervision, monitoring and evaluation of a nationwide scale-up of antiretroviral therapy in Malawi." *Bulletin of the World Health Organization* 84(4): 320–6.

Lock, M. (1995), *Encounters with Aging: Mythologies of Menopause in Japan and North America*, Berkeley and Los Angeles CA: University of California Press.

—(2001), "The tempering of medical anthropology: troubling natural categories." *Medical Anthropology Quarterly* 15(4): 478–92.

Long, D. (1996), "Milky Ways: Milk Kinship in Anthropological Literature and in a Turkish Village Community." Unpublished M. A. dissertation, University of Nijmegen, The Netherlands.

Lupton, D. (2012), "Infant embodiment and interembodiment: a review of sociocultural perspectives." *Childhood* 20(1): 37–50.

Lwanda, J. (2005), *Politics, Culture and Medicine in Malawi: Historical Continuities and Ruptures with Special Reference to HIV/AIDS*. Zomba, Malawi: Kachere Series.

Mabilia, M. (2006), *Breast Feeding and Sexuality. Behaviour, Beliefs and Taboos among the Gogo Mothers of Tanzania*. Oxford: Berghahn.

MacDonald, S. (2003), "Trafficking in history: multitemporal practices," in I. M. Greverus (ed.) *Shifting Grounds: Experiments in Doing Ethnography*. Münster: Lit, 93–116.

MacDonald, T. H. (2006), *Health, Trade and Human Rights*. Oxford: Radcliffe Publishing.

—(2012), "How I learned to be a breastfeeding dad." *Huffington Post*, http://www.huffingtonpost.com/trevor-macdonald/how-i-learned-to-be-a-bre_b_1452392.html (accessed September 9, 2014).

MacErlean, J. (1912), "Eoin Ó Cuileannáin, Bishop of Raphoe, 1625–1661." *Archivium Hibernicum: Catholic Historical Society of Ireland* 1: 77–121.

Machekanyange, Z. (1997), "Is breast milk still best?" *Africa Information Afrique*, September 8. Harare: Zimbabwe.

MacLachlan, M. and Namangale, J. J. (1997), "Tropical illness profiles: the psychology of illness perception in Malawi." *Public Health* 111: 211–13.

Maher, J. (2005), "A mother by trade: Australian women reflecting mothering as activity, not identity." *Australian Feminist Studies* 20(46): 17–29.

Maher, V. (1992), "Breast-Feeding in Cross-Cultural Perspective: Paradoxes and Proposals," in V. Maher (ed.) *The Anthropology of Breast-Feeding: Natural Law or Social Construct*. Oxford: Berg: 14–20.

—(ed.) (1992), *Il latte materno: I condizionamenti culturali di un comportamento*. Torino: Rosenberg & Sellier.

—(ed.) (2011), *Antropologia e diritti umani nel mondo contemporaneo*. Torino: Rosenberg & Sellier.

Mahon-Daly, P. and Andrews, G. J. (2002), "Liminality and breastfeeding: women negotiating space and two bodies." *Health and Place* 8: 61–76.

Malinowski, Bronisław (1922), Argonauts of the Western Pacific: An Account of Native Enterprise and Adventure in the Archipelagoes of Melanesian New Guinea. London: George Routledge & Sons, Ltd.

Maliwichi-Nyirenda, C. P. and Maliwichi, L. L. (2009), "Poverty and maternal health in Malawi," in T. W. Beasley (ed.) *Poverty in Africa*. Hauppauge NY: Nova Science.

Mannel, R., Martens, P., and Walker, M. (eds) (2008), *ILCA: Core Curriculum for Lactation Consultant Practice* (2nd edn). Sudbury, MA: Jones and Bartlett.

—(eds) (2013), *Core Curriculum for Lactation Consultant Practice* (3rd edn), Burlington MA: Jones and Bartlett Learning.

Marcus, G. E. and Cushman, D. (1982), "Ethnographies as texts." *Annual Review of Anthropology* 11: 25–69.

Marshall, J. L., Godfrey, M., and Renfrew, M. J. (2007), "Being a 'good mother': managing breastfeeding and merging identities." *Social Science and Medicine* 65: 2147–59.

Martin, E. (1987), *The Woman in the Body: A Cultural Analysis of Reproduction*. Boston: Beacon Press.

Mataya, R., Mathanga, D., Chinkhumba, J., Chibwana, A., Chikaphupha, K., and Cardiello, J. (2013), "A qualitative study exploring attitudes and perceptions of HIV positive women who stopped breastfeeding at six months to prevent transmission of HIV to their children." Malawi Medical Journal 25(1): 15–19.

Matheson, M. C., Allen, K. J., and Tang, M. L. K. (2012), "Understanding the evidence for and against the role of breastfeeding in allergy prevention." *Clinical and Experiment Allergy* 42(6): 827–51.

Matthews, E. (2002), *The Philosophy of Merleau-Ponty*. Montreal: McGill-Queen's University Press.

—(2006), *Merleau-Ponty: A Guide for the Perplexed*. London: Continuum.

Matthews Grieco, S. F. (1991), "Breast-feeding, wet-nursing and infant mortality in Europe (1400–1800)," in *Historical Perspectives on Breast-feeding*. Florence: UNICEF, Instituto degli Innocenti.

Mauss, Marcel (1923–4), *Forme et raison de l'échange dans les sociétés archaïques*, l'Année Sociologique, seconde série. Full text available for free at http:// classiques.uqac.ca/classiques/mauss_marcel/socio_et_anthropo/2_essai_sur_le_don/essai_sur_le_don.html (accessed August 21, 2014).

McCann, A. (2013), "Supporting families in milk sharing; what are the responsibilities of the childbirth professional?" Available from http://www.scienceandsensibility. org/?tag=human-milk-banks

Mccrea, A. (2007), "The Human Milk Bank: Cross Border Co-operation Looking After the Irish Premature Baby." *Irish Medical Journal*, www.imj.ie/Archive/Abstractsfro mtheIrishPeriNatalSociety2007.doc (accessed September 12, 2014).

McDade, T. W. and Worthman, C. M. (1998), "The weanling's dilemma reconsidered: a biocultural analysis of breastfeeding ecology." *Journal of Developmental and Behavioral Pediatrics* 19(4): 286–99.

McDonald, M. and Lambert, H. (2009), "Introduction," in M. McDonald and H. Lambert (eds) *Social Bodies*. Oxford: Berghahn Books: 1–17.

Mead, M. (1928), Coming of Age in Samoa: A Psychological Study of Primitive Youth for Western Civilisation. New York: William Morrow and Company.

—(1943), *The Problem of Changing Food Habits*. Washington DC: National Academy of Science.

—(1949), *Male and Female: A Study of the Sexes in a Changing World*. New York: William Morrow.

—(1970), "Working mothers and their children." *Manpower* 2(6): 3–6; reprinted (1970), *Childhood Education* 47(2): 66–71.

—(1972), *Blackberry Winter: My Earlier Years*. New York: Morrow and Company.

Merdji, M. (2006), "L'imaginaire du dégoût: une approche anthropologique de l'univers émotionnel de l'alimentation," in M. Kalika and P. Romaeler (eds) Recherches en management et organisation. Paris: Economica: 179–93.

Merdji, M. and Debucquet, G. (2008), "Manger la nature: le bon et le sain," in C. Fischler and E. Masson (eds) *Manger: Français, Européens et Américains face à leur alimentation*. Paris: Odile Jacob: 209–22.

Merleau-Ponty, M. (1981), *Phenomenology of Perception*. London: Routledge.

Miller, A. C. (2012), "On the margins of the periphery: unassisted childbirth and the management of layered stigma." *Sociological Spectrum* 32(5): 406–23.

Miller, A. C., and Shriver, T. E. (2012), "Women's childbirth preferences and practices in the United States." *Social Science and Medicine* 75(4): 709–16.

Ministère des Solidarités, de la Santé et de la Famille (2005), *Allaitement Maternel: Les Bénéfices pour la Santé de l'enfant et de sa mere*, les synthèses du programme

Modi, N. (2006), "Donor breast milk banking: unregulated requires evidence of benefit—editorials." *British Medical Journal* 333: 1133–4.

Mok, E., Multon, C., Piguel, L., Barroso, E., Goua, V., Christin, P., Perez, M. J., and Hankard, R. (2008), "Decreased full breastfeeding, altered practices, perceptions and infant weight change of prepregnant obese women: a need for extra support," *Pediatrics* 121: 1319–24.

Mol, A. (2003), *The Body Multiple: Ontology in Medical Practice*. Durham and London: Duke University Press.

—(2008), *The Logic of Care: Health and the Problem of Patient Choice*. New York and London: Routledge.

—(2010), "Care and its Values: Care in Practice," in A. Mol, M. Ingunn, and J. Pols (eds) *Care in Practice: On Tinkering in Clinics, Homes and Farms*. Bielefeld: transcript Verlag, pp. 215–34.

Mol, A., Moser, I., and Pols, J. (2010), "Care: putting practice into theory," in A. Mol, M. Ingunn, and J. Pols (eds) *Care in Practice: On Tinkering in Clinics, Homes and Farms*. Bielefeld: transcript Verlag: 7–26.

Moland, K. M. (2004), "Mother's milk an ambiguous blessing in the era of AIDS: the case of the Chagga of Kilimanjaro." *African Sociological Review* 8 (1): 83–99.

Moran, L. and Gilad, J. (2007), "From folklore to scientific evidence: breast-feeding and wet-nursing in islam and the case of non-puerperal lactation." *International Journal of Biomedical Science* 3(4): 251–7.

More, S. J. (2009), "Global trends in milk quality: implications for the Irish dairy industry." *Irish Veterinary Journal* 62 Supplement: 5–14.

Moss, T. (2013), "My plea for a better quality discussion on breastfeeding," Taramoss blog, February 15, 2013, http://taramoss.com/a-plea-to-improve-the-quality-of-debate-for-the-sake-of-our-health/ (accessed April 17, 2012).

Muers, R. (2010), "The ethics of breast-feeding: a feminist theological exploration." *Journal of Feminist Studies in Religion* 26(1): 7–24.

Mulford, C. (2012), "'Are We There Yet?' Breastfeeding as a Gauge of Carework by Mothers," in P. Hall Smith, B. Hausman, and M. Labbok (eds), *Beyond Health, Beyond Choice*. New Brunswick: Rutgers University Press: 169–79.

Murphy, E. (1999), "'Breast is best': infant feeding decisions and maternal deviance." *Sociology of Health and Illness* 21(2): 187–208.

Mustadrak Al Hakim (2010), www.Islamtoday, chapter 2, No. 196.

Muula, A. S. (2005), "What should HIV-AIDS be called in Malawi?" *Nursing Ethics* 21(2): 187–92.

Naouri, A. (2004), *Les pères et les mères*. Paris: Odile Jacob.

National Institute for Health and Clinical Excellence (NICE) (2009), *Survey of Donor Milk Banks in the UK*. Manchester: NICE.

—(NICE) (2010), *Donor Milk Banks: The Operation of Donor Milk Bank Services*. London: NICE, guidance.nice.org.uk/cg93.

Nduati, R. (1998), *HIV and Infant Feeding: A Review of HIV Transmission through Breast-feeding*. Geneva: UNICEF, UNAIDS, WHO.

Nduati R., Richardson, B. A., John, G., Mbori-Ngacha, D., Mwatha, A., Ndinya-Achola, J., Bwayo, J., Onyango, F. E., and Kreiss, J. (2001), "Effect of breast-feeding on mortality among HIV–1 infected women: a randomized trial." *Lancet* 357: 1651–5.

Nestlé Canada (2011), History. http://www.nestle.ca/en/aboutus/historique.htm. Last visited April 10, 2011, no longer available except on Internet Archive.

Nestlé Corporation (2011), History. http://www.nestle.com/AboutUs/History/ Pages/History.aspx (accessed April 24, 2014).

Nicholl, A., Newell, M., Praag, E. V., de Perre, P. V., Peckham, C. (1995), "Infant feeding practice and policy in the Presence of HIV–1 infection." *AIDS* 9: 107–19.

Niekerk, van A. and Zyl, van L. (1995), "The ethics of surrogacy: women's reproductive labour." *J. Med. Ethics*. 21: 345–9.

O'Brien, J. (1982), *Dear, Dirty Dublin: A City in Distress, 1899–1916*, Berkeley CA: University of California Press.

O'Reilly, E. and O'Donovan, J. (1817), *Sanas Gaoidhilge-Sagsbhearla, An Irish–English Dictionary … to which is annexed, a compendious Irish Grammar*. (There are several versions and the 1821 version is available on Google Books.)

Obladen, M. (2012), "Bad milk, part 1: antique doctrines that impeded breast-feeding." *Acta Paediatricia* 101: 1102–4.

OED. (2011), *Oxford English Dictionary*. http://www.oed.com/

Ortiz, F. (2012), "Breast Milk Banks: From Brazil to the World." Rio de Janeiro: Inter Press Service English News Wire, http://www.ipsnews.net/2012/09/breast-milk-banks-from-brazil-to-the-world/ (accessed September 14, 2014).

Osbaldiston, R. and Mingle, L. (2007), "Characterization of human milk donors." *Journal of Human Lactation* 23(4): 350–57.

Østergaard, L. R. and Bula, A. (2010), "They call our children Nevirapine babies: a qualitative study about exclusive breastfeeding among HIV positive mothers in Malawi." African Journal of Reproductive Health 14(3): 213–22.

Palmonari, A. and Speltini, G. (2008), "Allaitement, corps et contamination: notes sur les racines multiples de la connaissance sociale," in B. Madiot, E. Lage, and A. Arruda (eds) *Une approche engagée en psychologie sociale: l'œuvre de Denise Jodelet*. Paris: Erès: 199–205.

Pancino, C. (1984), *Il bambino e l'acqua sporca: storia dell'assistenza al parto dalle mammane alle ostetriche*. Milano: Franco Angeli.

Panczuk, J., Unger, S., O'Connor, D., and Lee, S. K. (2014), "Human donor milk for the vulnerable infant: a Canadian perspective." *International Breastfeeding Journal*, 9(4).

Pande, A. (2009), "'It May Be Her Eggs But it's My Blood': Surrogates and Everyday Forms of Kinship in India." *Qualitative Sociology* 32(4): 379–97.

—(2010), "Commercial surrogacy in India: manufacturing a perfect mother–worker. *Signs* 35(4): 969–92.

Parkes, P. (2004), "Milk kinship in Southeast Europe: alternative social structures and foster relations in the Caucasus and the Balkans." *Social Anthropology* 12: 341–58.

—(2005), "Milk kinship in Islam: substance, structure, history." *Social Anthropology* 13: 307–29.

—(2006), "Alternative social structures and foster relations in the Hindu Kush: milk kinship allegiances in the former mountain kingdoms of Pakistan." *Comparative Studies in Society and History* 43(1): 1–36.

Patel, T. (1994), *Fertility Behaviour: Population and Society in a Rajasthan Village.* Delhi: Oxford University Press.

—(2012), Interview with Dr. Nayana Patel, Fertility Specialist at Anand, Gujarat. October.

Perco, D. (2010), *Il latte prezioso: Belluno: Museo di Serravalla*, http://www.iborderline.net/rifugi-culturali/2010/08/il-latte-prezioso/ (accessed September 14, 2014).

Pilgrim, D. and Middleton, P. (2002), *Jim Crowe Museum of Racist Memorabilia.*

Pizzini, F. (1981), *Sulla scena del parto: luoghi, figure, pratiche.* Milano: Franco Angeli.

Pomata, G. (1980), "Madri illegittime tra Ottocento e Novecento. Cliniche e storie di vita." *Quaderni Storici* 44: 497–542.

Poulain, J. P. (2002a), *Sociologies de l'alimentation.* Paris: PUF.

—(2002b), *Manger aujourd'hui: attitudes, normes et pratiques.* Toulouse: Privat.

Powell, L. A., Redfern, R. C., Millard, A. R. and Gröcke, D. R. (2014), "Infant feeding practices in Roman London: evidence from isotopic analyses." Journal of Roman Archaeology 96: 89–110.

Preble, S. and Piwoz, E. G. (1998), *HIV and Infant Feeding: A Chronology of Research and Policy Advances and their Implications for Programs*, http://sara.aed.org/publications/cross_cutting/hiv_infant/html/infant.htm (accessed April 15, 2012).

Provencher, V., Polivy, J., and Herman, C. P. (2009), "Perceived healthiness of food: if it's healthy, you can eat more!" Appetite 52(2): 340–44.

Qadeer, I. (2009), "Social and ethical basis of legislation on surrogacy: need for debate." *Indian Journal of Medical Ethics* 6(1): 28–31.

Qadeer, I. and Reddy, S. (2013), "Medical tourism in India: perceptions of physicians in tertiary care hospitals." *Philosophy, Ethics, and Humanities in Medicine* 8(1): 20.

Randall, V. (2000), *The Politics of Childcare in Britain.* Oxford: Oxford University Press.

Rankin, S. H., Lindgren, T., Rankin, W. W. and Ng'oma, J. (2005), ",Donkey work: women religion and HIV-AIDS in Malawi." *Healthcare for Women International* 26: 4–16.

Rapp, R. (2000), *Testing Women, Testing the Fetus: The Social Impact of Amniocentesis in America.* New York: Routledge.

—"Gender, body, biomedicine: how some feminist concerns dragged reproduction to the center of social theory." *Medical Anthropology Quarterly* 15(4): 466–77.

Rea, M. F. (1990), "The Brazilian National Breast-Feeding Program: A Success Story." *International Journal of Gynecology and Obstetrics* 31: 79–82.

Reddy S. (2000), "Socio-economic dimensions of breast-feeding: a study in Hyderabad." *Health and Population: Perspectives and Issues* 23(3): 144–59.

—(2003), "Beliefs and practices related to parturition among the Konda Reddi tribe of Andhra Pradesh." *Man in India* 83(3–4): 315–36.

Reddy, S. and Qadeer, I. (2010), "Medical tourism in India: progress or predicament?" *Economic and Political Weekly* 45(20): 69–75.

Reed-Danahay, D. (1997). *Auto/Ethnography*. New York: Berg.

Regan, P. and Ball, E. (2013), "Breastfeeding mothers' experiences: the ghost in the machine." *Qualitative Health Research* 23(5): 679–88.

Renfrew, M. J., Craig, D., Dyson, L., McCormick, F., Rice, S., King, S. E., Williams, A. F. (2009), "Breastfeeding promotion for infants in neonatal units: a systematic review and economic analysis." *Health Technology Assessment* 13(40): 1–146.

Riggio, E. (2011), "Localizzare i diritti umani: le donne ridefiniscono i diritti nelle proprie comunità in India," in V. Maher (ed.) *Antropologia e diritti umani nel mondo contemporaneo*. Torino: Rosenberg & Sellier.

Rippeyoung, P. L. F. and Noonan, M. (2012), "Is breastfeeding truly cost free? Income consequences of breastfeeding for women." *American Sociological Review* 77(2): 244–67.

Rosato, M., Mwansambo, C. W., Kazembe, P. N., Phiri, T., Soko, Q. S., Lewycka, S., Kunyenge, B. E., Vergnano, S., Osrin, D., Newell, M. L., and de la Costello, A. M. (2006), "Women's groups' perceptions of maternal health issues in rural Malawi." *The Lancet* 368: 1180–8.

Rose, N. (1999) [1989], *Governing the Soul: The Shaping of the Private Self*. London: Routledge.

Rothman, B. K. (2006), "Marketing Maternity: Consumer Ideologies and the Making of Mothers," in W. Ernst (ed.) *Naturbilder und Lebensgrundlagen: Konstruktionen von Geschlecht*. Hamburg: Lit Verlag: pp. 107–19.

Rousseau, J.-J. (1762), *L'Émile ou De l'éducation*. La Haye.

Rudzik, A. E. F. (2012), "The experience and determinants of first-time breastfeeding duration among low-income women from Sao Paulo, Brazil." *Current Anthropology* 53(1): 108–17.

Rudzik, A. E. F., Breakey, A., and Bribiescas, R. G. (2014), "Oxytocin and Epstein-Barr virus: stress biomarkers in the postpartum period among first-time mothers from Sao Paulo, Brazil." *American Journal of Human Biology* 26(1): 43–50.

Ryan, K., Team, V., and Alexander, J. (2013), "Expressionists of the 21st century: the commodification and commercialization of expressed breast milk." Medical Anthropology 32(5): 467–86.

Ryan, K., Todres, L., and Alexander, J. (2011), "Calling, permission, and fulfillment: the interembodied experience of breastfeeding." *Qualitative Health Research* 21(6): 731–42.

Sahih Muslim, (2010), www.daruliftaa, Book 8, Hadeeth Number 342.

Salih, R. (2003), *Gender in Transnationalism: Home, Longing and Belonging among Moroccan Migrant Women*. London: Routledge.

SAMA (2009), "Assisted reproductive technologies: for whose benefit?" *Economic and Political Weekly* 44(18): 25–31.

Sandre-Pereira, G. (2003), "Amamentação e sexualidade [Breastfeeding and Sexuality]." *Estudos Feministas, Florianopolis* 11(2): 467–91.

Saravanan, S. (2010), "Transnational surrogacy and objectification of gestational mothers." *Economic & Political Weekly* 45(16): 26–9.

—(2013), "An ethnomethodological approach to examine exploitation in the context of capacity, trust and experience of commercial surrogacy in India." *Philosophy, Ethics, and Humanities in Medicine* 8(1): 10.

Sayad, A. (2002), *La doppia assenza: Dalle illusioni dell'emigrato alle sofferenze dell'immigrato*. Milano: Raffaello Cortina Editore.

Sbisà, M. (1992), *Come sapere il parto: storia, scenari, linguaggi*. Torino: Rosenberg & Sellier.

Scavenius, M., van Hulsel, L., Meijer, J., Wendte, H., and Gurgel, R. (2007), "In practice, the theory is different: a processual analysis of breastfeeding in northeast Brazil." *Social Science and Medicine* 64(3): 676–88.

Schanler, R. J., Lau, C., Hurst, N. M., and Smith, E. O. (2005), "Randomized trial of donor human milk versus preterm formula as substitutes for mother's own milk in the feeding of extremely premature infants." *Pediatrics* 116: 400–406.

Scheper-Hughes, N. (1992), *Death Without Weeping: The Violence of Everyday Life in Brazil*. Berkeley, CA: University of California Press.

—(2013), "Brazil: no more angel babies on the alto." *Berkeley Review of Latin American Studies*, http://clas.berkeley.edu/review/spring–2013?field_semester_year_tid=47

Scheper-Hughes, N. and Lock, M. M. (1987), "The mindful body: a prolegomenon to future work in medical anthropology." *Medical Anthropology Quarterly* 1(1): 6–41.

Schmied, V. and Lupton, D. (2001), "Blurring the boundaries: breastfeeding and maternal subjectivity." *Sociology of Health and Illness* 23(2): 234–50.

Sears, W. and Sears, M. (2001), *The Attachment Parenting Book: A Commonsense Guide to Understanding and Nurturing Your Baby*. London: Little, Brown and Company.

Sellen, D. W. (2001), "Comparison of infant feeding patterns reported for nonindustrial populations with current recommendations." *Journal of Nutrition* 131(10): 2707–15.

Shah, S. S. (1994), "Fosterage as a ground for marital prohibition in Islam and the status of human milk banks." *Arab Law Quarterly* 9(1): 3–7.

Shaikh, U. and Ahmed, O. (2006), "Islam and infant feeding." *Breastfeeding Medicine* 1(3): 164–7.

Shaw, R. (2004), "The virtues of cross-nursing and the 'yuk factor.'" *Australian Feminist Studies* 19(45): 287–99.

—(2007), "Cross-nursing, ethics, and giving breastmilk in the contemporary context." *Women's Studies International Forum* 30: 439–50.

Shaw, R. and Bartlett, A. (2010), *Giving Breastmilk: Body Ethics and Contemporary Breastfeeding Practice.* Toronto: Demeter Press.

Sherwood, J. (1988), *Poverty in 18th-century Spain: The Women and Children of the Inclusa.* Toronto: University of Toronto Press.

—(1993), "The milk factor: the ideology of breast-feeding and post partum illnesses 1750–1850." *CBMH/BCHM* 10: 25–47.

—(2010), *Infection of the Innocents: Wet nurses, Infants and Syphilis in France 1780–1900* Montreal: McGill-Queen's University Press.

Simmel, G. (1917), *L'individualisme moderne.* Paris: Payot.

SIN (2006), *Linee guida per la costituzione e l'organizzazione di una banca del latte umano donato.*

Smajdor, A. (2013), "Redefining reproduction." *Human Reproduction* 28: 65–6.

Smith, J. (2004), "Mothers' milk and markets." *Australian Feminist Studies* 19(45): 369–79.

Smith, J. and Forrester, R. (2013), "Who pays for the health benefits of exclusive breastfeeding?: an analysis of maternal time costs." *Journal of Human Lactation* 29(4): 547–55.

Smith, J. and Ingham, L. (2005), "Mother's milk and measures of economic output." *Feminist Economics* 11(1): 41–62.

Snyder, J. R. (1908), "The Breast Milk Problem." *Journal of the American Medical Association* 51: 1214.

Sobonya, S. (2013), "The Costs of Breastfeeding in the United States," Paper presented at the annual meetings of the American Anthropological Association, Chicago.

Solomons, B. (1934), "Report of the Rotunda Hospital." *Irish Journal of Medical Science* 6(104): 331–86.

Speller, V., Learmonth, A., and Harrison, D. (1997), "The search for evidence of effective health promotion." *BMJ* 315: 361–3.

Speltini, G. and Molinari, L. (1998), "L'allaitement et ses représentations," *Les cahiers internationaux de psychologie sociale* 39: 23–42.

Spencer, R. L. (2008), "Research methodologies to investigate the experience of breastfeeding: a discussion paper." *International Journal of Nursing Studies* 45(12): 1823–30.

Stearns, C. (2010), "The Breast Pump," in R. Shaw and A. Bartlett (eds) *Giving Breastmilk.* Toronto: Demeter: 11–23.

Stearns, C. A. (2013), "The embodied practices of breastfeeding: implications for research and policy." *Journal of Women Politics and Policy* 34(4): 359–70.

Strathern, M. (1992), *Reproducing the Future: Essays on Anthropology, Kinship and the New Reproductive Technologies.* Manchester: Manchester University Press.

—(ed.) (2000), *Audit Cultures: Anthropological Studies in Accountability, Ethics and the Academy.* London: Routledge.

Street, D. J. and Lewallen, L. P. (2013), "The influence of culture on breast-feeding decisions by African American and white women." *Journal of Perinatal Nursing* 27(1): 43–51.

Suizzo, M.-A. (2004), "Mother–child relationships in France: balancing autonomy and affiliation in everyday interactions." *Ethos* 32: 293–323.

Sullivan, S., Schanler, R. J., Kim, J. H., Patel, A. L., Trawetöger, R., Kiechl-Kohlendorfer, U., Chan, G. M, Blanco, C. L., Abrams, S., Cotton, C. M., Laroia, N., Ehrekranz, R. A., Dudell, G., Cristofalo, E. A., Meier, P., Lee, M. L., Rechtman, D. J., and Lucas, A. (2010), "An exclusively human milk-based diet is associated with a lower rate of necrotizing enterocolitis than a diet of human milk and bovine milk-based products." *The Journal of Pediatrics* 156: 562–7.

Sussman, G. D. (1982), *Selling Mother's Milk: The Wet-nursing Business in France 1715–1914.* Champaign, IL: University of Illinois Press.

Swanson, K. W. (2009), "Human milk as technology and technologies of human milk: medical imaginings in the early 20th-century United States." *WSQ: Women's Studies Quarterly* 37(1–2): 21–37.

Swanson, V., Nicol, H. McInnes, R., Cheyne, H., Mactier, H., and Callander, E. (2012), "Developing maternal self-efficacy for feeding preterm babies in the neonatal unit." *Qualitative Health Research* 22(10): 1369–82.

Sweetman, C. (2006), *How Title Deeds Make Sex Safer: Women's Property Rights in an Era of HIV.* United Kingdom: Oxfam International.

Tafseer, E. (1988), *Collected Quranic codes.* Beirut: Dr. Elkutub Elilmiya.

Tanderup, M., Reddy S., Patel, T., and Nielsen, B. B. (forthcoming), "Informed consent and medical decision-making in commercial gestational surrogacy: a mixed methods study in New Delhi, India." *Acta Obstetricia et Gynecologica Scandinavica.*

Tapias, M. (2006), "Always read and always clean?": competing discourses of breast-feeding, infant illness and the politics of mother-blame in Bolivia. *Body and Society* 12(2): 83–108.

Thairu, L. (2001), "'Infant feeding options for mothers with HIV: using women's insights to guide policies," in *Nutrition and HIV/AIDS.* UNAIDS, ACC/CCN Working Paper 20: 63–71.

Thorley, V. (2008), "Breasts for hire and shared breastfeeding: wet nursing and cross feeding in Australia, 1900–2000." *Health and History* 10(1): 88–109.

Thulier, D. (2009), "Breastfeeding in America: a history of influencing factors." *Journal of Human Lactation* 25(1): 85–94.

Tijou Traoré, A., Querre, M., Brou, H., Becquet, R., Leroy, V., Desclaux, A., and Desgrées Du Loû, A. (2009), "Roles regarding infant feeding within HIV+ couples." *Social Science and Medicine* 69(6): 830–37.

Titmuss, Richard (1970), *The Gift Relationship: From Human Blood to Social Policy.* London: Allen and Unwin. Reprinted and reissued with new chapters by J. Ashton and A. Oakley (eds) (1997), New Press.

Torres, J. M. C. (2013), "Breastmilk and labour support: lactation consultants' and doulas' strategies for navigating the medical context of maternity care." *Sociology of Health and Illness* 35(6): 924–38.

—(2014), "Medicalizing to demedicalize: lactation consultants and the (de)medicalization of breastfeeding." *Social Science and Medicine* 100: 159–66.

Torres, M. I. U., Lopez, C. M., Roman, S. V., Diaz, C. A., Cruz-Rojo, J., Cooke, E. F., and Alonso, C. R. P. (2010), "Does opening a milk bank in a neonatal unit change infant feeding practices? A before and after study." *International Breastfeeding Journal* 5(4), http://www.internationalbreastfeedingjournal.com/content/5/1/4

Tully, K. P. and Ball, H. L. (2013), "Trade-offs underlying maternal breastfeeding decisions: a conceptual model." *Maternal and child nutrition* 9(1): 90–8.

Tully, M. R. (2000), "A year of remarkable growth for donor milk banking in North America," *Journal of Human Lactation* 16(3): 235–6.

—(2001), "World congress on human lactation." *Journal of Human Lactation* 17(1): 51–3.

U.S. Department of Health and Human Services (2011), *The Surgeon General's Call to Action to Support Breast-feeding*. Washington DC: U.S. Department of Health and Human Services, Office of the Surgeon General, http://www.surgeongeneral. gov: 1–1961.

UNAIDS (2001), *Nutrition and HIV/AIDS: Nutrition Policy Paper no. 20*. Geneva: ACC/SCN.

—(2013), *Country profile, Burkina Faso: HIV and AIDS estimates (2012)*. Available at http://www.unaids.org/en/regionscountries/countries/burkinafaso/ (accessed January 23, 2014).

—(2014), Data on Malawi. http://www.unaids.org/en/regionscountries/countries/malawi/ (last accessed February 3, 2014).

UNAIDS, UNICEF, WHO (1997), *HIV and Infant Feeding: A Policy Statement Developed Collaboratively by UNAIDS, UNICEF and WHO*. Available at http://www.unaids.org/publications/documents/mtct/infantpole(f).html (accessed December 13, 2009).

UNDP (United Nations Development Program) (2006), *Human Development Report*. New York: Palgrave.

—(2010), *Human Development Report 2010—20th Anniversary Edition: The Real Wealth of Nations: Pathways to Human Development*. hdr.undp.org/en/reports/global/hdr2010/ (last accessed March 10, 2011); Malawi profile: http://hdrstats.undp.org/en/countries/profiles/MWI.html

—(2013), *Human Development Report 2013: Summary—The Rise of the South: Human Progress in a Diverse World*. http://hdr.undp.org/sites/default/files/hdr2013_en_summary.pdf (last accessed February 3, 2014).

UNICEF (2013), *Female Genital Mutilation/Cutting: A statistical overview and exploration of the dynamics of change*, New York: UNICEF.

—(2006), *The Baby Friendly Initiative*. www.babyfriendly.co.uk (accessed December 3, 2006).

—(2010), *Breast-feeding Practices by Age: Morocco*. Childinfo: Monitoring the Situation of Children and Women, Statistics by Area, http://www.childinfo.org/breast-feeding_morocco.html (accessed January 24, 2014).

UNICEF, UNAIDS, WHO, UNFPA, UNESCO (2010), *Children and AIDS: Fifth Stocktaking Report*. Geneva. Available at http://www.unicef.org/publications/index_57005.html (accessed January 24, 2014).

Updegrove, K. H. (2013a), "Donor human milk banking: growth, challenges, and the role of HMBANA." *Breastfeed Med* 8: 435–7.

—(2013b), "Nonprofit human milk banking in the United States." *Journal of Midwifery and Women's Health* 58(5): 1542–2011.

Van Esterik, P. (1988), "The Insufficient Milk Syndrome: Biological Epidemic or Cultural Construction," in P. Whelehan (ed.) *Women and Health: Cross Cultural Perspectives*. Granby MA: Bergin and Garvey: 97–109.

—(1989), *Beyond the Breast-Bottle Controversy*. New Brunswick NJ: Rutgers University Press.

—(1996a), "The cultural context of breastfeeding and breastfeeding policy." *Food and Nutrition Bulletin* 17(4): 422–31.

—(1996b), "Expressing ourselves: breast pumps." *Journal of Human Lactation* 12(4): 273–4.

—(2002), "Contemporary trends in infant feeding research." *Annual Review of Anthropology* 31: 257–78.

—(2008a), "Vintage breastmilk: exploring the discursive limits of feminine fluids," *Canadian Theatre Review* 137: 20–23.

—(2008b), "The Politics of Breastfeeding: An Advocacy Update," in Carole Counihan and P. Van Esterik (eds) Food and Culture: A Reader. New York: Routledge.

—(2010), "Breastfeeding and HIV/AIDS: Critical Gaps and Dangerous Intersections," in R. Shaw and A. Bartlett (eds) *Giving Breastmilk*. Toronto: Demeter Press.

—(2012), "Breastfeeding Across Cultures: Dealing with Difference," in P. Hall Smith, B. L. Hausman, and M. Labbok (eds) *Beyond Health, Beyond Choice: Breastfeeding Constraints and Realities*. New Brunswick: Rutgers University Press: 53–63.

Van Esterik, P. and Greiner, T. (1981), "Breastfeeding and women's work: constraints and opportunities." *Studies in Family Planning* 12(4): 184–97.

Van Wolputte, S. V. (2004), "Hang on to yourself: of bodies, embodiment, and selves." *Annual Review of Anthropology* 33: 251–69.

Venancio, S. I., Escuder, M. M. L., Saldiva, S. R. D. M., and Giugliani, E. R. J. (2010), "Breastfeeding practice in the Brazilian capital cities and the Federal District: current status and advances." *Jornal de pediatria* 86(4): 317–24.

Verdier, Y. (1979), *Façons de dire, façons de faire: la laveuse, la couturière, la cuisinière*. Paris: Gallimard.

Victora, C. G., Barros, F. C., Horta, B. L., and Lima, R. C. (2005), "Breastfeeding and school achievement in Brazilian adolescents." *Acta Paediatrica* 94(11): 1656–60.

Vora, K. (2014), "Experimental sociality and gestational surrogacy in the Indian ART clinic." *Ethnos* 79(1): 63–83.

Waldby, C. (2002), "Biomedicine, tissue transfer and intercorporality." *Feminist Theory* 3(3): 239–54.

Waring, M. (1988), *If Women Counted*. San Fransisco: HarperCollins.

Warner, J. (2006), *Perfect Madness: Motherhood in the Age of Anxiety*. London: Vermilion.

Washburn, R. (2014), "Measuring personal chemical exposure through biomonitoring: the experiences of research participants." *Qualitative Health Research*, published online before print, February 18, 2014, DOI: 10.1177/1049732314521899.

Watson, M. L. (1941), "Our frozen milk." *The American Journal of Nursing* 41 (6): 672–4.

Weaver, G. (2006), 'Response to Modi.' BMJ.com. http://www.bmj.com/cgi/eletters/333/7579/1133#150815 (accessed May 10, 2010).

—(2008), Director of the oldest milk bank in the UK, Queen Charlotte's Milk Bank, and the chair of the United Kingdom Association for Milk Banking (UKAMB). Personal communication.

Weber, M. (1956), *Economie et société: les catégories de la sociologie (Tome 1)*. Paris: Plon.

White, E. (1999), *Breast-feeding and HIV-AIDS: The Research, the Politics, the Women's Responses*. Jefferson NC: McFarland.

WHO (1981), *International Code on the Marketing of Breastmilk Substitutes*. Geneva.

—(2003), *Global Strategy for Infant and Young Child Feeding*. Geneva: WHO.

WHO (2003a), *HIV and Infant Feeding: Framework for Priority Action*. Geneva: WHO.

—(2003b), *HIV and Infant Feeding: Guidelines for Decision-Makers*. Geneva: WHO.

—(2003c), *HIV and Infant Feeding: A Guide for Health-care Managers and Supervisors*. Geneva: WHO.

—(2006), *HIV and Infant Feeding Update (Based on 2000 and 2006 Technical Consultations)*. Geneva: WHO.

—(2007), *HIV Transmission through Breastfeeding: A review of Available Evidence— Update (Original Review 2003, Updated 2005)*. Geneva: WHO.

—(2009a), *HIV and Infant Feeding Revised Principles and Recommendations RAPID Advice*. Geneva: WHO.

—(2009b). *WHO Country Cooperation Strategy 2008–2013: Malawi*. Brazzaville: WHO Regional Office for Africa.

—(2009c), *HIV/AIDS Data and Statistics*. http://www.who.int/hiv/data/en/

—(2010a), *Guidelines on HIV and Infant Feeding 2010*. Geneva: WHO.

—(2010b), *World Health Statistics 2001: Data Tables for Malawi*. Downloaded from http://www.who.int/whosis/whostat/2010/en/index.html (last accessed May 6, 2011).

—(2014), *Global Health Observatory Data Repository: Country Data for Malawi from 2002*. http://apps.who.int/gho/data/node.country.country-MWI?lang=en (last accessed February 3, 2014).

WHO Statement (2001), "Effect of Breast-feeding on Mortality among HIV-infected Women," in UNAIDS *Nutrition and HIV/AIDS: Nutrition Policy Paper no. 20*. Geneva ACC/SCN

WHO, UNAIDS, UNICEF (2010), *Towards Universal Access: Scaling Up Priority HIV/AIDS Interventions in the Health Sector. Progress Report 2010*. Available at http://www.who.int/hiv/pub/2010progressreport/report/en/index.html (accessed December 1, 2010).

WHO and UNICEF (1989), *Joint Statement on the Protection, Promotion and Support of Breast-feeding*. Geneva.

WHO, UNICEF, UNFPA, UNAIDS (2003), *HIV and Infant Feeding: Guidelines for Decision Makers*. Geneva, WHO. Available at http://www.unfpa.org/public/home/publications/pid/2457 (accessed January 24, 2014).

Wickes, I. G. (1953a), "A history of infant feeding: part I—primitive peoples: ancient works: Renaissance writers." *Archives of Disease in Childhood* 28(138): 151–8.

—(1953b), "A history of infant feeding Part III." *Archives of Disease in Childhood* 9: 416–22.

Wiessenger, D. (2012), "It's All About Research," *WABA MSTF—E-newsletter V10N1*. http://www.waba.org.my/whatwedo/gims/english.htm (accessed April 17, 2014).

Williams, F. (2012a), *Breasts: A Natural and Unnatural History*. New York: Norton.

—(2012b), "Just what's inside those breasts?" npr.org (accessed April 17, 2014).

Wolf, J. H. (1999), "'Mercenary hirelings' or 'a great blessing'?: doctors' and mothers' conflicted perceptions of wet nurses and the ramifications of infant feeding in Chicago 1870–1960." *Journal of Social History* 33(1): 97–120.

—(2001), *Don't Kill Your Baby: Public Health and the Decline of Breastfeeding in the 19th and 20th centuries*. Columbus OH: Ohio State University Press.

Wolf, J. B. (2010), "Against Breastfeeding – Sometimes," in J. Metzl and A. Kirkland (eds) *Against Health: How Health Became the New Morality*. New York: New York University Press.

—(2011), *Is Breast Best? Taking on the Breastfeeding Experts and the New High Stakes of Motherhood*. New York and London: NYU Press.

Wolfenstein, M. (1955), "French Parents Take their Children to the Park," in M. Mead and M. Wolfenstein *Childhood in Contemporary Cultures*. London: University of Chicago Press, 99–117.

Worden, M. (2007), "Food for thought?" *Journal of Neonatal Nursing* 13(1): 4–5.

World Health Organization and UNICEF (2003), *Global Strategy for Infant and Young Child Feeding*. Geneva: World Health Organization.

Yang, C. P. (1993), "History of lactation and breast cancer risk." *American Journal of Epidemiology* 138(2): 1050–56.

Zeitlin, J., Mohangoo, A., and Delnord, M. (eds) (2013), *The European Perinatal Health Report: Health and Care of Pregnant Women and Babies in Europe in 2010*. Europe: Euro Peristat.

Ziegler J. B., Coper D. A., Gold J., and Johnston R. (1985). "Postnatal transmission of AIDS-associated retrovirus." *Lancet*, 20: 1896–98.

Zizzo, G. (2009), "Lesbian families and the negotiation of maternal identity through the unconventional use of breastmilk." *Gay and Lesbian Issues and Psychology Review* 5(2): 96–109.

—(2013), "Perceptions and negotiations of 'failure' in an Australian breast milk bank," in T. Cassidy (ed.) *Breastfeeding:* Global Practices, Challenges, Maternal and Infant Health Outcomes. New York: Nova Publishers: 77–92.

Index

Lightning Source UK Ltd.
Milton Keynes UK
UKOW06f0008220616

276816UK00001B/50/P